Philosophy and Medicine

Founding Editors
H. Tristram Engelhardt Jr.
Stuart F. Spicker

Volume 146

The Philosophy and Medicine series is dedicated to publishing monographs and collections of essays that contribute importantly to scholarship in bioethics and the philosophy of medicine. The series addresses the full scope of issues in bioethics and philosophy of medicine, from euthanasia to justice and solidarity in health care, and from the concept of disease to the phenomenology of illness. The Philosophy and Medicine series places the scholarship of bioethics within studies of basic problems in the epistemology, ethics, and metaphysics of medicine. The series seeks to publish the best of philosophical work from around the world and from all philosophical traditions directed to health care and the biomedical sciences. Since its appearance in 1975, the series has created an intellectual and scholarly focal point that frames the field of the philosophy of medicine and bioethics. From its inception, the series has recognized the breadth of philosophical concerns made salient by the biomedical sciences and the health care professions. With over one hundred and twenty five volumes in print, no other series offers as substantial and significant a resource for philosophical scholarship regarding issues raised by medicine and the biomedical sciences.

Emily E. Anderson
Editor

Ethical Issues in Community and Patient Stakeholder–Engaged Health Research

Springer

Editor
Emily E. Anderson
Neiswanger Institute for Bioethics,
Stritch School of Medicine
Loyola University Chicago
Maywood, IL, USA

ISSN 0376-7418 ISSN 2215-0080 (electronic)
Philosophy and Medicine
ISBN 978-3-031-40378-1 ISBN 978-3-031-40379-8 (eBook)
https://doi.org/10.1007/978-3-031-40379-8

This Springer imprint is published by the registered company Springer Nature Switzerland AG
The registered company address is: Gewerbestrasse 11, 6330 Cham, Switzerland

We dedicate this book to
All those who have served as research participants, research partners, and research advocates
Your contributions to improve the research process and the health and well-being of patients and communities are inspiring.

Acknowledgments

Many thanks to Jake Young for his indispensable assistance in preparing this book for publication, to all the authors for contributing content on important topics despite the challenges of the pandemic, and to Holly A. Taylor, Emma Tumilty, and Michael McCarthy for your additional support.

Contents

Editor and Contributors

About the Editor

Emily E. Anderson PhD, MPH, is Professor of Bioethics at Stritch School of Medicine, Loyola University Chicago. Early in her career, she coordinated community-based public health studies, leading to a lifelong interest in the ethics of engaging community and patient stakeholders in research. She is co-author (with Amy Corneli) of *100 Questions (and Answers) About Research Ethics* and creator of CIRTification, a free online human research protections training program for community research partners (https://ccts.uic.edu/tools/cirtification/).

Contributors

Emily E. Anderson Neiswanger Institute for Bioethics, Stritch School of Medicine, Loyola University Chicago, Maywood, IL, USA

Lisa Ballance Office of the Vice President for Research and Innovation, Virginia Commonwealth University, Richmond, VA, USA

Adina Black Community-Campus Partnerships for Health (CCPH), Raleigh, NC, USA

Adam Bourne Australian Research Centre for Sex, Health and Society, La Trobe University, Melbourne, VIC, Australia

Stephanie Solomon Cargill Albert Gnaegi Center for Health Care Ethics, Saint Louis University, Saint Louis, MO, USA

Dolores Castañeda Center for Healthy Work. School of Public Health, University of Illinois Chicago, Chicago, IL, USA

Paige Castro-Reyes Community-Campus Partnerships for Health (CCPH), Raleigh, NC, USA

Jule Chapman Sex Workers United Against Violence (SWUAV), Vancouver, BC, Canada

Tommy Chou Department of Psychiatry and Human Behavior, Brown University, Providence, RI, USA

Weight Control and Diabetes Research Center, The Miriam Hospital, Providence, RI, USA

Melissa Chrusfield Greater Lawndale Healthy Work Council, Chicago, IL, USA

Andrea L. DaViera Department of Psychology, University of Illinois at Chicago, Chicago, IL, USA

Emily M. A. Doerksen Centre of Genomics and Policy, McGill University, Montreal, QC, Canada

James M. DuBois Center for Clinical and Research Ethics, Division of General Medical Sciences, Washington University School of Medicine, Saint Louis, MO, USA

Brendan Durkin Boston College, Boston, MA, USA

Andrew Evans Reilly Center for Science, Technology, and Values, University of Notre Dame, Notre Dame, IN, USA

Micah Fialka-Feldman Taishoff Center, School of Education, Syracuse University, Syracuse, NY, USA

Stacy L. Frazier Department of Psychology, Florida International University, Miami, FL, USA

Phoebe Friesen Department of Equity, Ethics, and Policy, Department of Social Studies of Medicine, McGill University, Montreal, QC, Canada

Melody S. Goodman Department of Biostatistics, School of Global Public Health, New York University, New York, NY, USA

Sylvia Gonzalez Center for Healthy Work, School of Public Health, University of Illinois Chicago, Chicago, IL, USA

Alexis Grant WestEd, San Francisco, CA, USA

Alize E. Gunay Department of Family Medicine and Bioethics, McGill University, Montreal, QC, Canada

Adrian Guta School of Social Work, University of Windsor, Windsor, Canada

Elisa A. Hurley Boston, MA, USA

Jeni Hebert-Beirne School of Public Health, University of Illinois Chicago, Chicago, IL, USA

Adlaide Holloway Greater Lawndale Healthy Work Council, Chicago, IL, USA

Linda Kahn Department of Family Medicine, Jacobs School of Medicine and Biomedical Science, University at Buffalo, Buffalo, NY, USA

Latajah Lassus Clark Atlanta University, Atlanta, GA, USA

Nicolas D. Leech-Crier Transformative Health & Justice Research Cluster, University of British Columbia, British Columbia Mental Health and Substance Use Services, PHS Community Services Society/Vancouver Coastal Health Mobile Overdose Prevention Unit, Megaphone Magazine, Vancouver, BC, Canada

Jennifer Plascencia Lopez Community Health Sciences, School of Public Health, University of Illinois Chicago, Chicago, IL, USA

Samona Marsh Sex Workers United Against Violence, Vancouver, BC, Canada

Katherine McDonald Falk College of Sport and Human Dynamics, Syracuse University, Syracuse, NY, USA

Jim McLeod Hives for Humanity, Vancouver, BC, Canada

Gianna McMillan Bioethics Institute, Loyola Marymount University, Los Angeles, CA, USA

Lisa Mikesell School of Communication and Information, Rutgers University, New Brunswick, NJ, USA

Maghboeba Mosavel Department of Health Behavior and Policy, School of Population Health, Virginia Commonwealth University, Richmond, VA, USA

Barbara Mintzes School of Pharmacy and Charles Perkins Centre, Faculty of Medicine and Health, The University of Sydney, Sydney, NSW, Australia

Jacob Myers Boston University, Boston, MA, USA

Scott D. Neufeld Psychology Department, Brock University, St. Catherines, ON, Canada

Peter A. Newman Factor-Inwentash Faculty of Social Work, University of Toronto, Toronto, ON, Canada

Lisa Parker School of Pharmacy and Charles Perkins Centre, Faculty of Medicine and Health, The University of Sydney, Sydney, NSW, Australia

Briona Phillips Department of Health Behavior and Policy, School of Population Health, Virginia Commonwealth University, Richmond, VA, USA

Kristyn A. Pierce Department of Pediatrics, NYU Langone Health, New York, NY, USA

Angela Potochnik Department of Philosophy, University of Cincinnati, Cincinnati, OH, USA

Al Richmond Community-Campus Partnerships for Health (CCPH), Raleigh, NC, USA

Elizabeth Ripley School of Medicine, Virginia Commonwealth University, Richmond, VA, USA

Millicent Robinson School of Social Work, University of North Carolina, Chapel Hill, NC, USA

Ariel Schwartz Institute on Disability, University of New Hampshire, Durham, NH, USA

Nancy Shore Community-Campus Partnerships for Health (CCPH), Raleigh, NC, USA

Social Work, University of New England, Portland, ME, USA

Ryan Spellecy Center for Bioethics and Medical Humanities, Medical College of Wisconsin, Milwaukee, WI, USA

Vetta Sanders Thompson Brown School, Washington University in St. Louis, Saint Louis, MO, USA

Laurene Tumiel-Berhalter Department of Family Medicine, Jacobs School of Medicine and Biomedical Science, University at Buffalo, Buffalo, NY, USA

Part I
Theory

Chapter 1
Introduction: What We Talk About When We Talk About the Ethics of Engaging Patient and Community Stakeholders in Health Research

Emily E. Anderson

Research ethics as an academic discipline has developed over the last 50 or so years as part of the broader field of bioethics. The focus of academic research ethics has been primarily, but not exclusively, on the ethical inclusion and protection of human research participants in clinical biomedical research, and to a somewhat lesser extent, in behavioral and social sciences research. Respect for persons, beneficence, and justice, considered the guiding principles for ethical research, are outlined in the seminal *Belmont Report* (National Commission for the Protection of Human Subjects of Biomedical and Behavioral Research, 1979) and inform U.S. federal regulations for human research (45 CFR 46; 21 CFR 50, 56). Since the publication of the *Belmont Report,* a robust literature has developed, with research ethics scholars debating application of these principles to ethical challenges raised by specific research designs, settings, and emerging technologies. Research ethics has addressed, for example, phase I clinical trials with healthy volunteers, placebo-controlled studies in low-resource settings, emergency research with individuals who cannot provide informed consent, cluster randomized trials, and genome-wide association studies.

More recently, research ethicists have begun to consider questions of patient and community stakeholder engagement (Anderson & Spellecy, 2021; Mikesell et al., 2013; Spellecy & Anderson, 2021). These analyses focus on a wide range of issues, are informed by different disciplinary frameworks and norms, and both overlap with and diverge from traditional research ethics in interesting and important ways. This volume aims to bring together, in one place, scholarship on the ethics of stakeholder

E. E. Anderson (✉)
Neiswanger Institute for Bioethics, Stritch School of Medicine, Loyola University Chicago, Maywood, IL, USA
e-mail: emanderson@luc.edu

E. E. Anderson (ed.), *Ethical Issues in Community and Patient Stakeholder–Engaged Health Research*, Philosophy and Medicine 146,
https://doi.org/10.1007/978-3-031-40379-8_1

engagement in research. Here, ethics, patient and community stakeholders, and health-related research are all conceptualized broadly.

Research that engages patient and community stakeholders poses unique ethical challenges, not because of research design or nascent technology but because such research includes additional actors, each with their own perspectives, values, interests, goals, and lived experiences (Clinical and Translational Science Awards Consortium, 2011). Importantly, for the considerations of ethics, the accountability of academic researchers to patient and community research partners differs in important ways from their accountability to research participants, and thus requires consideration of additional guiding principles and revised frameworks. In turn, these patient and community research partners are also accountable to research participants and to other members of the communities from which these participants are recruited. There are unique considerations given the geographic, social, and emotional proximity of these research partners to participants and the fact of their community membership.

In conceptualizing this volume, I aimed to include scholarship that considers these additional actors, goals, and obligations from a broad range of disciplinary perspectives, across different kinds of research topics and methods, and from the perspectives of engaged patient and community stakeholders, academic researchers, and research ethicists. To that end, this volume includes reflections on theory (Part I) and practice (Part II) as well as analyses of unique ethical considerations (Part III) and challenges for the regulatory oversight of patient and community-engaged health research (Part IV).

The chapters in Part I, "Theory," review a variety of conceptual frameworks that inform patient and community stakeholder-engaged research. In Chap. 2, "Theorizing Participatory Research," Andrew Evans and Angela Potochnik review theoretical resources for conceptualizing and designing participatory research projects, focusing on why scientists conduct participatory research, why community members participate, and the value of such research. In Chap. 3, "An Evolving Ethical Framework for Patient and Community-Engaged Research," Lisa Mikesell proposes a preliminary ethical framework for patient and community-engaged research, taking into account the multiple roles that different stakeholders can occupy, the limits of traditional, dominant ethical frames, and emerging scholarship. In Chap. 4, "Beyond Good Intentions: Principles for Anti-racist Community-Engaged Research," Alexis Grant and Andrea L. DaViera describe a history of oppressive and exploitive research practices and outline guiding principles to ensure that community-engaged research is not just respectful and non-exploitive but explicitly anti-racist. In Chap. 5, "Demystifying How Academic-Community Partnerships Use Reflexivity and Praxis to Promote Participatory Research Principles of Equity and Justice," Jeni Hebert-Beirne, Sylvia Gonzalez, Melissa Chrusfield, Adlaide Holloway, Jennifer Plascencia Lopez, and Dolores Castañeda discuss inherent power imbalances in research partnerships and present guidelines for intentional reflexivity to promote attention to equity and justice that they have used with the Greater Lawndale Health Work project in Chicago, Illinois. In Chap. 6, "Reflexivity: A Strategy for Ethics- and Values-Driven Community Partnerships in Mental Health," Tommy Chou and Stacy L. Frazier expand on reflexivity and provide another model for academic-community research partnerships to structure reflection and mindfulness.

The chapters in Part II, "In the Field," focus on practical issues in patient and community stakeholder-engaged research and share stories from the front lines. In Chap. 7, "How Do You Define Community and Why Is it Important?," Laurene Tumiel-Berhalter and Linda Kahn address the challenges of defining different types of communities and the importance of understanding their complexities, using examples from their research in Buffalo, New York. In Chap. 8, "Community Researchers and Ethical Considerations: Burdens in the Field," Maghboeba Mosavel and Briona Phillips describe challenges associated with physical, social, and emotional proximity that community researchers who conduct participant recruitment, data collection, and data dissemination may experience, drawing on their experience on multiple projects in Cleveland, Ohio, Petersburg, Virginia, and South Africa. In Chap. 9, "Community-Engaged Research with People with Developmental Disabilities: A Conversation with Community Researchers about their Ethical Inclusion," Brendan Durkin, Micah Fialka-Feldman, Jacob Myers, Ariel Schwartz, and Katherine McDonald share insights for fostering respect and meaningful inclusion in research with communities of people with developmental disabilities. In Chap. 10, "Community Conversations about Culturally Responsive Health Research for African American Communities," Adina Black, Millicent Robinson, Paige Castro-Reyes, Al Richmond, Latajah Lassus, and Nancy Shore share findings from listening sessions with African Americans in North Carolina that highlight the importance of earning trust, building genuine relationships, and understanding the historic and contemporary factors that influence decisions regarding research participation. In Chap. 11, "The Power of Personal Narrative: My Experience with SACHRP, the FDA, and Bioethics," Gianna McMillan reflects on her experience as the mother of a research participant and a patient advocate who started sharing her story to impact research policy.

In Part III, authors consider the unique ethical considerations that arise in patient and community-stakeholder engaged research. In Chap. 12, "Patient Advocacy Organizations and Conflicts of Interest in Research," Lisa Parker and Barbara Mintzes discuss how industry funding of patient organizations can affect research activities and call for more transparency. In Chap. 13, "Representing and Protecting: Gatekeepers in Community-Engaged Research," Ryan Spellecy presents considerations that arise when community and patient organizations or representatives serve as research gatekeepers, monitoring and in some cases even determining what research does and does not get conducted with their communities. In Chap. 14, "Paying Research Participants and Community and Patient Research Partners: An Engaging Ethical Issue," Lisa Ballance and Elizabeth Ripley discuss ethical and regulatory considerations for appropriate compensation for both research participants and research partners and outline emerging best practices. In Chap. 15, "Rethinking Risks and Benefits in Stakeholder-Engaged Research: Lessons from HIV, Substance Use, and Sexual Health Research with Marginalized Communities," Adrian Guta, Peter A. Newman, and Adam Bourne draw from their own experience to describe the risks and benefits in stakeholder-engaged research and how these might be weighed differently than in traditional human research. In Chap. 16, "Data Decisions and Ethics: The Case of Stakeholder-Engaged Research," Melody S. Goodman, Kristyn A. Pierce, James M. DuBois, and Vetta Sanders Thompson outline considerations for data ownership, deciding how data are used, and deciding what gets published.

The chapters in Part IV address important issues in research ethics oversight. In Chap. 17, "Applying the *Belmont* Principles to Stakeholder-Engaged Research: Adaptions and Limitations," Elisa A. Hurley describes both the flexibility and the limitations of applying *Belmont's* framework to stakeholder-engaged research. In Chap. 18, "Stakeholder Engagement and (the Limits of) IRB Review," Stephanie Solomon Cargill analyzes the tensions that can occur between IRBs and researchers conducting patient and community-engaged studies and proposes some solutions. In Chap. 19, "Community Research Ethics Oversight: Place, Experience, and Expertise," Alize E. Gunay, Phoebe Friesen, and Emily M. A. Doerksen describe place-based and community-led research ethics governance initiatives that aim to elevate community voice in discussions surrounding research conduct. In Chap. 20, "Introducing the Downtown Eastside Community Research Ethics Workshop: Notes on a Process for Community Ethics Review," Scott D. Neufeld, Jule Chapman, Nicolas D. Leech-Crier, Samona Marsh, and Jim McLeod describe their experience developing and piloting one such initiative in Vancouver, British Columbia, Canada.

There are different ways to characterize scholarship on the ethics of patient and community-engaged research that has emerged to date. In my own review, I have identified five key themes. The first theme is that engagement can make research more ethical. The second theme is the value of stakeholder voice in defining what is ethical. The third theme is the development of specific ethical principles and guidance *for* engagement. The fourth theme is that the fact of engagement changes how we the application of traditional research ethics guidance and requirements. The fifth theme is that engagement can transform traditional research ethics principles and frameworks. To conclude this introduction to the volume, I briefly describe each of these themes below. The chapters in this volume span these themes, providing a robust, holistic, and multi-disciplinary – albeit, of course, incomplete – analysis of the ethics of patient and community stakeholder-engaged health research.

Health researchers initially embraced patient and community stakeholder engagement as a means of protecting research participants and communities from potential harms. Patient and community stakeholder engagement, when done thoughtfully and with intention, can add ethical value to research studies, making them safer, beneficial, and fairer (Wallerstein & Duran, 2017). Thus, stakeholder engagement is often framed as "more ethical"; for communities that have been exploited by researchers, engagement is arguably ethically *required*. This value added can be described as both intrinsic (e.g., "the right thing to do") and instrumental (e.g., necessary for trust). It is often noted that research ethics was born of scandal (Reverby, 2012). Some of the most infamous research scandals, from last century and in the more recent past, have involved some form of deception. These include the Public Health Service-funded study of syphilis in poor African American men in rural Alabama (Jones, 2008), the Willowbrook study that involved deliberately infecting cognitively impaired children with hepatitis (Robinson & Unruh, 2008), and the first-in-human gene transfer study that led to the death of Jesse Gelsinger (Wilson, 2010). Involving patient and community stakeholders in research planning and implementation shines the light on researcher behavior, thus minimizing the potential for deception or misunderstanding. Patient and community engagement can also foster trust, which is necessary to recruit participants, especially in communities or groups where past dubious behavior of researchers or research institutions has led to mistrust or distrust (Shavers et al., 2000).

Beyond transparency and trust, engagement provides voice and representation, which are necessary for important ethical determinations, such as whether a research study is valuable from the perspective of those being studied, whether the risks of a study are reasonable in relation to the potential benefits, or whether the procedures, risks, and potential benefits are adequately described in an informed consent form. Many chapters in this volume highlight the critical role of stakeholder voices in defining what is ethical in research. For example, McMillan (Chap. 11) reflects on her experience contributing to research ethics policy. Black and co-authors (Chap. 10) share findings from listening sessions with community members who have participated in research. Ballance and Ripley (Chap. 14) emphasize the importance of including stakeholder perspectives in decisions about payment to research participants and research partners. Guta, Newman, and Bourne (Chap. 15) articulate how community research partners may define risks and benefits differently than academic research partners. Goodman and co-authors (Chap. 16) emphasize how stakeholder partners should be involved in decisions about data use and sharing. Neufeld and co-authors (Chap. 20) provide an example of community research review, a mechanism for elevating community voice in research.

The authors of all chapters in this volume, whether explicitly or implicitly, take the position that considering the perspectives of patient and community stakeholders contributes to ethical research. However, they also take the position that stakeholder engagement can be done superficially, thoughtlessly, or even recklessly, and that engagement done poorly does not only disrespect but can even cause harm to stakeholders and communities (Brown et al., 2021). Stakeholder engagement in research is a process – a long and resource intensive process – the best practices for which have ethical dimensions and thus require specific guidance (Clinical and Translational Science Awards Consortium, 2011; Israel et al., 1998; Wallerstein & Duran, 2017). Several chapters in this volume address the unique ethical responsibilities that academic researchers have when engaging patient and community partners in research. Durkin and co-authors (Chap. 9) discuss what it means for researchers to treat community research partners respectfully. Hebert-Beirne and colleagues (Chap. 5) and Chou and Frazier (Chap. 6) describe their experiences of dynamic reflection in order to promote equity and power sharing. Mosavel and Philips (Chap. 8) discuss specific risks to and strategies for protecting community research partners working in the field.

A fourth theme in scholarship on patient and community stakeholder-engaged research involves the application of existing ethical and regulatory guidance to the unique aspects of engaged work. Stakeholder-engaged research also requires rethinking traditional research ethics concepts such as conflicts of interest, discussed by Parker and Mintzes (Chap. 12), or protection from potential risk of harm, discussed by Guta, Newman, and Bourne (Chap. 15) and Mosavel and Phillips (Chap. 8).

A final theme that has emerged from recent scholarship is that the theory and practice of engagement has the potential to radically transform the way we – all stakeholders in the health research community – think about ethics and the responsible conduct of research. Patient and community stakeholder engagement in health-related research has grown exponentially in the last three decades, as has its acceptance not simply as a legitimate approach but as a "key ingredient" of ethical research. This growth has been accompanied by changes in how the health research community thinks about ethics. The expansion of stakeholder engagement has stimulated reassessment of the criteria by which research studies are evaluated, the norms that define ethical research, and the regulations and mechanisms that exist to promote ethical research and protect research participants. Revision of these criteria, norms, and regulations is impending, as the scientific community is incrementally re-conceptualizing their understanding of the obligations of researchers and institutions to research participants and local communities. Examples of this can be seen in recent debates about the extent of researchers' obligations to share both individual results and aggregated findings with participants and share data with other scientists. Chapters in this volume address the deficiencies of the *Belmont* framework (Hurley, Chap. 17), describe the tension between the federal research regulations for institutional review board (IRB) review and stakeholder-engaged research (Cargill, Chap. 18), propose new models for evaluating the ethics of research (Gunay and co-authors, Chap. 19; Neufeld and co-authors, Chap. 20) and propose new frameworks for determining the ethical responsibilities of researchers (Mikesell, Chap. 3; Grant and DaViera, Chap. 4).

In introducing the chapters in this volume, I would also like to make a note about terminology. Research that engages patient and community stakeholders includes a range of approaches such as community-based participatory research (CBPR), patient centered outcomes research (PCOR), participatory action research (PAR), and others. Thus, authors in this volume use different terminology to describe their particular approaches, but all under the wide umbrella of "community and patient stakeholder-engaged research." Authors also use the terms "partners," "stakeholders," and "community researchers" to respectfully refer to research collaborators not employed by traditional academic research institutions, not formally trained in research, and/or hired as research personnel primarily because of shared characteristics with research participants rather than prior research work experience.

Health research is broadly inclusive of clinical biomedical research, public health and health promotion research, nursing research, allied health research, and social science research aimed at improving human health and well-being. In inviting contributions, I aimed to include authors working in as many different areas of health research as I could. I also aimed to be inclusive of a wide range of research approaches, methods, disciplines, and communities. Of course many are missing (voices from indigenous communities, scholars writing about the ethics of genetic research with identifiable communities, and considerations of research in humanitarian crises are just a few examples that immediately come to mind).

Lastly, in inviting contributions I aimed to include as many patient and community stakeholder perspectives as possible. Of course, the structures of academic publication make this challenging, and writing a book chapter – especially during a global pandemic – might be viewed as a luxury not all can afford. However, several chapters provide models of stakeholder partner inclusion in authorship. For those interested in the ethics of engaged research, I want to conclude with a final challenge: to continue to re-think the usual way of doing research.

References

Anderson, E. E., & Spellecy, R. (2021). Research that engages community and patient partners. In A. S. Iltis & D. MacKay (Eds.), *Oxford handbook of research ethics*. Oxford.

Brown, B., Taylor, J., Dubé, K., Kuzmanović, D., Long, Y., & Marg, L. (2021). Ethical reflections on the conduct of HIV research with community members: A case study. *Journal of Empirical Research on Human Research Ethics, 16*(1–2), 65–77.

Clinical and Translational Science Awards Consortium, Community Engagement Key Function Committee Task Force on the Principles of Community Engagement. (2011). *Principles of community engagement*. US Government Printing Office.

Israel, B. A., Schulz, A. J., Parker, E. A., & Becker, A. B. (1998). Review of community-based research: Assessing partnership approaches to improve public health. *Annual Review of Public Health, 19*(1), 173–202.

Jones, J. H. (2008). The Tuskegee syphilis experiment. In *The Oxford textbook of clinical research ethics* (pp. 86–96). Oxford University Press.

Mikesell, L., Bromley, E., & Khodyakov, D. (2013). Ethical community-engaged research: A literature review. *American Journal of Public Health, 103*(12), e7–e14.

National Commission for the Protection of Human Subjects of Biomedical and Behavioral Research. (1979). *The Belmont Report: Ethical principles and guidelines for the protection of human subjects of research*. https://www.hhs.gov/ohrp/regulations-and-policy/belmont-report/read-the-belmont-report/index.html#xethical.

Reverby, S. M. (2012). Ethical failures and history lessons: The US Public Health Service research studies in Tuskegee and Guatemala. *Public Health Reviews, 34*(1), 1–18.

Robinson, W. M., & Unruh, B. T. (2008). The hepatitis experiments at the Willowbrook State School. In *The Oxford textbook of clinical research ethics* (pp. 80–85). Oxford University Press.

Shavers, V. L., Lynch, C. F., & Burmeister, L. F. (2000). Knowledge of the Tuskegee study and its impact on the willingness to participate in medical research studies. *Journal of the National Medical Association, 92*(12), 563.

Spellecy, R., & Anderson, E. E. (2021). Patient and community engagement. In E. Bankert, B. Gordon, E. Hurley, & S. Shriver (Eds.), *IRB management and function*. Jones and Bartlett.

Wallerstein, N., & Duran, B. (2017). The theoretical, historical and practice roots of CBPR. In *Community-based participatory research for health: Advancing social and health equity* (pp. 17–29). Wiley.

Wilson, R. F. (2010). The death of Jesse Gelsinger: New evidence of the influence of money and prestige in human research. *American Journal of Law & Medicine, 36*(2–3), 295–325.

Emily E. Anderson, PhD, MPH is Professor of Bioethics at Loyola University Chicago's Stritch School of Medicine. Early in her career she coordinated community-based public health studies, leading to a lifelong interest in the ethics of engaging community and patient stakeholders in research. She is co-author (with Amy Corneli) of *100 Questions (and Answers) About Research Ethics* and creator of CIRTification, a free online human research protections training program for community research partners (https://ccts.uic.edu/resources/cirtification/).

Chapter 2
Theorizing Participatory Research

Andrew Evans and Angela Potochnik

2.1 Introduction

Scientific research involving public participation is nothing new. Participatory research on the environment and living world was conducted as early as the 1880s. These projects mostly consisted of the public collecting data on birds and the weather (Bonney et al., 2009). In the 1960s and 1970s, participatory research on butterflies was conducted in the UK and on spiderwort flowers near nuclear reactors in Japan (Kimura & Kinchy, 2019). Another early example of participatory research is the long-running work of the Cornell Lab of Ornithology, in which members of the public help to collect data on bird breeding habits, courtship behaviors, habitats, color morphs, and more (Bonney et al., 2009; Eitzel et al., 2017). Kimura and Kinchy (2019) highlight several more recent projects, such as studies on the impact of fracking on communities in Pennsylvania and New York, the detection of radiation in Japan, and the monitoring of genetically engineered crops in Mexico.

Some trace the beginning of participatory research back to Kurt Lewin's "action research" (1946) and the associated "participatory action research." This early version of participatory research was connected to social activism and "undertaken with or by—not *on* or *for*—society's marginalized peoples" (Macaulay, 2017, 256). This tradition and focus on marginalized groups is also tied to Paulo Freire's

A. Evans (✉)
Reilly Center for Science, Technology, and Values, University of Notre Dame, Notre Dame, IN, USA
e-mail: aevans23@nd.edu

A. Potochnik
Department of Philosophy, University of Cincinnati, Cincinnati, OH, USA
e-mail: potochaa@ucmail.uc.edu

E. E. Anderson (ed.), *Ethical Issues in Community and Patient Stakeholder–Engaged Health Research*, Philosophy and Medicine 146,
https://doi.org/10.1007/978-3-031-40379-8_2

theories and his influential work, *Pedagogy of the Oppressed* (1970). Other terms for participatory research include citizen science, community-based participatory research, community science, and critical participatory action research. Different terminology is associated with different scientific disciplines and, often, different forms of public participation. Participatory research ranges from large-scale ecology monitoring programs, to localized studies of health outcomes carried out with community leadership, to research designed from the ground up with community-identified social change as the outcome. We follow Dunlap et al. (2021) and use the term "participatory research," or PR, as an umbrella term for any scientific research involving public participation (See Vaughn & Jacquez, 2020 for a fuller discussion of the variety of terminology and participatory practices).

The purpose of this chapter is to survey theoretical resources for conceptualizing and designing participatory research projects. In the next section, we introduce two competing formulations of the goal of PR: *social change* and *knowledge gathering*. We then consider subtler questions about why scientists conduct participatory research and why community members participate, as well as the value of such research. In the following section, we apply this theoretical framework to challenges that participatory research faces and provide some guiding questions for the development, implementation, and analysis of participatory research projects. Next, we consider different typologies of participatory research. One typology categorizes projects by level of community member involvement (Shirk et al., 2012), while others take the virtues of participation into account (Kimura & Kinchy, 2016; Dunlap et al., 2021). Lastly, we explore how these theoretical resources apply to participatory research occurring in health contexts. PR approaches are perhaps particularly promising in health research, given the research focus on human subjects and the relevance of the research to stakeholder concerns.

2.2 What's the Point of Participatory Research?

In order to gain perspective on participatory research, it may be useful to ask what goal or goals are furthered by including the public in the research process. Because PR occurs in a variety of contexts, each focused on different phenomena with different aims of prediction, explanation, or action, there is reason to think its goals may vary with some of these differences.

Cooper and Lewenstein (2016) and Eitzel et al. (2017) introduce a helpful way to characterize two distinct strands of participatory research: one focused on *social change* and the other focused on *knowledge gathering*. The first strand primarily comes from the work of Alan Irwin (1995). This approach sees participatory research as a form of democratic participation and an effort towards systemic change. As Irwin (1995) puts it, "We now have 'science for the people'; in other words, the various attempts (both practical and theoretical) to place technical expertise at the direct service of people" (5).

The PR examples mentioned above on fracking, radiation, and genetically engineered crops, drawn from Kimura and Kinchy (2019), were all spurred by concerned community members and designed to serve the interests of the community. Therefore, these are examples of PR as social change. For example, in 2012, communities in Pennsylvania and New York began monitoring their own water quality in response to fracking in the area. Water monitoring groups were created that forged partnerships with academic researchers and professional scientists. This research prompted government agencies to take action on water quality (Kimura & Kinchy, 2019). The purpose of this effort was not only to gather knowledge but also to protect the health and safety of community members. Action research and participatory action research are also in the tradition of PR as social change. These forms of research put primary emphasis on the role of the community members pushing for reform.

The second strand characterizes the value of participatory research as stemming from the ability to collect large amounts of data. This is exemplified by the approach of Rick Bonney and colleagues at the Cornell Lab of Ornithology (2009). For years, the lab has recruited public participants to assist scientists in answering research questions about birds. This has resulted in data about bird distribution patterns, how the environment impacts breeding, how infectious diseases spread in animal populations, and how acid rain affects birds. In addition to data collection, the lab aims to educate the public on birds—pursing both "scientific and educational outcomes" (Bonney et al., 2009, 978). Despite this commitment to educating the public, a major goal of the lab is clearly to harness the power of public participation to gather more data than would be possible using traditional research methods:

> Studying large-scale patterns in nature requires a vast amount of data to be collected across an array of locations and habitations over spans of years or even decades. One way to obtain such data is through citizen science, a research technique that enlists the public in gathering scientific information. (Bonney et al., 2009, 977)

These two different orientations to public participation in scientific research—social change and knowledge gathering—result in different features and standards for success. Ottinger (2017) also emphasizes the distinction between these two orientations and points out how the locus of authority differs between them. Whereas the goal of knowledge gathering motivates the preservation of authority for scientists, the goal of social change motivates disrupting traditional authority structures and empowers the included members of the public to lead—and lead in a way that generates both social and scientific change. Ottinger stresses that the more conservative knowledge gathering approach risks diverting resources and attention from the more radical approach that can change both science and society.

We also see a difference between the two strands of PR in terms of whose perspectives they emphasize. Members of the public participating in PR can be expected to have different intentions, aims, and agendas than the scientists pursuing PR (cf. Dunlap et al., 2021). Projects that pursue social change will benefit from taking on perspectives of the participating public in order to achieve community goals. PR projects aimed at knowledge gathering, in contrast, are more often scientist-driven, since knowledge gathering is central to the aim of traditional scientific research. That said, it is nonetheless possible for PR with the goal of social change to preserve scientists' authority and prioritize their perspectives; conversely, PR with the goal of knowledge gathering can take seriously the participating public's priorities.

Finally, note that these two PR goals of social change and knowledge gathering are not mutually exclusive and may not be at odds. It is possible for research projects to both further the scientific aim of generating knowledge and contribute to social change—indeed, sometimes pursuing certain types of scientific knowledge furthers a social agenda. As mentioned above, the efforts in New York and Pennsylvania to study the impact of fracking aimed to obtain data about water quality as well as to pressure the government to improve water quality. In our view, it is helpful to think of participatory research in terms of these two strands or goals of social change and knowledge gathering identified by Cooper and Lewenstein (2016) and Eitzel et al. (2017). These strands relate to distinct traditions of PR, are associated with different priorities, and may impact the power dynamics of the collaboration between researchers and participants.

Let us now take a closer look at the specific purposes of participatory research and how those might relate to one another. As one might imagine, the recognized purposes of participatory research vary across disciplines and research traditions, as reflected in the terminological variety we have already noted. Citizen science expands scientific projects by leveraging the power of citizens; community-based participatory research leverages the participation of community members for the good of those communities; action research aims at practical, often sociopolitical, goals. Finer delineations of types of purposes within these traditions can help identify different kinds of values produced by participatory approaches, as well as challenges posed by conflicting agendas among researchers, participants, or the combination of the two.

Returning to PR as social change and PR as knowledge gathering, we can see that the former is *sociopolitical* in nature, while the latter is *epistemic*. Dunlap et al. (2021) similarly distinguish between epistemic, practical, and ethical goals of participatory research. Their category of ethical goals is similar to what we have termed sociopolitical goals, while practical goals is a helpful third category. Dunlap et al. also point out that the same features of PR might satisfy multiple different goals. Amassing more scientific data, for example, is a way that PR serves a common epistemic goal but might also promote the practical goal of increasing the chance of publication, and this increase in the amount of data or data points might also serve the ethical or sociopolitical goal of, say, improving health outcomes.

We think it is useful to further break down the category of sociopolitical or ethical goals. Research goals can be *political* in nature, that is, goals that are politically valanced given current societal norms. These might be perceived as politically partisan and be controversial, such as the goal of ending fracking. *Societal* goals, in contrast, are broad social goals that are widely shared, such as improving health or educational outcomes. Finally, *communal* goals are sociopolitical or ethical goals that benefit some particular, often local, community. An example of a communal goal for PR is improving the water quality in Flint, Michigan. We summarize these

Table 2.1 We propose these five categories of goals that participatory research may aim to advance, based in part on the discussions of Cooper and Lewenstein (2016), Eitzel et al. (2017), and Dunlap et al. (2021)

Categories of PR goals	Description of goals
Epistemic	Goals that further knowledge, such as improving research questions, increasing data, and improving accuracy of findings
Practical	Goals that improve an individual's life, or practice of life. For example, publication success, educational enrichment, or being a part of a research community
Communal	Goals of a specific (often local) community as defined by community stakeholders, such as improved water quality in a particular city or improved healthcare access for transgender adults
Societal	Broad social goals that are widely shared, such as improving health or educational outcomes
Political	Goals that are politically valanced or the priority of which is disputed, such as ending fracking or decreasing reliance on coal and oil

categories of potential goals participatory research might aim to advance in Table 2.1.

We have suggested that a given participatory research project can simultaneously pursue different types of goals, and the same features of PR projects might advance multiple goals of different types. It is also possible, or even likely, that different stakeholders in a PR project—especially researchers and public participants—will prioritize different types of goals (Dunlap et al., 2021). The setting of goals and prioritization among them reflects the perspective and values possessed by an individual or community. Dunlap et al. (2021) call this the "perspectival nature of values" (286). An example of the significance of perspective for goal setting is how the influence of the participating public can promote social change in PR. Members of the public motivated to participate in scientific research are often motivated by communal, societal, or political goals. We can also see divergence in terms of practical goals. For scientists involved in PR, publication of their research is likely a practical goal. In contrast, public participants are more likely to value other forms of recognition (for example, having their contribution publicized on the project website), practical impacts of the research, or their own personal enrichment.

However, we cannot draw sweeping conclusions about types of goals pursued by scientists vs. public participants. While it may be that scientists often have epistemic and practical goals for their research, this need not be the case. A scientist may aim to affect social change with their research, and a public participant may genuinely want to contribute to knowledge gathering. Researchers and public participants may share a goal that benefits society at large. The point is simply that the goals of any PR project depend on and are defined by who is involved. As Dunlap et al. (2021) note, "What counts as a virtue and how important it is compared to other virtues depends on who is evaluating it and what their larger goals and values are" (287).

2.3 Addressing the Challenges of Participatory Research

Articulating categories of PR goals and how these can vary with perspective clarifies concerns that have been raised about PR. A standard objection is that PR is too tainted by advocacy (Elliott & Rosenberg, 2019; Kimura & Kinchy, 2019). This criticism expresses skepticism about the political goals of PR from a perspective that privileges epistemic goals. The categorization of PR goals we have introduced makes it possible to replace this objection with more helpful specific questions about individual PR projects: What, if any, is the project's political goal, and does pursuit of that goal improperly impinge on the epistemic attributes of the research? For example, a project on the impacts of climate change run by activists clearly has a political goal and may be criticized for being epistemically biased. Would a different goal (say, societal or practical) lead to a different research approach, and if so, what benefits and drawbacks would there be to that alternative approach? Another criticism of PR is that it results in volunteers doing research that should be the government's responsibility, shifting responsibility for health and safety onto the community itself (Kimura & Kinchy, 2019). This challenge indicates that two societal goals can be at odds (e.g., government accountability vs. public knowledge of water quality).

A related but distinct concern sometimes raised about PR, especially when the inclusion of the participating public is limited to data collection, is that the quality of data is lower than it would have been if professional scientists had collected it. Kovaka (2021) points out that, in a survey by Burgess et al. (2017), many scientists cited data quality as a concern with PR. Kovaka compellingly argues that attending to the specific goals of any given research project enables us to appreciate the compensatory advantages of participatory approaches—such as breadth of data and variety of circumstances for data collection, investment in the research, and more—that offset any limitations in data quality. Of course, when data accuracy is critically important, a PR approach with a large number of data collectors may not be well suited to the project given risks to reliability. But in other cases, public participation may improve data quality, thus our emphasis on attending to the particular goals of PR projects. There have been efforts to understand the impact of community participant involvement on data collection, quality, and analysis. For example, in a qualitative study where university researchers and service-user researchers collected and interpreted data on mental healthcare experiences, additional analysis was conducted to identify and understand differences between the two groups' interpretation (Gillard et al., 2010).

Attending to the perspectival nature of goals also offers a helpful interpretation of concerns that have been raised about the power dynamics of PR. In some projects, despite public involvement, scientists remain in charge:

> Scientists primarily value volunteers' contributions to the extent that the information participants collect can be compiled into large data sets. Conceptualizing citizen scientists as "volunteers" seems to put them in a role that is perpetually subordinated to "real" scientists. (Kimura & Kinchy, 2019, 64)

This potential power imbalance between scientists and public participants can be articulated in terms of which goals—or more to the point, whose goals—a PR project serves. Scientists and the participating public may well have divergent goals for the project, and if the scientists have more power than the participating public, their goals may be advanced to the detriment of the public participants' goals.

We cannot fully address these challenges here. Rather, we emphasize that it is important to critically examine the types of goals furthered by PR, how those goals relate to one another, and who possesses those goals. This analysis can guide productive engagement with such challenges as well as determination of when participatory approaches are called for and what variety of participation is appropriate.

Inspired by this promise, here is a goal-based series of questions that may be useful to consider and perhaps even explicitly discuss when designing, implementing, and analyzing a PR project:

1. What are the primary goals of the research project from the scientists' perspective(s)?
2. What are the primary goals of the research project from the participants' perspective(s)?
3. From the scientists' perspective(s), what is the main reason for including the public in the project?
4. From the public participants' perspective(s), what is the main reason for working with scientists to pursue their goals?
5. What is the relationship between public participants' goals and the scientists' goals? To what extent can both be achieved, and how can achievement of all goals be maximized? What methods are in place to achieve goals?
6. What is the relationship between public participants and scientists in the project? How are matters of power and privilege addressed? Is this done adequately?

Questions 1 and 2 concern the motivation of the project from the perspective of all participants. More explicitly attending to both questions can ensure that details of project design, especially the extent and form of public participation, further the goals of both scientists and the public. Questions 3 and 4 explore why public participation is appropriate for the project and what motivates scientists and public participants to be part of the project. Finally, Questions 5 and 6 explicitly interrogate the interactions and power dynamics between scientists and public participants.

2.4 Types of Participatory Research

The previous discussions of the goals of participatory research suggest that participatory methods can be useful in different regards (epistemic, practical, political, societal, communal) and that the goals of a participatory research project may vary with perspectives, especially of scientists vs. participating public. In this section, we draw from three typologies for participatory research approaches developed by Shirk et al. (2012), Kimura and Kinchy (2016), and Dunlap et al. (2021) to articulate a perspective-driven approach to categorizing types of PR projects. Such a categorization can clarify similarities and differences among PR projects. This can also highlight decision points in the development of a participatory research project by making more explicit how the project could have developed differently along some dimension(s). When designing a PR project, we suggest using all three typologies in the following order: start by using the Dunlap et al. (2021) typology to identify divergence in goals, then use the Kimura and Kinchy (2016) typology to determine the intended virtues or payoffs of the project, and end with the Shirk et al. (2012) typology to determine the level of public participation. We end by extending our list of questions to consider when developing and implementing a project.

As discussed above, Dunlap et al. (2021) highlight the perspectival nature of PR goals. As a starting point for PR categorization, they ask: What are the goals of the participating public and scientists, and to what extent do these diverge? When the goals of the participating public and scientists are well aligned, then either party can guide the research design and execution, with the other party included as expertise, ability, and interests dictate. Often, this scenario plays out with the professional scientists conceiving of, planning, and designing the research, with public participation in data gathering and/or data analysis. This arrangement works well for the Cornell Lab of Ornithology, where scientists and interested members of the public share the goals of protecting birds and educating the public about birds. Professional scientists are well positioned to structure the research, while the participating public has strength in numbers and geographic distribution to support data collection and outreach efforts.

However, as we have noted, the goals of public participants often deviate from those of professional scientists. In such cases, we concluded in the prior section that it is essential to ascertain the goals of the participating public, ensure these are met by research design, and address conflicts caused by power differentials. In the present context, note that when goals diverge, ensuring public participants' goals are met by the research design also tends to require the inclusion of public participation earlier in research design, often at the stages of determining specific research questions and methods. This approach is common in some traditions of PR, including community-based participatory research and action research, but less common in citizen science traditions. We should also note that in some cases of PR as social change, public participants initiate and lead the research process, as in the example discussed above of water monitoring in New York and Pennsylvania (Kimura & Kinchy, 2019). In situations like this, public participant goals will take precedence over the goals of scientists (if scientists are involved in the research at all).

Once the goals of the participating public and scientists are identified and alignment or divergence among them ascertained, this information can be used to specify the particular aims of the research. Different specific aims of explanation, prediction, or action motivate different features of the methods and design of scientific research (Potochnik, 2015). This is where the categorization put forward by Kimura and Kinchy (2016) can be useful. Their typology of PR considers widely recognized *virtues*, including but not limited to: increasing scientific data; improving the participating public's scientific literacy and engagement (mentioned above); building community capacity for action; improving the relationships between scientists and the public; and driving policy change. These virtues span the types of goals we identified in the previous section: epistemic, practical, communal, societal, and political. The participating public's and scientists' specific goals for a PR project will determine which of these virtues are prioritized, which in turn shapes other aspects of the project.

One important consideration of any PR project is the nature of public participation: To what parts of the project does the public contribute, and to what extent? This aspect of PR projects is (or at least should be) influenced by the virtues the project aims towards, which we have suggested are shaped by the professional scientists' and participating public's goals. This chain of considerations starts with participants' possibly divergent goals for the research project, moves to the question of the virtues or payoffs of the project and approach, and finally asks: what form of participation is warranted?

Shirk et al. (2012) categorize participatory approaches according to the extent of public participation, which is helpful at this juncture. Here, we have ordered Shirk et al.'s categories in increasing degree of influence by the participating public. *Contributory* projects are fully designed by scientists and members of the public only contribute to implementing the research, often in data collection. *Collaborative* projects are also designed by scientists but allow the public to have some control over research questions. In *co-created* projects, at least some members of the public participate in all aspects of the research, including design and management. *Contractual* projects occur when communities contract scientists to conduct research on their behalf. Finally, in *collegial* contributions, members of the public conduct independent research with varying degrees of recognition by the scientific establishment. This categorization provides a neat separation of PR projects into types, ordered by degree of public participants' control of the project. Although it might be tempting to think that control is the important variable in PR approaches, we hope it is clear that goals and virtues should also be considered as part of the broader analysis we have developed here. When designing PR projects, we suggest proceeding from a consideration of goals (and possible divergence in goals) to a consideration of payoffs or virtues, and only then to a consideration of the necessary degree of participation.

Continuing with the approach we adopted in the previous section, we end this section with some questions about the type of involvement public participants and scientists should have in a PR project, based on consideration of aims:

7. In what ways should the relationship between scientists' goals and public participants' goals each shape the research agenda?
8. Whose expertise is relevant, and in what ways, to the pursuit of these goals?
9. What are the ultimate virtues or payoffs for the project, and are these reflected in the shared goals between scientists and public participants?
10. At what PR project stage(s) should scientists be involved? At what PR project stage(s) should public participants be involved? How does this set up further the ultimate goals of the project?

Question 7 is related to Question 5 at the conclusion of the previous section, regarding the relationship between public participants' goals and scientists' goals. However, Question 7 is slightly different, asking how the various goals influence the specifics of the research design. Question 8 encourages reflection about how the expertise of the scientists and public participants is important for pursuing the specific constellation of goals for the PR project. Question 9 connects goals to payoffs, making sure that the goals for the project actually align with expected outcomes. Finally, Question 10 prompts project designers to reflect on what role scientists and public participants should play in the project, given the considerations of previous questions.

2.5 Participatory Research in Health Contexts

In this section, we apply the theoretical resources we have introduced above to health contexts and include a discussion of the unique ethical challenges of participatory health research. Often, PR in health contexts is referred to as "biomedical," as in, "biomedical citizen science." But this term is linked to specific medical contexts like research hospitals and associated with the reductionist "medical model" of health. In this section, we adapt our umbrella term "participatory research" and speak of "participatory health research," including not only traditional biomedical research that involves public participation but also research done by individuals in their own homes or by groups of non-professionals in the community.

There are a variety of approaches under the umbrella of participatory health research. "Community-based participatory research" (CBPR), an approach discussed above, is common in public health contexts. The orientation of CBPR is to treat the community as a partner rather than the subject of research (Shore, 2007). CBPR falls under the umbrella of PR as social change since its goals are often social, communal, or political in nature. In contrast, "research as coproduction" is a term used by Gillard et al. (2012) for health research in which service users and university researchers work together, not with the goal of social change, but instead with the goal of knowledge gathering. "Biohacking," refers to the practice of do-it-yourself biology, for example, people tinkering with biotechnology in their home or at a community laboratory (Trejo et al., 2021). "Grinders" are people who experiment on their own bodies, via body modification, often with the goal of enhancement (Trejo et al., 2021). In "self-tracking studies," people track their daily health data either individually or in collaboration with others, usually using an internet-based platform (Wiggins & Wilbanks, 2019). Lastly, "survivor research" stands in contrast to CBPR, which is a collaboration between scientists and public participants, as well as biomedical citizen science, which is primarily individual-driven. An example of survivor research is that conducted by mental health service users who reject the way psychiatry operates and seek an alternative (Ormerod et al., 2018).

An example of CBPR is the LU-Salud project conducted by researchers in psychology, education, and medicine at the University of Cincinnati. This study sought to better understand health issues in the local Latino community. Academic researchers recruited Latino community members, conceived of as "co-researchers," who collaborated at each stage of the research (Vaughn et al., 2017). The co-researchers helped design surveys and then led efforts to disseminate the surveys in the targeted community. As data were collected, regular meetings of the academic researchers and community co-researchers helped all parties stay informed throughout the process. At the end of the study, the co-researchers contributed to the interpretation of data (Vaughn et al., 2017). This PR project involved shared researcher and public participant goals of improved health outcomes in the targeted community that are communal in nature, alongside perhaps other subsidiary epistemic and practical goals. These communal goals were best served through significant community involvement.

In contrast, Gillard et al. (2010) provide an example of "research as coproduction" in which university researchers and service-user researchers conducted a qualitative study on the experience of psychiatric detention. All parties took part in the development, implementation, and interpretation of the interviews. Though this study is similar in structure to the LU-Salud study, its goals were not necessarily social change but instead the coproduction of knowledge.

Unlike both CBPR and "research as coproduction," biohacking, research conducted by grinders, and self-tracking studies are all typically driven by individual rather than shared goals. These practices are sometimes referred to collectively as "biomedical citizen science" and are characterized by their autonomous and individualized nature (Trejo et al., 2021). Interestingly, citizen science traditions discussed above are typically driven by professional researchers, while biomedical citizen science of this form is typically driven by public participants, with professional researchers only involved in the margins, if at all. This is not to say that there is no community aspect to these practices; biohacking and grinder groups gather to promote and collaborate on projects. However, even then, the research is primarily individual-driven.

One example of biomedical citizen science is the self-tracking of health data by people sometimes called "lifehackers" (Trejo et al., 2021). Wiggins and Wilbanks (2019) distinguish between forms of lifehacking that have varying levels of social collaboration. In 'N-of-1' studies, individuals track their "diets, environments, sleep, medicines, bathroom habits, and more…" independently without collaborating with others. In contrast, 'N-of-we' communities exist for lifehackers to share results and tips with each other. These communities employ N-of-1 methods, but exchange information with each other. A third model is 'N-of-many-1s' studies, which are top-down operations in which professional institutions standardize and aggregate self-tracking data. This is the least autonomous of the three types of self-tracking studies (Wiggins & Wilbanks, 2019) and thus bears the greatest resemblance to researcher-driven citizen science in other fields.

"Survivor research" exists in opposition to the power structures of establishment psychiatry and so bears resemblance to the antipsychiatry and Mad Pride movements. The "Survivor Researcher Network Manifesto" explicitly describes this movement as having roots in "survivor activism" that "seeks to challenge the psychiatric system" (Ormerod et al., 2018, 4). The purpose of the Survivor Researcher Network is to connect service users who want to conduct mental health research that is independent, and often critical of, academic psychiatric research. Despite the fact that both survivor research and CBPR push for social change, survivor research is distinct in that it exists outside the mainstream of healthcare and has a particular focus on mental health issues.

In general, participatory health research faces the same challenges that exist for all types of PR, such as power dynamics. Participatory health research is also sometimes criticized as biased or tainted by advocacy. This is especially the case in CBPR and forms of action research, since goals are often framed in terms of community improvement and social change. However, some challenges are specific to participatory health research. In health contexts, the line between public participant and human subject can be blurred. In forms of PR that target non-human subjects, this is not an issue; when PR projects test food for radiation, it is clear that the food is the subject of research, and the public participants are engaging as scientists. However, in health contexts, the bodies and/or viewpoints of participants can do double duty as the subject of scientific inquiry and participants in the process of inquiry. For example, in the LU-Salud study, community members played an active role in the development and implementation of the research, but ultimately the data being collected represented the beliefs, needs, and behaviors of other community members. So, while some community members played the role of co-researcher, others played the role of human subject. Grinders have autonomy over what is done to their body, yet it is still their body that is being experimented on. In this way, grinders are both scientist and human subject. Ultimately, involvement in participatory health research can be empowering. In reference to CBPR, one interviewee in Shore's (2007) study said, "participants [become] actors in the process rather than just objects, and by giving them some control over the process, it potentially creates the kind of knowledge that will be more useful to them" (34).

Since participatory health research can involve intervening on human bodies, safety concerns may arise. Institutional Review Boards (IRBs) are administrative bodies whose review is required for any institutionally sponsored research in order to protect the rights of human subjects. IRBs decide what is allowable according to ethical standards. These boards are often viewed with suspicion in biohacking and grinder communities (Trejo et al., 2021). When practices like biohacking and body modification are conducted without institutional support or involvement, no such ethical or regulatory oversight exists. Trejo et al. (2021) conducted a qualitative study that observed attitudes about ethical oversight in biomedical citizen science communities. They found that these communities highly value their bodily autonomy and consider practices like body modification their right. Options like obtaining IRB approval were generally unpopular not just because of the value these groups place on autonomy, but also because it is expensive and time consuming to acquire IRB approval. Instead, community members tended to prefer ethical oversight that occurred from within their community or individual ethical self-reflection (Trejo et al., 2021). In this context, it is helpful to consider the specific goals motivating a PR project. Any initiatives by professional researchers and their institutions to constrain, shape, or regulate projects, such as institutional recognition, financial resources for the research, access to intellectual or practical resources from the institution, or something else, will be most likely to succeed if they meaningfully further the public participants' research goals. Consideration of the specific goals for the research and the public participation in, or leadership of, that research is key.

Participatory health research that involves data mining poses risks. These risks are particularly salient for lifehackers who track their daily health data. Most of these studies require the use of large data-sharing networks like Facebook, Fitbit, or 23andMe, which carry some risk of data breaches or misuse of data by corporations (Wiggins & Wilbanks, 2019) and raise questions about who really benefits from these studies. Even though much of this research is driven by individual participants' interests, their reliance on corporations and institutions for data tracking puts them at risk of exploitation (Wiggins & Wilbanks, 2019).

The theoretical resources introduced earlier in the chapter can be applied to these challenges that are specific to participatory health research. More generally, the goal-based consideration of PR projects that we have introduced provides resources for understanding the array of participatory health research approaches and the distinctive contributions and challenges of each. We have suggested that PR goals can be divided into five categories: epistemic, practical, political, societal, and communal. Because goals are perspectival in nature, it is important to identify when goals diverge between stakeholders. CBPR projects often aim towards communal and political goals. They seek to benefit the local community and push for social change. Biohackers and grinders, on the other hand, usually have practical goals such as learning about science, body enhancement, or expressing bodily autonomy, and therefore the projects benefit the individuals that implement them. When more than one stakeholder is involved, goals can diverge. For instance, scientists conducting participatory health research may have primarily epistemic goals that conflict with the practical, communal, or political goals of participants. Determining the goals of a project, who prioritizes which goals, and where goals diverge is thus enlightening for participatory health research.

The typologies introduced above can also inform understanding of participatory health research in all its forms. Using Shirk et al.'s (2012) typology, for example, we can identify biohacking and body modification projects as collegial contributions—since they involve community members doing science independent of institutional influence. CBPR, on the other hand, tends towards the production of collaborative or co-created research depending on the level of community involvement. LU-Salud is co-created because community members participated in setting the research questions and the designing of surveys. Survivor research may be seen as a form of collegial contribution, although this tradition has formed in opposition to establishment psychiatry.

Finally, as this discussion suggests, the series of questions that we introduced are useful for participatory health research as well. It is important to understand how and why public participants and academic researchers alike are involved in the research, how they benefit, and what the shared goals of the project are. Further it is important to determine how goals result in outcomes and what role scientists and public participants each play in that process. In fact, these questions become even more urgent in health contexts. Because the line can be blurry between public participant and human subject, and because some participatory health research occurs fully outside the governance of institutional structures, the risk of exploitation is higher. A study that appears or even intends to be working with a community towards common goals may actually exploit participants for labor and data collection. Indeed, this pitfall has been all too common in the history of participatory research. Therefore, it is vital for the goals and interests of public participants to be explicitly identified and protected, which requires significant attention to power structures, thoughtful research design, and more.

2.6 Conclusion

Participatory research is a big tent—so it is at once important and challenging to describe the relevant terminology, concepts, and theoretical resources. In this chapter, we began by introducing a handful of examples of PR and varieties in its execution. We discussed two strands of participatory research that have been identified by Cooper and Lewenstein (2016) and Eitzel et al. (2017): *social change* and *knowledge gathering*. We highlighted the perspectival nature of goals and the importance of considering the divergence of goals between stakeholders. We also introduced three typologies that exist for categorizing participatory research projects and suggested a method of applying all three, working from attending to the goals of professional researchers and public participants, to identifying the virtue(s) of the PR project, to finally identifying the extent of public participation that can further the specific goals at hand. This resulted in a list of questions that might be used to guide the development, implementation, and analysis of PR projects. We ended by applying these concepts to participatory health research and identifying specific challenges that this form of PR faces. We hope that the theoretical resources introduced in this chapter prove helpful to the design, implementation, and theorizing of participatory research.

Acknowledgements We want to thank everyone who has been helpful in the writing of this chapter. This includes especially the University of Cincinnati Center for Public Engagement with Science research and discussion group, from which many of these ideas emerged. We also want to thank Emily Anderson for inviting us to contribute to this volume. Thank you to Maggie Su and an anonymous reviewer as well for helpful comments. Finally, we want to thank the organizers and participants of the Bioethics, Citizen Science, and Human Subject Protection Conference at Cincinnati Children's Hospital and Medical Center in September 2021, where Potochnik gave a presentation with some ideas that have made their way into this chapter.

References

Bonney, R., Cooper, C. B., Dickinson, J., Kelling, S., Phillips, T., Rosenberg, K. V., & Shirk, J. (2009). Citizen science: A developing tool for expanding science knowledge and scientific literacy. *American Institute of Biological Sciences, 59*(11), 977–984.

Burgess, H. K., DeBey, L. B., Froehlich, H. E., Schmidt, N., Theobald, E. J., Ettinger, A. K., HilleRisLambers, J., Tewksbury, J., & Parrish, J. K. (2017). The science of citizen science: Exploring barriers to use as a primary research tool. *Biological Conservation, 208*, 113–120.

Cooper, C. B., & Lewenstein, B. V. (2016). Two meanings of citizen science. In D. Cavalier (Ed.), *The rightful place of science: Citizen science*. Arizona State University Press.

Dunlap, L., Corris, A., Jacquart, M., Biener, Z., & Potochnik, A. (2021). Divergence of values and goals in participatory research. *Studies in History and Philosophy of Science, 88*, 284–291.

Eitzel, M. V., Cappadonna, J. L., Santos-Lang, C., Duerr, R. E., Virapongse, A., West, S. E., Kyba, C. C. M., Bowser, A., Cooper, C. B., Sforzi, A., Metcalfe, A. N., Harris, E. S., Thiel, M., Haklay, M., Ponciano, L., Roche, J., Ceccaroni, L., Shilling, F. M., Dörler, D., Heigl, F., Kiessling, T., Davis, B. Y., & Jiang, Q. (2017). Citizen science terminology matters: Exploring key terms. *Citizen Science: Theory and Practice, 2*(1), 1–20.

Elliott, K. C., & Rosenberg, J. (2019). Philosophical foundations for citizen science. *Citizen Science: Theory and Practice, 4*(1), 1–0. https://doi.org/10.5334/cstp.155

Freire, P. (1970). *The pedagogy of the oppressed*. Herder and Herder.

Gillard, S., Borschmann, R., Turner, K., Goodrich-Purnell, N., Lovell, K., & Chambers, M. (2010). 'What difference does it make?' Finding evidence of the impact of mental health service user researchers on research into the experiences of detained psychiatric patients. *Health Expectations, 3*(2), 185–194.

Gillard, S., Simons, L., Turner, K., Lucock, M., & Edwards, C. (2012). Patient and public involvement in the coproduction of knowledge: Reflection on the analysis of qualitative data in a mental health study. *Qualitative Health Research, 22*(8), 1126–1137.

Irwin, A. (1995). *Citizen science: A study of people, expertise, and sustainable development*. Routledge.

Kimura, A. H., & Kinchy, A. (2016). Citizen science: Probing the virtues and contexts of participatory research. *Engaging Science, Technology, and Society, 2*, 331–361

Kimura, A. H., & Kinchy, A. (2019). *Science by the people: Participation, power, and the politics of environmental knowledge*. Rutgers University Press.

Kovaka, K. (2021). Evaluating community science. *Studies in History and Philosophy of Science, 88*, 102–109.

Lewin, K. (1946). Action research and minority problems. *Journal of Social Issues, 2*(4), 34–46.

Macaulay, A. C. (2017). Participatory research: What is the history? Has the purpose changed? *Family Practice, 34*(3), 256–258. https://doi.org/10.1093/famora/cmw117

Ormerod, E., Beresford, P., Carr, S., Gould, D., Jeffreys, S., Machin, K., Poursanidou, D., Thompson, S., & Yiannoullou, S. (2018). Survivor researcher network manifesto. *Survivor Researcher Network*. https://survivorresearcher.net/wp-content/uploads/2021/04/2018_SRN_MANIFESTO.pdf. Accessed 30 July 2023.

Ottinger, G. (2017). Reconstructing or reproducing? Scientific authority and models of change in two traditions of citizen science. In D. Tyfield, R. Lave, S. Randalls, & C. Thorpe (Eds.), *The Routledge handbook of the political economy of science*. Routledge.

Potochnik, A. (2015). The diverse aims of science. *Studies in History and Philosophy of Science, 53*, 71–80.

Shirk, J. L., Ballard, H. L., Wilderman, C. C., Phillips, T., Wiggins, A., Jordan, R., McCallie, E., Minarchek, M., Lewenstein, B. V., Krasny, M. E., & Bonney, R. (2012). Public participation in scientific research: A framework for deliberate design. *Ecology and Society, 17*(2), 29.

Shore, N. (2007). Community-based participatory research and the ethics review process. *The Journal of Empirical research Ethics: An International Journal, 2*(1), 31–42.

Trejo, M., Canfield, I., Bash Brooks, W., Pearlman, A., & Guerrini, C. (2021). 'A cohort of pirate ships': Biomedical citizen scientists' attitudes toward ethical oversight. *Citizen Science: Theory and Practice, 6*(1), 1–15.
Vaughn, L. M., & Jacquez, F. (2020). Participatory research methods—Choice points in the research process. *Journal of Participatory Research Methods, 1*(1).
Vaughn, L. M., Jacquez, F., Zhen-Duan, J., Graham, C., & Marschner, D. (2017). Latinos Unidos por la Salud: The process of developing an immigrant community research tam. *Collaborations: A Journal of Community-based Research and Practice, 1*(1), 2.
Wiggins, A., & Wilbanks, J. (2019). The rise of citizen science in health and biomedical research. *The American Journal of Bioethics, 19*(8), 3–14.

Andrew Evans is visiting assistant professor of Health, Humanities, and Society at the University of Notre Dame Reilly Center for Science, Technology, and Values. Their research is on the philosophy of mental health, bioethics, and socially engaged philosophy of science. They received their PhD in Philosophy and MA in Mental Health Counseling from University of Cincinnati.

Angela Potochnik is professor and director of the Center for Public Engagement with Science. Her research addresses the nature of science and its successes and the relationships between science and the public. She is the author of *Idealization and the Aims of Science* (2017) and coauthor of *Recipes for Science* (2018), an introduction to scientific methods and reasoning. She earned her PhD from Stanford University in 2007.

Chapter 3
An Evolving Ethical Framework for Patient and Community-Engaged Research

Lisa Mikesell

3.1 Introduction

Health researchers today employ several forms of engaged research including but not limited to community-based participatory research (CBPR) (Wallerstein et al., 2018), patient-centered research (Johnson & Smalley, 2020), citizen science (Hecker et al., 2019), and participatory action research (Keahey, 2020). The processes and practices of engaging patients and community vary across research contexts. In some studies, patients and communities serve in rather limited roles, while in others they are extensively involved in decision-making throughout the entire research process (Brown, 2021). Subsequently, I refer to this work collectively as "engaged research" and attempt to develop a preliminary ethical framework that I hope can be applicable and adaptable across this continuum of engagement (Carman et al., 2013), since there is no one-size-fits-all approach to engaged research (Patient Centered Outcomes Research Institute, 2018).

Despite variability in how engagement is both conceptualized and realized in practice, patient and community involvement in different forms has become widespread and is recommended by many organizations and health research funders as good research practice (Oliver, 2006). Commonly cited benefits of engaged research include community buy-in and increased participation, improved patient and community understanding of the research process and materials, and improved health care quality (Carman et al., 2013; Merker et al., 2022). In addition to these tangible benefits, it has also been suggested that patient/community engagement is an ethical approach to research that is important in and of itself. For example, engaged research is often framed as an ethical response to past research misconduct (Buchanan et al.,

L. Mikesell (✉)
School of Communication and Information, Rutgers University, New Brunswick, NJ, USA
e-mail: lisa.mikesell@rutgers.edu

E. E. Anderson (ed.), *Ethical Issues in Community and Patient Stakeholder–Engaged Health Research*, Philosophy and Medicine 146,
https://doi.org/10.1007/978-3-031-40379-8_3

2007; Flicker et al., 2007) because it incorporates patient and community perspectives, is sensitive to participants' experiences and needs, often aims to share power and decision making, and is oriented to community building (Israel et al., 2010; Strong et al., 2009).

Despite these ethical priorities, however, engaged research poses new ethical challenges (Kass, 2001; Wilson et al., 2018), many of them arising because of the altered roles of and relationships between academic investigators and patient/community investigators who are now collaborating in more extensive ways (Bromley et al., 2015). Traditionally a member of a patient population or community participated in research as a "human subject," which is a well-defined and limited role. As Bromley et al. (2015) describe, the role is *context dependent* in that subjects agree to participate in a study that takes place in a particular context, such as a laboratory or clinic. It is *task focused* because involvement in the study is limited to well-defined activities to support the provision of specific kinds of data. Lastly, it is *time limited* in that a subject's role, and thereby the researcher-subject relationship, is terminated when data collection ends. These limits to the subject role with respect to context, task, and time have similarly limited the requirements of ethical oversight: institutional review boards (IRBs) and research ethics boards (REBs) focus exclusively on how to protect individual human subjects when they provide data for a researcher-designed and researcher-controlled study (Boser, 2007).

Engaged research reconceptualizes the role of individuals in research as "participants," and even "partners." This reconceptualization addresses growing concerns about the traditional passive "subject" who is expected to comply with researchers' agendas. In contrast, these new roles recognize the agency and expertise of patients and community members who are involved in a wide range of tasks and activities supporting research. Along with these role expansions, engaged investigators also recognize research as a "site of struggle" that requires reflection on how "the ethical enactment of research is enshrined in hegemonic institutions and decision-making that promote a generic, biomedical model of ethical inquiry" (van Zyl & Sabiescu, 2020, p. 2; see also Guta et al., 2010). While these renewed roles as participants and partners positively reshape research processes and the relationships that support them, they also raise new ethical challenges.

Recognizing unique ethical challenges and developing frameworks to address them is crucial. Engaged research is often assumed to be ethical simply because it involves patients/community members more integrally in the scientific process. For example, a literature review on the ethics of CBPR—an approach described by Israel et al. (1998) as "a collaborative approach to research that equitably involves, for example, community members, organizational representatives, and researchers in all aspects of the research process" (p. 177)—found that authors rarely "mention that conducting CBPR does not automatically ensure the ethics of the work" (Mikesell et al., 2013, p. e12). This is presumably because "the principles involved in conducting ethical CBPR are largely synonymous with the principles of CBPR itself" such as trust, collaboration, shared power and decision-making, transparency, and mutual respect (p. e12).

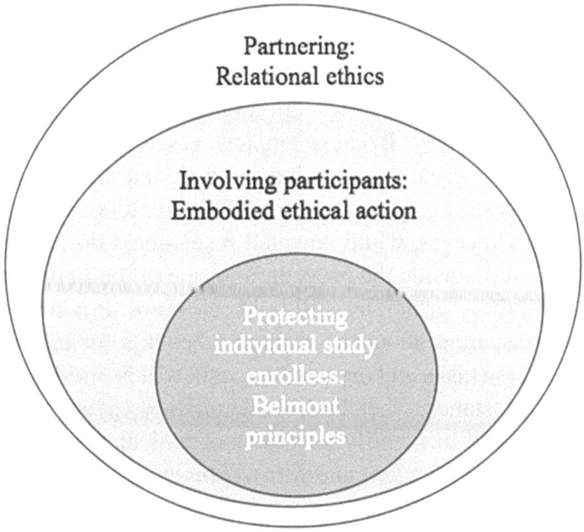

Fig. 3.1 Considering the *Belmont* principles, embodied ethical action, and relational ethics to protect study enrollees, involve participants, and build and maintain partnerships in engaged research

This chapter describes an emerging—and evolving—preliminary ethical framework for patient and community-engaged research, taking into account the multiple roles that individuals involved in engaged research often occupy: enrolled individual (traditionally the "subject" role), participant, and partner (see Fig. 3.1). This framework acknowledges a tension in engaged research, as researchers often simultaneously work to uphold the dominant ethical frames embedded in our scientific institutions that direct research practices while also recognizing that these frames are flawed. Accordingly, this framework is meant as a starting place that will demand ongoing refinement. This is due in part to the fact that I was initially trained as an academic researcher and that training may bias my perspective in ways I have yet to realize. Additionally, engaged researchers seem to be still coming to terms with how to balance the ethics of scientific integrity and the institutionally-ingrained traditional ethical principles for research with ethical considerations related to supporting the well-being and interpersonal relationships that develop across all those impacted by a research project, not only "human subjects."

3.2 Protecting *Enrolled Individuals* and Their Data: *Belmont* Principles and the "Subject" Role

The *Belmont Report* outlines three principles guiding the ethical protection of individuals who participate in research that engaged investigators continue to value (see Bromley et al., 2015): respect for persons, beneficence, and justice. *Respect for persons* stipulates that individuals should be treated as autonomous decision makers regarding their participation in research. *Beneficence* requires researchers to maximize benefits and minimize harms by carefully considering the risk-benefit ratio of participating in a study. Lastly, the principle of *justice* requires that risks and benefits of research be fairly distributed across society so that one group of people does not bear most of the risk while other groups benefit from their sacrifices (National Commission for the Protection of Human Subjects of Biomedical and Behavioral Research, 1979). Because engaged research significantly expands the role of individuals in research, some have questioned the continued relevance of the *Belmont* principles for engaged research (Gilbert, 2006; Shore, 2007; see Chap. 17, this volume). However, while engaged researchers do frequently encounter novel ethical dilemmas outside the procedural scope of the *Belmont* principles (see next two sections), these principles still hold relevance. It is important in any research study to be transparent about the risks and benefits for individuals who participate in data collection tasks and explain how data will be used and protected (Chen et al., 2006).

For instance, when both academic (n = 15) and community (n = 14) investigators were asked to identify attributes of ethical engaged research, most (75.9%) mentioned *the protection and fair treatment of those enrolled and their data* (Bromley et al., 2015). This suggests that enrolled individuals whose primary task is to provide data for the study are still perceived to require special ethical protections that the *Belmont* principles help outline. The third most commonly identified attribute (identified by 37.9% of practitioners) was that *the study is IRB, HIPAA, and Belmont compliant* (Bromley et al., 2015), again suggesting that for engaged researchers, the *Belmont* principles still hold significance. However, engaged investigators do not perceive individuals who participate in research studies, even when their role is limited to data provision, as "subjects." It has been argued that the term itself suggests a form of exploitation by which individuals are obligated to comply with researchers directing the study (Ammerman et al., 2003). Outdated expectations of obligation and passive engagement in research are precisely what engaged research aims to overcome. Thus, while the data provision tasks of enrolled individuals still require important ethical oversight, investigators more thoughtfully recognize that individuals, even in this rather restricted role, bring expertise and knowledge to the table. To that end, many engaged researchers take care to provide summaries of results to individuals who may have provided data for a study and share and solicit feedback from them about study findings.

Importantly, the *Belmont* principles take on extended meaning when applied thoughtfully, because engaged research requires investigators to carefully consider the impact of research on the communities and patient populations to which those individuals providing data belong (Mikesell et al., 2013). That is, engaged researchers consider not only the agency and autonomy of enrolled individuals but extend this principle to carefully consider *community autonomy*. This entails valuing community needs, interests, values, and strengths; voluntary community participation in research (which aligns with engaged researchers' orientation to conduct research *with* rather than *on* or *for* communities (Wells & Jones, 2009)); and recognition of all parties' work. Similarly, beneficence extends beyond individuals as researchers consider how risks and benefits should be evaluated for the community at large. This requires considering, for example, how research findings may be internalized by the broader community and the potential harms that might occur if data were repurposed without community permission (Monahan & Steward, 2003). Lastly, the principle of justice is perceived to extend in meaning to *social and community justice*, requiring negotiations with the community to prioritize community benefits of research and consideration of how the burdens of participation and research benefits are equitably distributed.

Extending the *Belmont* principles to community-engaged research thus requires a significant shift in how the principles are applied as well as careful consideration of the challenges that may arise for investigators when moving beyond the scope of the principles' original intent. Such application has been addressed through the involvement of patients and community members in the research process, not only as enrolled individuals who provide data, but as "participants" who are often involved in many or all stages of the research process.

3.3 Engaging *Participants*: Embodied Ethical Action

In engaged research, patient and community members often take on an expanded role, not only engaging in well-defined research tasks to provide data but participating in integral ways in the design and oversight of the project. For example, they may identify relevant areas of exploration that are important to patients/communities, select or modify measures, develop recruitment efforts and community outreach initiatives, assist in data analysis and interpretation, and help disseminate findings to patients/communities. In these ways and others, patients and community members enact a "participant" role as integral and valued members of the research team.

These more engaged participant roles reshape the ethical landscape for engaged researchers. For instance, ethical challenges arising from these new roles and relationships can include managing insider-outsider tensions, determining community representation, managing multiple roles of those who are involved on the project, and challenges with community commitment (Mikesell et al., 2013). Accordingly, many investigators recognize that ethics requires "a heightened attentiveness to the ethical implications of all research activities," an approach that has been described as "embodying ethical action" (Bromley et al., 2015). This approach is described by engaged researchers as "meeting the highest ethical standards in *each action and interaction* through exacting ethical choices" (p. 902, emphasis added) and is understood to evolve throughout the lifecycle of a project and thus require "continuous ethical awareness" (p. 902). Accordingly, embodying ethical action requires concern for knowledge production as required for sound science as well as responsibility for and accountability to the entire team, even when that responsibility requires addressing participant and community concerns that may not be directly connected to study procedures or outcomes (see Chaps. 6 and 8 , this volume).

Although recognizing their limitations, engaged investigators still draw on the *Belmont* principles to frame notions of embodied ethical action. In one study, engaged investigators described embodied ethical action as requiring a more expansive consideration of how the *Belmont* principles are relevant for participants and also identified the challenges that such expansion brings (Bromley et al., 2015). For instance, respect for persons is understood to extend to *all* participants. Historically, ethical oversight by IRBs prioritized protections for enrolled individuals only, but through the lens of embodied ethical action, ethical considerations now apply to everyone on the research team. This approach thus further prioritizes respect for *everyone* involved in the project, including individuals providing data, participants designing the study, those collecting and analyzing the data, those helping with project management, etc. Participants may include enrolled individuals; patients; community members, organization leaders and other stakeholder advisors contributing to a variety of research and engagement tasks; graduate and undergraduate students; and other co-researchers. Ethical oversight is as important for considering how the primary investigator(s) of the study treats and trains graduate student researchers as it is for considering how informed consent is obtained from enrolled individuals providing data.

The embodied ethical approach is not without challenges. In considering how to embody the *Belmont* principles, investigators should reflect on the changing personal relationships between team members and community members—for example, if participants involved in study oversight and data collection have long-standing personal relationships with those enrolled in the study—to identify the potential for coercion, unfair treatment, or breach of confidentiality (Clark et al., 2010). Embodied ethical action also calls for application of the principle of beneficence beyond knowledge production tasks to assess benefits and harms for a range of project-related activities. This includes, for instance, how to "achieve substantive research roles" for participants in research tasks and decision-making (Bromley et al., 2015, p. 904) and how to "manage conflicting priorities that compete with research activities" (p. 903). Participants come with varying expertise and differing desires for involvement in a project. How project leadership identifies participants' expertise and how research teams utilize varying expertise may not be straightforward, and transparency regarding the approaches to these decisions is required. Similarly, participants may bring or develop expertise and priorities that do not immediately align with the priorities of the initially agreed upon research agenda, and this may require ongoing dialogue as well as project modifications and reconceptualization. Reconsidering beneficence requires that participants' time and effort is valued and appropriately compensated (see Chap. 14, this volume). This requires funding that enables not only tasks related to data collection and analysis but tasks directly supporting interactions and familiarity among members of the team and members of the community (Mayan & Daum, 2016). Ideally, compensation would also extend to training and professional development activities.

Lastly, an embodied ethical approach allows for the negotiation of justice whereby participants are called to thoughtfully respond to the possible reluctance of patient and community members to engage in research and still remain aligned with the study vision over time (Bromley et al., 2015). For example, the realities of the pressures and responsibilities of patient/community investigators outside of the project means that participants may "get on and off the bus" (Ferré et al., 2010). They may initially agree to participate but later limit their participation or withdraw for periods of time altogether and then return. Additionally, while many forms of engaged research have been described in idealistic terms—*equal* participation and participant involvement in *all* phases of the research—the wisdom and lived experiences of community and patient investigators and the training and expertise of academic researchers may mean that equal participation in all phases is not always feasible or desired by participants.

The challenges associated with extending the *Belmont* principles to participants on the team highlight the need for ongoing dialogue to foster understanding of and demonstrate respect for differing cultural values, belief systems, lived experiences, and priorities. In this respect, engaged work moves beyond the roles participants play in progressing the research project's aims and initiatives and considers the *partnerships* that develop among all investigators and stakeholders who may be directly and indirectly involved with and impacted by the project.

3.4 Building and Maintaining *Partnerships*: Relational Ethics

Although the *Belmont* principles remain relevant, there is recognition that they alone are not sufficient to fulfill the ethical requirements of engaged research, even when extended to patient populations/community as described above. Indeed, others have articulated that the *Belmont* principles are simply the bare minimum for upholding ethical standards (Bromley et al., 2015). The initial intention was to provide oversight for traditional research involving "human subjects," which is time, task, and context limited. Thus, the *Belmont* principles merely provide a foundational schema, one with which academic investigators are familiar and on which patient/community investigators, who may be new to research, can be trained (which is usually required by academic institutions). Accordingly, these principles may impose constraints on how embodied ethical action is realized in practice because they may encourage practitioners to treat ethics less as an evolving, situated process and more as a list of requirements. These principles alone, even when thoughtfully extended in their application, seem insufficient, because those involved with the research project are often not only individual enrollees providing data or participants on the team contributing to project aims but also research *partners*.

Partnerships require more than the ethical oversight of project tasks that allow for a rigorous and valid scientific process (which is an equally important ethical imperative for most experienced academic and community investigators alike) (Mejlgaard et al., 2020). Partnerships also require more than oversight of engagement tasks that build functional and productive interactions among team members and enable a project to run smoothly. They require the cultivation of collaborative and mutually beneficial relationships and invested dialogue, the recognition of self and other, the achievement of intersubjectivity, accountability for past research misconduct, and the understanding of how this work can be reparative. Developing and maintaining collaborative and trusting partnerships where partners invest in each other as well the project entails the adoption of "relational ethics," which provides the foundations for ethical engaged health research.

Relational ethics aligns with embodied ethical action because it similarly recognizes that relationships are central to engaged research and that ethics is situated, negotiated, requires constant attention, and exists beyond the institutional ethical paradigm. However, it also explicitly emphasizes a strong orientation to humanistic values such as human rights, trust, dignity, respect, and intellectual humility (Wilson et al., 2019). Relational ethics attends to the power dynamics between patients/community and institutions that are often assumed to be static in traditional research. Accordingly, such an approach can reveal power dynamics that may be problematic for patients/community and/or academic researchers that would have likely gone unnoticed or have been poorly dealt with in the past when institutional ethics was the only framework providing guidance (Clark et al., 2010).

More than two decades ago, King et al. (1999) described research as deeply relational and put forth a "relationships paradigm," recognizing that "all research is 'cross-cultural'" (p. 1), because it necessarily entails relationships among many stakeholders, each operating within a unique culture, including researchers, researchers in training, academic institutions, community organizations, community members, funders, governments, and enrolled individuals. Given that research misconduct still occurred after the U.S. Common Rule and the Nuremburg Code, their goal was "to find new ways to consider and address ongoing moral problems in all human subjects research" (p. 1) in order to "facilitate human subjects research that is sensitive and responsible as well as scientifically fruitful" (p. 2). They identified complex ethical cases that required additional attention such as how much influence funders should have on the direction of research and how, despite having procedures, the process of informed consent was still flawed. Although their focus remained on the role of "human subjects," their new paradigm "emphasize[d] relationships, interactions, power, responsibility, and contextual and historical considerations in examining moral issues" (p. 5). While the importance of relational ethics in research was proposed many years ago, we have yet to codify principles or guidelines that make it a priority for most research, whether engaged or not.

More recently, Wilson et al. (2019), when developing an ethical framework for engaged research with vulnerable populations, recognize how "bioethics [still] conceptualizes the moral agent as individualistic, unembedded in relationships and unencumbered by social, economic, or political circumstances or identities that shape moral deliberations—in theory yielding a generic moral agent" (p. 92). Accordingly, they argue that ethical engaged research must allow partners "to account for the relationships and cultural contexts within which individuals are embedded" (p. 92). Thus, a relational ethical approach requires thoughtful recognition of the contexts in which individuals, participants, and partners on our projects live and work.

Adding to the notion of relational ethics and drawing on Ellis (2007), Hodgetts et al. (2021) describe relational ethics in the following manner: "Rather than concentrating on epistemological concerns about what sort of knowledge should be produced, relational ethics 'requires researchers to act from our hearts and minds, acknowledge our interpersonal bonds to others, and to take responsibility for actions and their consequences'" (p. 2). Hodgetts et al. (2021) further identify a "tripartite framework" of principles associated with social justice that guides their relationship-centered work on homelessness: (1) *moral inclusion*, which "relates to the positioning of persons or groups who are often marginalized within the scope of justice as being worthy of fair treatment"; (2) *moral complexity*, which "reflects the realization that arbitrary poles of 'good' and 'bad,' as often defined by authoritative institutions, are not always clearly demarcated or mutually exclusive states in actuality;" and (3) *procedural fairness*, which "refers to the fairness of the procedures that are enacted to determine socially just outcomes" (pp. 2–3, see also Drew, 2015). Thus, from a relational ethics perspective, the maintenance of interpersonal relationships is at the ethical center of engaged health research. But even beyond this, relational ethics calls for the careful consideration of how society, institutions, and other sites of authority position the patients and communities researchers work with and how those sites' established procedures—whether knowingly or not—unjustly create obstacles and support inequitable outcomes.

Relational ethics (as demonstrated in Fig. 3.1) is foundational to engaged research and equally applies to those who occupy the roles of enrolled individuals and participants on projects. For example, even when serving in more limited roles, enrolled individuals and participants are not just treated as data providers or laborers required to make a project run but as people with voices and experiences. Researchers are responsible for re-presenting these to the world through how we write and talk about them in our publications and presentations (Narayan, 1997). Partners are people who bring expertise, understanding of sociocultural contexts, and relationships with patients and community, which all provide insights and learning opportunities for the entire team, for project outcomes, and for every team member's sense of belonging and acceptance within the research community being developed. Of course, these partnerships will likely bring tensions, differences of opinion, and interpersonal strife. However, starting a project with a relational ethics approach can help address the ethical challenges that will most surely arise.

3.5 Discussion

Academic researchers have inherited the *Belmont* principles as they inform institutional ethical requirements and required training for all project team members. Even as engaged research alters the roles of and relationships between academic investigators and patients/community members, the continued relevance of these principles remains strong. Perhaps because of their institutional embeddedness, these principles provide a schema through which many engaged investigators view the new research roles and relationships that characterize their work. However, these principles no long exclusively *define* the ethics of their work as they have been considerably expanded and applied to both the community at large and to all participating members of the investigative team (Khodyakov et al., 2016).

There is also recognition that engaged research requires something more than the *Belmont* principles, even in their expanded form. Given the variety of approaches to engaged research (from citizen science to CBPR), it is difficult to know if, as a community of practice (Kuhn, 2002), we might reach consensus about what an ethical framework should look like for all kinds of engaged work. Some practitioners value an integration of institutional and relational ethics, and some want a complete overhaul. That is, some argue that engaged research requires an *additional* lens through which to address ethical concerns—one that complements the *Belmont* principles that have traditionally guided scientific processes. They believe that researchers should aim to balance research integrity, institutional ethics, and relational ethics. Others, however, argue that engaged research calls for a *different* lens altogether, since the constraints placed upon investigators tend to enforce "pre-packaged principles, protocols, and ready-made forms to sign, typically overlooking or ignoring the divergent points of view that may stem from participants" and partners (van Zyl & Sabiescu, 2020, p. 2).

Regardless of where one lands in this debate, most agree that engaged research requires attention to *relational ethics* that looks beyond the boundaries of the project and project-related tasks and recognizes that people and relationships matter beyond their instrumental value to achieving project aims. Relational ethics requires researchers to genuinely care for others and each other, invest in others' lived experiences, and understand how those experiences matter for both the outcomes of the project and for the betterment and well-being of enrolled individuals, research team members, and communities and patient populations. It requires that we consider the social justice and reparative requirements of research, especially with communities that have suffered horrendous ethical violations and mistreatment. Lastly, it requires that we engage in respectful practices that recognize the humanity and dignity of enrolled individuals, participants, and partners.

Given the range of approaches to engaged research, the framework proposed here accounts for institutional requirements for research integrity and human subjects protection while also recognizing the limits of these principles in their application to participants, partners, and the broader community. Accordingly, this framework aims to capture the realities of engaged research ethics, which may be meaningful to researchers and projects in different ways. For some, these realities may provide an understanding of the layers of ethics that are required of this work and may thus offer insights about how to integrate the institutional requirements that impose practical constraints with our moral obligations to engage in relational ethics. Perhaps for others, this framework explicates the traditional, normative orientation to ethics that is both deeply ingrained in our institutional contexts and also fundamentally evolving. The framework may thus provide insights about how to supplant the institutionalized system and contribute to the important counter discourses that demand new attention to the moral underpinnings of health research (Mackenzie & Stoljar, 2000; Maclean, 2009). This framework is notably more descriptive of the ethical landscape of engaged research than prescriptive; this was intentional as I wanted to capture the wide-ranging orientations of engaged researchers and the potential compatibility and conflicts that may simultaneously exist in our current ethical paradigms. As King et al. (1999) remarked when developing a new relationships paradigm, new paradigms "do not just appear. They evolve out of older ones, and those who attempt to implement and justify them must struggle with what to keep from earlier systems and how to defend their rejection of the rest" (p. 5).

Acknowledgements I would like to thank my early collaborators and mentors—especially Elizabeth Bromley, Dmitry Khodyakov, Ken Wells, and Loretta Jones—who introduced me to community-based participatory research and helped me more thoughtfully explore the ethics of this work.

References

Ammerman, A., Corbie-Smith, G., St George, D. M. M., Washington, C., Weathers, B., & Jackson-Christian, B. (2003). Research expectations among African American church leaders in the PRAISE! Project: A randomized trial guided by community-based participatory research. *American Journal of Public Health, 93*(10), 1720–1727. https://doi.org/10.2105/ajph.93.10.1720

Boser, S. (2007). Power, ethics, and the IRB: Dissonance over human participant review of participatory research. *Qualitative Inquiry, 13*(8), 1060–1074. https://doi.org/10.1177/1077800407308220

Bromley, E., Mikesell, L., Jones, F., & Khodyakov, D. (2015). From subject to participant: Ethics and the evolving role of Community in Health Research. *American Journal of Public Health, 105*(5), 900–908. https://doi.org/10.2105/AJPH.2014.302403

Brown, N. (2021). Scope and continuum of participatory research. *International Journal of Research and Method in Education, 45*(2), 200–211. https://doi.org/10.1080/1743727X.2021.1902980

Buchanan, D. R., Miller, F. G., & Wallerstein, N. (2007). Ethical issues in community-based participatory research: Balancing rigorous research with community participation in community intervention studies. *Progress in Community Health Partnerships, 1*(2), 153–160. https://doi.org/10.1353/cpr.2007.0006

Carman, K. L., Dardess, P., Maurer, M., Sofaer, S., Adams, K., Bechtel, C., & Sweeney, J. (2013). Patient and family engagement: A framework for understanding the elements and developing interventions and policies. *Health Affairs, 32*(2), 223–231. https://doi.org/10.1377/hlthaff.2012.1133

Chen, D. T., Jones, L., & Gelberg, L. (2006). Ethics of clinical research within a community-academic partnered participatory framework. *Ethnicity & Disease, 16*(Suppl 1), S118–S135.

Clark, N., Hunt, S., Jules, G., & Good, T. (2010). Ethical dilemmas in community-based research: Working with vulnerable youth in rural communities. *Journal of Academic Ethics, 8*, 243–252. https://doi.org/10.1007/s10805-010-9123-y

Drew, N. (2015). Social and emotional wellbeing, natural helpers, critical health literacy and translational research: Connecting the dots for positive health outcomes. *Australian Psychiatry, 23*, 620–622. https://doi.org/10.1177/1039856215604979

Ferré, C. D., Jones, L., Norris, K. C., & Rowley, D. L. (2010). The healthy African American families (HAAF) project: From community-based participatory research to community-partnered participatory research. *Ethnicity & Disease, 20*(102), S2-1-8.

Flicker, S., Travers, R., Guta, A., McDonald, S., & Meagher, A. (2007). Ethical dilemmas in community-based participatory research: Recommendations for institutional review boards. *Journal of Urban Health, 84*(4), 478–493. https://doi.org/10.1007/s11524-007-9165-7

Gilbert, S. G. (2006). Supplementing the traditional institutional review board with an environmental health and community review board. *Environmental Health Perspectives, 114*(10), 1626–1629. https://doi.org/10.1289/ehp.9005

Guta, A., Wilson, M. G., & Flicker, S. (2010). Are we asking the right questions? A review of Canadian REB practices in relation to community-based participatory research. *Journal of Empirical Research on Human Research Ethics, 5*(2), 35–46. https://doi.org/10.1525/jer.2010.5.2.35

Hecker, S., Haklay, M., Bowser, A., Makuch, Z., Vogel, J., & Bonn, A. (2019). *Citizen science: innovation in open science, society and policy*. UCL Press.

Hodgetts, D., Rua, M., Groot, S., Hopner, V., Drew, N., King, P., & Black, D. (2021). Relational ethics meets principled practice in community research engagements to understand and address homelessness. *Journal of Community Psychology*, 1–13. https://doi.org/10.1002/jcop.22586

Israel, B. A., Shultz, A. J., Parker, E. A., & Becker, A. B. (1998). Review of community-based research: Assessing partnership approaches to improve public health. *Annual Review of Public Health, 19*, 173–202. https://doi.org/10.1146/annurev.publhealth.19.1.173

Israel, B. A., Coombe, C. M., Cheezum, R. R., Shulz, A. J., McGranaghan, R. J., Lichtenstein, R., Reyes, A. G., Clement, J., & Burris, A. (2010). Community-based participatory research: A capacity-building approach for policy advocacy aimed at eliminating health disparities. *American Journal of Public Health, 100*(11), 2094–2102. https://doi.org/10.2105/AJPH.2009.170506

Johnson, L. B., & Smalley, J. B. (2020). Engaging the patient: Patient-centered research. In K. L. Hall, A. L. Vogel, & R. T. Croyle (Eds.), *Strategies for team science success: Handbook of evidence-based principles for cross-disciplinary science and practical lessons learned from health researchers* (pp. 135–148). Springer.

Kass, N. E. (2001). An ethics framework for public health. *American Journal of Public Health, 91*(11), 1776–1782. https://doi.org/10.2105/ajph.91.11.1776

Keahey, J. (2020). Sustainable development and participatory action research: A systematic review. *Systemic Practice and Action Research, 34*, 291–306. https://doi.org/10.1007/s11213-020-09535-8

Khodyakov, D., Mikesell, L., Schraiber, R., Booth, M., & Bromley, E. (2016). On using ethical principles of community-engaged research in translational science. *Translational Research, 171*, 52–61. https://doi.org/10.1016/j.trsl.2015.12.008

King, N. M. P., Henderson, G. E., & Stein, J. (1999). *Beyond regulations: Ethics in human subjects research*. University of North Carolina Press.

Kuhn, T. (2002). Negotiating boundaries between scholars and practitioners. *Management Communication Quarterly, 16*(1), 106–112. https://doi.org/10.1177/0893318902161008

Mackenzie, C., & Stoljar, N. (2000). *Relational autonomy: Feminist perspectives on autonomy, agency, and the social self*. Oxford University Press.

Maclean, A. (2009). *Autonomy, informed consent and medical law: A relational challenge*. Cambridge University Press.

Mayan, M. J., & Daum, C. H. (2016). Worth the risk? Muddled relationships in community-based participatory research. *Qualitative Health Research, 26*(1), 69–76. https://doi.org/10.1177/1049732315618660

Mejlgaard, N., Bouter, L. M., Gaskell, G., Kavouras, P., Allum, N., Bendsten, A.-K., Charitidis, C. A., Claesen, N., Dierickx, K., Domaradzka, A., et al. (2020). Research integrity: Nine ways to move from talk to walk. *Nature, 586*, 358–360. https://doi.org/10.1038/d41586-020-02847-8

Merker, V. L., Hyde, J. K., Herbst, A., Solch, A. K., Mohr, D. C., Gaj, L., Dvorin, K., & Dryden, E. M. (2022). Evaluating the impacts of patient engagement on health services research teams. *Journal of General Internal Medicine, 37*, 33–41. https://doi.org/10.1007/s11606-021-06987-z

Mikesell, L., Bromley, E., & Khodyakov, D. (2013). Ethical community-engaged research: A literature review. *American Journal of Public Health, 103*(12), e7–e14. https://doi.org/10.2105/AJPH.2013.301605
Monahan, A., & Steward, D. E. (2003). The role of lay panelists on grant review panels. *Chronic Diseases in Canada, 24*(2–3), 70–74.
Narayan, K. (1997). How native is a 'native' anthropologist? In L. Lamphere, H. Ragone, & P. Zavella (Eds.), *Situated lives: Gender and culture in everyday life* (pp. 23–41). Routledge.
National Commission for the Protection of Human Subjects of Biomedical and Behavioral Research. (1979). *The Belmont report: Ethical principles and guidelines for the protection of human subjects research.* US Department of Health, Education, and Welfare.
Oliver, S. (2006). Patient involvement in setting research agendas. *European Journal of Gastroenterology & Hepatology, 18*(9), 935–938.
Patient-Centered Outcomes Research Institute (PCORI). (2018). *The value of engagement.* Posted October 30, 2018. https://www.pcori.org/engagement/value-engagement. Accessed 13 Aug 2022.
Shore, N. (2007). Re-conceptualizing the Belmont report. *Journal of Community Practice, 14*(4), 5–26. https://doi.org/10.1300/J125v14n04_02
Strong, L. L., Israel, B. A., Schultz, A. J., Reyes, A., Rowe, Z., Weir, S. S., & Poe, C. (2009). Piloting interventions within a community-based participatory research framework: Lessons learned from the health environments partnership. *Progress in Community Health Partnerships, 3*(4), 327–334. https://doi.org/10.1353/cpr.0.0094
van Zyl, I., & Sabiescu, A. (2020). Toward intersubjective ethics in community-based research. *Community Development, 51*(1), 1–20. https://doi.org/10.1080/15575330.2020.1777178
Wallerstein, N., Duran, B., Oetzel, J., & Minkler, M. (Eds.). (2018). *Community-based participatory research* (3rd ed.). Jossey-Bass.
Wells, K., & Jones, L. (2009). Research' in community-partnered, participatory research. *JAMA, 302*(2), 320–321. https://doi.org/10.1001/jama.2009.1033
Wilson, E., Kenny, A., & Dickson-Swift, V. (2018). Ethical challenges in community-based participatory research: A scoping review. *Qualitative Health Research, 28*(2), 189–199. https://doi.org/10.1177/1049732317690721
Wilson, W. D., Jackson, F. H., & Harrell, J. R. (2019). Framework for ethical community engagement (ECE) with underserved populations in the rural south: A help for bioethics and healthcare promotion. *Journal of Health Care for the Poor and Underserved, 30*(4), 91–104. https://doi.org/10.1353/hpu.2019.0120

Lisa Mikesell is an associate professor in the School of Communication and Information and associate faculty at the Institute for Health, Health Care Policy and Aging Research. Integrating her backgrounds in mental health services and communication scholarship, her work uses mixed methods to enhance patient and community engagement, improve patient-provider communication, and identify and implement practices of patient-centeredness to foster trusting healthcare relationships.

Chapter 4
Beyond Good Intentions: Principles for Anti-racist Community-Engaged Research

Alexis Grant and Andrea L. DaViera

The goal of research is to understand, explore, or describe the world around us. While this may be seen as a morally pure intention, historically research has been an exclusionary practice in which data are extracted from people and communities to benefit researchers and their institutions through funding, publications, and credit for discovery. Such exclusionary and extractive research practices have disproportionately harmed racialized and historically-excluded groups. Racism continues to undermine the actualization of society's full potential; racism not only wastes social capital and human resources, it also stifles research quality and impact. In this chapter, we describe the need for anti-racist, community-engaged research. To be anti-racist is distinct from being "not-racist" and is marked by active efforts to address racism and its effects (Kendi, 2019). To call for anti-racist research also implies a recognition that research is inherently racist and that researchers have a responsibility to try to reform their own practice and dismantle those ingrained aspects of systemic racism that have led to disproportionate burdens of risk, inequities in health outcomes, and access to care.

In recent years, there has been an increasing emphasis on community engagement as a remedy for the historical harms of biomedical and behavioral research. Community-engaged research includes a variety of methods and approaches but can be defined broadly as "the process of working collaboratively with groups of people affiliated by geographic proximity, special interests, or similar situations with respect to issues affecting their well being" (Balls Berry & Acosta-Pérez, 2017).

A. Grant (✉)
WestEd, San Francisco, CA, USA
e-mail: agrant@wested.org

A. L. DaViera
Department of Psychology, University of Illinois at Chicago, Chicago, IL, USA
e-mail: adavie6@uic.edu

E. E. Anderson (ed.), *Ethical Issues in Community and Patient Stakeholder–Engaged Health Research*, Philosophy and Medicine 146,
https://doi.org/10.1007/978-3-031-40379-8_4

While many would agree that community-engaged research is a means to address historical abuse, unethical treatment, and exploitation in the fields of health, medicine, psychology, education, and others, community-engaged methods alone cannot ensure that research is anti-racist. Community engagement is characterized by practices that can be observed, whereas anti-racist research is defined by the extent to which it aims to address the impacts of racism.

Wanting to engage in anti-racist research requires a critical perspective of racism and the other interlocking systems of oppression that undergird systemic inequities in health, research, and beyond. Racism in research is not a metaphor or artifact of history alone—it is material, as we will explain throughout this chapter. Anti-racist research is both a goal and a product; it is an action and an orientation. To this end, we introduce a working definition of anti-racist community-engaged research.

We define anti-racist, community-engaged research as *research that decolonizes knowledge production through the participation of groups of people affiliated by geographic proximity, special interests, or similar situations working to actively change and/or dismantle the intersectional, interlocking oppressive systems that affect well-being.*

In this chapter, we will first begin our discussion by framing institutional positionality, awareness of which is essential for anti-racist work. We will then present four principles of anti-racist, community-engaged research: it is grounded in a socio-ecological perspective, centers intersectionality, is emancipatory, and strives to be decolonial in both research practice and outcomes. This chapter is informed by an understanding of institutional racism, individual power and privilege, and critical race theory (CRT), which defines anti-racist tenets, modes of knowledge production, and systemic transformation (Ford & Airhihenbuwa, 2018; Crenshaw et al., 1995). As an extension of CRT, we also center intersectionality as a guiding lens for anti-racist, community-engaged research.

4.1 Start Here: Awareness of Institutional Positionality

The first step in conducting anti-racist community-engaged research is to be aware of participating institutions' histories of colonization and oppression. Many academic, political, and governmental institutions have a legacy of racist, colonialist displacement as well as modern-day racist policies and practices. Every Ivy League university in the United States, with the exception of Cornell University, was founded with profits from the slave trade, used slave labor, or profited from slavery in some other way (Brophy, 2016; Wilder, 2014). The founders and early presidents of Harvard, Dartmouth, Yale, Princeton, Columbia, University of Pennsylvania, and Brown University were slaveowners and/or directly participated in slave trading (Wilder, 2014). In their early days, medical institutions including Dartmouth, University of Pennsylvania, and Columbia University used slaves' corpses and bodies for experimentation (Wilder, 2014; Democracy Now, n.d.). Even institutions that were not founded by slaveowners still benefited from colonialism. For example, our own institution, the University of Illinois system, opened in 1868 after raising $648,767 from the sale of 477,710 acres of the land of the Three Fire Peoples: the Ojibwe, Odawa, and Bodewadmi (Illinois, 2018). The construction of the Chicago campus in 1963 required over 8000 people and 630 businesses in one of the city's few integrated neighborhoods to move or close (University of Illinois Chicago, 2016). The continued expansion of University of Illinois Chicago's (UIC's) campus (along with UI Health, a large public hospital) continues to displace people and businesses and drives up property values in the area, causing gentrification (Marx, 1997). Institutions may "acknowledge" past harms without any material changes to rebuild communities. Meanwhile, communities remember the real harm caused by these institutions, resulting in historical and structural trauma that affects their current health and economic conditions. Our positionality as researchers cannot be separated from the institutions we represent. We do not have space here to elaborate on racist practices in the recruitment of participants, students, and faculty, in teaching, in employment practices, or in delivering health care. Such examples from public health, healthcare, and academic institutions are discussed elsewhere (Washington, 2006; Corburn, 2007; Abel, 2004). Awareness of this full history of institutional practices of colonization and oppression is essential to a commitment to anti-racist research. Yet, awareness alone is not enough. Community-engaged researchers must embrace their role as agents of institutional change to dismantle racism at their institutions (Sabati, 2019). If we care about health equity, we have to hold our institutions accountable for past and present harms. Furthermore, as will be discussed below, the awareness of one's own positionality is important when researchers interact with a community that may have suffered harm from their institution.

4.2 Principles of Anti-racist Community-Engaged Research

1. *Anti-racist research is grounded in a socio-ecological approach that treats racism as a root cause of health inequities.*

Anti-racist research begins with a guiding theory or logic model, so we must proactively consider how our models treat race and racism (Chicago Beyond, 2019; Stern et al., 2021). The concept of race was created by Enlightenment thinkers, but it is now established that race and "biogeographical ancestry" have no biological or genetic basis (Perez-Rodriguez & de la Fuente, 2017). Thus, the use of race as a default variable in health research is problematic and careless (Stolley, 1999; Matsui et al., 2020; Neblett, 2019; Bastos et al., 2010; Perez-Rodriguez & de la Fuente, 2017; Lewontin, 2005; Boyd et al., 2020). If racism is a determinant of health inequities, we should consider the *why* and *how* of collecting data on racial identity. In data collection and analyses, we should stop treating race as a biological factor or as a proxy for ethnicity, culture, skin color, discrimination, or racism; all of these concepts can be measured better in ways other than by asking for someone's race (Kagawa Singer et al., 2016; Neblett, 2019). In our analyses, we must identify assumptions underlying the evaluation of differences between groups. "Risk" is socially defined and disproportionately distributed across populations (Fine & Ruglis, 2009). In this sense, *racism*—not race—is the risk factor. Additionally, we should consider how we use "white" as a referent group, replicating the notion that non-white groups are "other" (Hardeman & Karbeah, 2020). The continuation of these practice reinforces the misconception—aligned with white supremacy—that health disparities are primarily the fault of racial minorities. By changing how we use and analyze race, our research can become more anti-racist.

In the case of intervention research, a socioecological approach that recognizes the influence of a variety of determinants on a single behavior should include structural determinants of health. The logic model for the research should show how the primary intervention addresses the system that allows for and perpetuates health disparities, and not just the behavior of an individual or a household (Bailey et al., 2017; Clarke et al., 2013; Gordon-Larsen, 2006; Neblett, 2019; Stern et al., 2021). We might consider mapping social etiologies linking racism to ethnically-defined (not racially-defined) populations—or even better, populations defined by the presence and impacts of structural racism (Ford & Airhihenbuwa, 2018; Ford & Harawa, 2010). An integration of socioecological models is modeled by Stern et al. (2021), who consider how attachment theory from the field of psychology is relevant to discussions of racism. Attachment theory incorporates how individuals experience and react to being threatened, refers to interpersonal dynamics, and describes behavior that takes place in a context where systemic racism and discrimination exist. They consider a socioecological, critical, and intersectional framework for their research and describe its potential impact on their participants, research team, methods, and context. Although it may seem methodologically complex to include racism as a research variable, there are useful CRT-derived frameworks and methodologies (Ward et al., 2019; Matsui et al., 2020; Kaufman, 2008; Paul-Emile, 2014; Obasogie, 2013; Gilbert & Ray, 2016; Doll et al., 2018; Boyd et al., 2020; Galan et al., 2020; Williams & Mohammed, 2013).

2. *Anti-racist research embraces intersectionality.*

Anti-racist research must take an intersectional approach, which is rooted in hundreds of years of Black Feminist scholarship, activism, and struggle (Buchanan & Wiklund, 2021; Buchanan et al., 2020; Combahee River Collective, 1977; Collins & Bilge, 2020; hooks, 1981; Crenshaw, 1989). Intersectionality is a critically needed framework for anti-racist research because it guides understanding of how multiple systems of power (such as racism and colonialism) interconnect, co-create, and reinforce each other (Hankivsky, 2012; Bauer, 2014; Hancock, 2007; Bowleg, 2012; Alexander-Floyd, 2012; Crenshaw, 1989). At minimum, a working definition of intersectionality includes the following components: (1) all individuals have intersecting social identities; (2) embedded in these identities are differential access points to privilege and power; and (3) these identities and their differential positions of power are shaped by social context (Else-Quest & Hyde, 2016). In order to be anti-racist, one must recognize how race interacts with multiple aspects of identity including gender, sexuality, ethnicity, (dis)ability, and more (Kendi, 2019.)

More importantly, scholars advocate that we move beyond the focus on "multiply marginalized" communities (Moradi & Grzanka, 2017). Instead, intersectionality proposes that we take a systems level approach and recognize that systems of power and oppression are interlocking, such that they co-create and maintain each other (Buchanan & Wiklund, 2021). For example, racism and capitalism coalesce to form *racial capitalism,* which can be described as "the centrality of race in structuring social and labor hierarchies in capitalist economies" (McClure et al., 2020, 1245). McClure and colleagues demonstrated how racial capitalism drives racialized COVID-19 disparities via viral spread in labor industries with overrepresentation of infections among Black, Indigenous, racialized and immigrant populations, particularly in health care, food and agriculture, construction, nursing homes, and carceral settings. This overrepresentation is not by chance, but results from how racial capitalist hierarchies structure who deserves which types of employment, working conditions, and pay.

How we "do" intersectionality-informed research requires attention, as intersectionality affects many steps of the research process (Cole, 2009; Agénor, 2020; Bauer, 2014). In operationalizing constructs and developing theoretical models, we must recognize the multiple axes along which social identities are unique. Methodologically, we must describe the heterogeneity of groups (Ford & Harawa, 2010; Hardeman & Karbeah, 2020) and examine data at multiple intersections of social identity, such as race, gender, socioeconomic class, sexual orientation, and citizenship status (Alhasan et al., 2020). Much health and social sciences research collects race data according to the Office of Management and Budget (OMB) and NIH reporting mandates. However, we argue that these mandated categories conflate meaningful ethnic, cultural, and structural variation of social groups (see Table 4.1 for a summary and critique). When collecting race data, we suggest that researchers familiarize themselves with the community with which they seek to work and to ask community members how they define themselves. This can be accomplished by introducing a single open-ended question in addition to the required OMB measure: "How do you describe your race or ethnicity?"

While it is important to ask questions about social identity that are inclusive of intentionality, most intersectionality research only focuses on statistical interactions of sociodemographic variables (Grzanka, 2020; Bowleg, 2012). This is what some would call "weak" intersectionality (Dill & Kohlman, 2021; Grzanka, 2020). Building a stronger base of intersectionality-informed research would contend with the "structural realities" (Bowleg & Bauer, 2016) that underpin both the decisions we make in research and the problems we study. For example, a research study examining health equity might oversample Black men and women to allow for the detection of race and gender differences in statistical analyses (Else-Quest & Hyde, 2016). However, this solution may obscure the impact of incarceration on health equity, as it is well-documented that incarcerated individuals are disproportionately Black due to racial inequities in the criminal legal system (Brewer & Heitzeg, 2008;Bowleg & Bauer, 2016). Intersectionality would suggest that we take a critical, sociohistorical approach to how we measure race and other sociodemographic markers. Data collection could include measures that capture additional forces that

Table 4.1 Office of Management and Budget race codes critiques

NIH OMB Race Codes (Last Revised 1997) (Office of Extramural Research, 2001)	**Critical considerations:** *These race codes consider the groups as a monolith, clouding the rich ethnic diversity and histories within groups*
American Indian or Alaska Native. A person having origins in any of the original peoples of North and South America (including Central America), and who maintains tribal affiliation or community attachment	"American Indian" is a misnomer. It is difficult to capture the diversity of people indigenous to North America with one title. "Native American" includes different nations across the continent, each with their own definition of citizenship, culture, and histories. Further, indigenous people have experienced barriers to claiming indigenous ancestry and may not identify as indigenous even if they are
Asian. A person having origins in any of the original peoples of the Far East, Southeast Asia, or the Indian subcontinent including, for example, Cambodia, China, India, Japan, Korea, Malaysia, Pakistan, the Philippine Islands, Thailand, and Vietnam	This generalization represents social groups that are vastly heterogeneous in terms of language and nationality, reflecting different histories of imperialism and colonialism and consequently, different statuses across economic mobility, religion, and citizenship
Black or African American. A person having origins in any of the black racial groups of Africa. Terms such as "Haitian" or "Negro" can be used in addition to "Black or African American"	Black and African American are not synonymous. Black is a race, the attribution of which is based on skin color. Black includes individuals whose ethnicity may be from any country. African American is an ethnicity reflecting a specific history of American slavery
Hispanic or Latino. A person of Cuban, Mexican, Puerto Rican, South or Central American, or other Spanish culture or origin, regardless of race. The term, "Spanish origin," can be used in addition to "Hispanic or Latino"	This term is non-specific and includes individuals with ancestry spanning continents. Latin American and Hispanic are distinct and diverse ethnicities, each with their own histories of colonialism and imperialism. Latin American countries have their own ethnic groups not captured by the term "Hispanic/Latino"
Native Hawaiian or Other Pacific Islander. A person having origins in any of the original peoples of Hawaii, Guam, Samoa, or other Pacific Islands	Pacific Islands each have their own culture, nationality, and history with colonialism that informs how individuals' health is influenced by their ethnicity
White. A person having origins in any of the original peoples of Europe, the Middle East, or North Africa	This gross over-generalization ignores how these groups hold different roots in racism, colonialism, and imperialism, and resistance against them

impede health equity, such as experiences with the criminal legal system. However, when confronted with structural realities that go beyond what we can "control" in quantitative analyses, we suggest that researchers consider more mixed- and qualitative methods (Abrams et al., 2020; Bowleg & Bauer, 2016).

Moreover, we must also strive to be accountable to the scholarship of those who have come before us (Bauer, 2014; Agénor, 2020; Abrams et al., 2020). In fact, failing to do so may cause unintentional negative effects and further perpetuate the very harms that we seek to address. Moradi and Grzanka (2017) put forth seven guidelines regarding using intersectionality as a field of study, research approach, and critical praxis. See Table 4.2 for an adapted summary of these guidelines and our own practical examples of how each could be achieved.

Anti-racist research that applies intersectional approaches must also be critically reflexive (Hankivsky, 2012) and generate "knowledge reflexively through critically analyzing previous actions; this knowledge then informs subsequent actions toward transformative change" (Lykes et al., 2018). Reflexivity includes awareness of how one's values, positionality, biases, and status influence the research process and one's impact on the research community (Case, 2017). Reflexivity is necessary to create meaningful collaboration, intentional power sharing, and decision making – critical features of community-engaged research. As discussed at the beginning of this chapter, reflexivity begins with an awareness of oneself and the history, perceived power, and material resources of one's institution (see Chap. 6, in this volume). One way to engage in reflexivity is to self-study (Bullough & Pinnegar, 2001), for example, using empirical and ethnographic techniques to systematically examine one's own experience. This could be as simple as maintaining a research journal where one logs key reflections of identity and how it impacted one's research or practice or could involve more sophisticated and intentional techniques of autoethnography (Ellis et al., 2011). Ultimately, it is not enough to merely confess one's power and privilege; acknowledgement ultimately has no impact on equity (Lensmire et al., 2013). Privilege cannot be revoked or reduced, regardless of how one feels about it (Memmi, 2013; Loomba, 2015). We all stand somewhere on axes of social privilege, based on our sociodemographic lineages, such as race, class, educational attainment, as well as privilege associated with our job, title, or position. In anti-racist research, we must consider *how* to use our power.

3. *Anti-racist research is emancipatory.*

Emancipation is a process developed "to free oneself from restraint, control, or the power of someone else, especially to free oneself from any kind of slavery" (Merriam-Webster, 2021). In order to be emancipatory, research must be designed for the participation of marginalized or overlooked groups. This means that a distinguishing characteristic of anti-racist community-engaged research is that it creates spaces and opportunities for meaningful participation of the community. In order to address racist systems, research must prioritize meaningful participation of those impacted by racist ideas and policies.

Anti-racist research must approach participatory methods with care. This means ensuring authentic and diverse representation, recognizing that no community is monolithic (again, with an intersectional lens). The only way to actively dismantle the conditions that produce racialized harm is not to do research "on" historically marginalized communities, but to do research "with" them (Fine, 2013; Gaudry, 2011; Chicago Beyond, 2019). Participatory methods can be implemented poorly and tokenize rather than empower minorities (Dzidic & Bishop, 2017). Thus, as we discuss participation, we must give attention to power and privilege as individuals (Hardeman et al., 2016; Ratele & Malherbe, 2020) and as members of an institution (Boyd et al., 2020; Galan et al., 2020; Brown et al., 2019; Chicago Beyond, 2019).

Table 4.2 Guidelines for using intersectionality as a field of study, research approach, and critical praxis

Guidelines adapted from Moradi and Grzanka (2017)	Practical examples
Understand and reference the Black Feminist scholarship and activism that historically and continually begets intersectionality	Read diverse academic and nonacademic literature on origins and theories of intersectionality and incorporate this historical understanding in your research and how you approach community. A few examples include *How We Get Free and the Combahee River Collective,* edited by Keeanga-Yamahtta Taylor (2017), bell hooks hallmark book *Ain't I a Woman: Black Women and Feminism* (1981), and *Intersectionality* edited by Collins and Bilge (2020) Also see Buchanan et al.'s (2020) description of intersectionality's historical underpinnings. The authors argue that *intersectional cultural humility* (as opposed to "cultural competence") is necessary to generate genuine compassion and empathy without being able to fully "know" the experiences of the oppressed (Buchanan et al., 2020)
Engage in re-imagining epistemic orientations to incorporate critical tools and perspectives in research	Evaluate how biases and values of epistemology may affect the ability to conduct intersectionality research. For example, *QuantCrit* is a CRT perspective about quantitative methodology that recognizes how racism shapes and produces quantitative data and analysis (Suzuki et al., 2021; Garcia et al., 2018; Gillborn et al., 2018) Explore, describe, measure, and observe how researcher positionality influences the research process. For example, maintain a research journal or engage in some form of empirical self-study Engage your research with interdisciplinary coalitions of scholars, activists, and communities specialized in that content knowledge. For example, the Youth Justice Research Collaborative (Public Science Project, 2021) housed at the Public Science Project at the City University of New York brought together youth, researchers, legal experts, and activists to challenge discriminatory criminal legal policies that drive youth incarceration
Recognize that intersectionality applies to all people and reject stereotypical prototypes of intersectionality	When doing intersectional research, focus on more than just the interaction of race and gender identity. Incorporate critiques and measures of other social identities and their relation to power, such as sexual orientation, (dis)ability status, nationality, immigration status, and work status, to name a few Conduct intersectional research and interventions with social groups that are privileged in addition to those that are historically marginalized for the purpose of resisting oppression. For example, Dancis and Coleman (2022) describe findings from a university-based anti-racism intervention for White students, the Systemic Racism Curriculum Project (Coleman et al., 2019). They suggest that this curriculum helped students alter their worldviews to better understand and challenge systemic racism

(continued)

Table 4.2 (continued)

Guidelines adapted from Moradi and Grzanka (2017)	Practical examples
Adapt and integrate measures and theories across disciplines to capture intersectional identity and experience	Integrate theories across disciplines (e.g., critical race theories, disability justice theories, feminist theories) that each must contend with intersectionality. For an example, see Stern et al. (2021) When measuring a phenomena or outcome of interest, use single-axis measures (e.g., focusing on one social group) in addition to those created for groups at the intersections. For an example, Balsam and colleagues developed a measurement scale that assesses multiple minority-based microaggressions and stress for people of color who also identify as LGBTQ (Balsam et al., 2011)
Stop using conceptualizations and terminology that focus solely on marginalized identities and instead focus on latent oppressive systems and social inequalities	Reconceptualize sociodemographic categories (e.g., race, gender) as independent variables and main predictors as opposed to control variables (Helms et al., 2005) Instead of suggesting that race is a risk factor for health disparities, name the social inequality that produced that disparity—*racism*. "Gatekeepers" such as journal editors should encourage this reconceptualization Use language that situates the health disparity or problem at the systems rather than individual level. For example, instead of believing that "African Americans don't trust medical research," consider how medical research institutions have not earned African Americans' trust
Expand the purpose and evaluation of research to also include meaningful community engagement and systems-level social change	Reflect on the degree to which your research process and products support community engagement and systematic social change Consider the difference between research "about" social justice compared to research that reveals social injustice and promotes equity. For example, Rosenberg et al. (2017) analyzed racial disparities in public health research funding and found that funding for issues affecting white Americans (e.g., ischemic heart disease) vastly outnumbered that affecting more Black Americans (e.g., firearm-associated homicide). They call for an equitable distribution of funding resources Measure or evaluate the social and political impact of your research in addition to scholarly impact. For example, track how many think tanks or advocacy groups cite your work, if it is discussed in news articles or community organizations, or how many leaders reply to an email summarizing your study findings

(continued)

Table 4.2 (continued)

Guidelines adapted from Moradi and Grzanka (2017)	Practical examples
Consider how research and activism can be a cyclical, generative process that is committed to social justice	Intersectional scholarship should imbue intersectional activism and vice versa. Make and attend to calls to action to challenge the systemic forces that you study Activism should be more than an implication of your research and should be a part of the research process itself For example, Crenshaw's #SayHerName and the international #MMIW (Missing and murdered Indigenous women) campaigns extend intersectional scholarship to activism. Both campaigns reveal how interlocking systems of historical and current oppression dehumanize Black, Indigenous, and racialized women. Watch the #SayHerName TedTalk (Crenshaw, 2016)

A common participatory approach is to include people from the community as part of the research team. In anti-racist research, the contributions of all partners are recognized as meaningful—the academic researcher may be an expert of theories and methods, but community researchers are experts in the context, subject matter, and lived experience. In these partnerships, researchers should consider their positionality and role as more of a facilitator or friendly outsider, a guest of the community (Greenwood & Levin, 1998; Gaudry, 2011). The value of community members as part of the research process can be conveyed through compensation as well as through language. For example, instead of a title of "community researcher," one might say "co-researcher" or "researcher who is from the community," in contrast to "academic researcher" rather than simply "researcher." Or one could attribute the title of researcher to all those who are fulfilling the role of researcher and conceptualize roles as researchers based on people's area of expertise, rather than where each researcher is institutionally situated. For example, a community member hired as part of the research team to specifically help with recruitment might be called the "recruitment specialist" or "community liaison." Although it may be a small change, in the work to be anti-racist, language matters and is a powerful tool to change attitudes and assumptions—for example, that a community researcher contributes less or has less impact on a research team.

Emancipatory research should prioritize dissemination of results to those who participated in research and will be impacted by its findings so that the results can be used to enact change. Teams should present findings in formats that are easily used by the community for subsequent action or inquiry. For research to be anti-racist, we must move beyond traditional book chapters and journal articles and instead engage in alternative forms of dissemination, such as short magazine articles, zines, websites, social media posts, pamphlets, videos, podcasts, etc. (Neblett, 2019). To support change in the community, we must prioritize dissemination of research findings in spaces and settings that traditionally oppress or silence marginalized groups to bring more visibility to those groups—such as forums with public figures and politicians, major news outlets, or social media campaigns. We should also engage these groups in project design to generate and frame results in ways that are useful to them. Furthermore, all dissemination activities or communications regarding one's research or the study population should place narratives and data about special populations in the social, political, and historical context from which they came (Hartman, 1997). The prioritization of dissemination to decision-makers requires "extra work" on the researchers' part, but it is meaningful because it is a step towards challenging power dynamics that shape the reality of participants. Within these recommendations, use participatory methods to identify specific dissemination methods and products most appropriate for the community and topic.

Emancipatory research also gives participants and communities tools for capacity building for action and change. Research outcomes should include increasing participants' capacity to solve problems, develop skills, exercise self-determination, and wield power for decision-making and policy-making in the institutions that impact them (McKnight & Kretzmann, 2012; Decorby-Watson et al., 2018; Morgan, 2006). McKnight provides resources on asset based community development (McKnight & Kretzmann, 2012). Others recommend capacity building strategies for individuals through skills and knowledge building (Nowell & Harrison, 2011; Decorby-Watson et al., 2018) and coalition building for communities (Kendall et al., 2012; Zakocs & Edwards, 2006) or community organizing (Minkler, 2012). Communities should also be supported to make use of study data. This can be achieved through co-ownership of research data with partners, a community organization, or collective outside of the university that represents participants, codified in legal agreements and memorandums of understanding (Chicago Beyond, 2019).

To further consider how power inequities exist in research, we recommend a guidebook created by Chicago Beyond entitled, "Why am I Always Being Researched? Available at https://chicagobeyond.org/researchequity/. This guidebook outlines seven inequities in research that stand in the way of impact and are held in place by power dynamics: access, information, validity, ownership, value, accountability, and authorship (Chicago Beyond, 2019).

4. *Anti-racist research aims to be decolonial in its practice and impact.*
In alignment with socio-ecological, intersectional, and emancipatory frameworks, anti-racist community-engaged research should strive to be decolonial (Janes, 2016; Collins et al., 2018; Wallerstein et al., 2017; Gaudry, 2011) because racism is an outcome of colonialism (Horne, 2020; Tuck & Yang, 2012; Da Silva, 2007). In this section, we aim to describe briefly what it would mean to see a decolonial shift in anti-racist community-engaged research practice and impact. We highly encourage readers to engage deeply with critical texts written by indigenous and critical scholars, as we do not have space to cover the depth of this work in this brief chapter (Tuck & Yang, 2012; Patel, 2014; Singh et al., 2018; Daza & Tuck, 2014; Dei & Lordan, 2016; Smith, 2018; Riddell et al., 2017; Boonzaier & van Nieker, 2019; Kelley et al., 2013; Koster et al., 2012; Brayboy et al., 2012). In addition to frameworks and resources for doing ethical community-engaged research with indigenous communities, consider what we propose as preliminary material connecting anti-racism and anti-coloniality.

As we stated at the beginning of this chapter, to call for anti-racist research is to accept that research is inherently racist. Likewise, we call for decolonial research in acknowledgement that research is inherently colonialist. "Data as land" captures the idea that academia collects data from colonized and complexly oppressed peoples via an extractive research process (Gaudry, 2011) that allows the researcher to "own" the data and therefore construct cultural narratives about those people and use it as a tool for violence (Patel, 2014; Singh et al., 2018, 386). Incorporating de/anti/post-colonial and indigenous frameworks, Singh et al. (2018) present two principles to guide anti-oppressive techniques of data collection and researcher training: to make the power dynamic between the researcher-researched "other" explicit, and to aim to humanize the researched "other." These are critical pillars of decolonial research because the parallels between *colonizer-colonized* and *researcher-researched* are similar. This is not by chance, but because mainstream, Eurowestern research still relies on extraction to prosper (Gaudry, 2011; Patel, 2014; Tuck & Yang, 2012).

Before we address how to be decolonial in our impact, we must consider the ways colonial logics are present in mainstream, Eurowestern health and social sciences research. Colonial logics include the ways in which researchers "at-risk" and "asterisk" indigenous peoples (Tuck & Yang, 2012; Patel, 2014). "At-risking" indigenous peoples conceptualizes them solely as a marginalized group barely in existence, neglecting and therefore isolating indigenous resilience and resistance. "Asterisking" or homogenizing and codifying indigenous groups as "other" creates blurred ethnocultural categories that similarly lead to indigenous erasure. Furthermore, the positivist epistemologies of health and social sciences and the focus on "objectivity" reflects the desire to create distance between the researcher and the researched "other." Together, these factors pathologize indigenous groups and makes them invisible, which leads to further mistreatment (Haozous et al., 2014; Tuck & Yang, 2012). Another colonial logic underlying mainstream research is the tendency to ask questions that solely focus on how historically and currently colonized groups are not conforming or thriving in institutions built for and by settlers (Singh et al., 2018).

How do we move beyond recognizing the presence of colonial logics in research to actively trying to undo them in our practice? As discussed earlier in this chapter, reflexivity is an essential piece of anti-racist research. We can take it a step further by considering how we can enact "everyday actions" (Singh et al., 2018, 386) of decoloniality to disrupt Eurowestern-centrism in research. Singh et al. (2018) emphasize these steps in community-based researcher training and data collection. In their community-based RCT, the ROSES program, they created an anti-oppressive curriculum to train researchers on "research as a site of resistance, not a justification for oppression," and "research as humanizing through restoring critical compassion and complex personhoods" (387). This training aids researchers in their capacity to develop critical perspectives necessary for decolonial practice. This is accompanied by supportive and compassionate research supervision that aids in developing critical awareness of how Eurowestern hegemony has both manifested the social inequity that shapes our research problem and our relations to the communities with which we work. This awareness does not negate the inevitable embodied sorrow that some will feel when they realize how their positions of power are linked to histories of violence. Therefore, Singh et al. (2018) emphasize that we must normalize this discomfort, and to know that just because we cannot experience the lived reality of the researched "other," we can still develop solidarity with them.

In data collection, we must design our approaches to be attentive to community needs. For example, Singh et al. (2018) describe how data collection and consent/assent processes should be community and participant-centered instead of researcher-centered. This may mean traveling to participants' homes for data collection, providing or compensating childcare, allowing for family discussion of the research opportunity, and other ways to make participation in research accessible. Furthermore, just as we must be flexible in how we physically enter the lives of participants, and we must be transparent in explaining the "hidden social contract" (Singh et al., 2018, 389) between the researcher and the participant. That is, through the transaction of consent/assent and data collection, the participant receives a short-term incentive in the form of a financial compensation for their time, lost work hours, childcare, transportation, etc., while researchers gain immensely more resources in the longer term through published manuscripts which may support achievement of future grants, employment, and influence. Singh et al. (2018) share how a transparent approach to data collection can extend the amount of time needed to collect data, for example if the potential participant needs to talk the situation through with a friend or family member. This approach may also lead to refusal of participation and thus no data collection. Importantly, this approach prioritizes the needs of the participant and community.

Above all, anti-racist and anti-colonial research holds researchers accountable through formal or informal agreements with community members (Morton Ninomiya & Pollock, 2017). Researchers are trained to be accountable to many things—funding agencies, peer review processes, tenure review, and more—yet we are not trained to be accountable to the communities, resources, data, relationships, and land that provides us scholarship and success. While we could blame our mentors, institutions, or broad society for not having a system of accountability in place, as anti-racist practitioners, we can start with accountability to ourselves and extend this to our team and institutions. To be accountable to communities broadly would mean that researchers start all research with an agreement that is to be honored, across short- and long-term impacts of research and our institutions. One might begin a research project with a public or open forum with community members or other stakeholders, having a conversation about what the research is, why it is impactful or important, and what the expected outcomes or outputs should be. With an approach like this, individual researchers and the research group as a whole can invite accountability from the community if or when they have impacts or outcomes from the research, whether expected or unexpected. A forum like this also gives the community some discretion over what happens with their data and allows them to dictate involvement in the study. In addition, a conversation with the community allows them to judge the value of the knowledge produced or effectiveness of the research (a component of anti-racist work), rather than judging the research solely by typical academic metrics.

Lastly, we must do research with a purpose, and strive to undo the violence of racism and coloniality. While that may seem like a daunting goal, we argue that there are ways that health and social science scholars can work toward this goal by doing research that validates and humanizes oppressed peoples and using material resources to uplift their communities. Most researchers do not generally think they perpetrate the violence of Eurowestern, settler-colonial domination through individual actions; however, this harm continues because of continued collective inaction, masked behind veneers of objectivity. We undo this by doing the opposite. As representatives of our institution, we should be advocates for unveiling and rectifying injustices, giving reparations, and bestowing land and data sovereignty to the indigenous and local communities. We can do this by using our education and research tools to advocate for these goals, raising understanding and awareness of these issues, and using participatory and action research techniques to identify how land and data sovereignty can happen in reality.

4.3 Conclusion: More than Intent

Anti-racist research is measured by its impact, not its intent. If research is anti-colonial and anti-racist, it should benefit the community, above all. Not only should the community gain knowledge that is useful to them, but the research process should be used to achieve equity, challenge power structures, change policy, or advance changes in the material livelihoods of communities affected by racism. To help researchers evaluate the potential impact of their research, we have created a list of questions for reflection to evaluate if and how research is anti-racist (Table 4.3). These questions are designed to help researchers engage in critical reflection on their own research practice to provide the impetus for doing anti-racist, community-engaged research.

An anti-racist community engaged researcher is one that sees socioecological, intersectional, emancipatory, and decolonial approaches as necessity. A number of resources provide specific guidance on integrating equity throughout the research process, from conceptualization to analysis and dissemination, specific to populations or topics (Wallerstein et al., 2017; Chicago Beyond, 2019; Grzanka, 2020). These principles we provide are not meant to be a checklist but rather indicators of anti-racist research. Conducting anti-racist research is not a "one size fits all" approach but one tailored to the context of the location, population, and power dynamics, both past and present. Above all else, *anti-racist research is necessarily critical of our institutions and of ourselves and is accountable to the communities with whom we do research.* We hope that with the examples provided, readers are equipped to deeply reflect and consider how to transform research practices and processes to be anti-racist. To do anti-racist research, the entire team must be ready and willing to bring the principles of antiracism into every aspect of their work (Lensmire et al., 2013).

Table 4.3 Is this research anti-racist? Questions for reflection

Before starting: To be anti-racist, you must be aware of your positionality within an institution	How has my institution historically functioned as a tool of racism and white supremacy? In its founding? During the slave trade, Jim Crow, and civil rights eras? In more recent decades? How does my institution continue to perpetuate systems of oppression within the research process? In IRB processes or requirements? In policies/structures for compensation and incentives to participants? In practices related to hiring researchers, research staff, or paying consultants? How does my institution continue to perpetuate systems of oppression outside of the research process? In hiring practices? In student recruitment and retention? In teaching? In its partnership with private organizations? In allocating internal funds? What is the history of research in this community? For this organization? For these participants? How is my institution perceived by the community?
Anti-racist research is grounded in a socio-ecological approach	What are the assumptions of the approach I plan to use? How could this approach reinforce privilege of those who already have power? Does my research treat racism as a dominant social force and a fundamental cause of health inequality? How is my outcome discussed in relation to racism? Is racism treated as a risk factor? Does it put blame or responsibility for poor health outcomes on a minority group, or on the system? Does it explain why or how racism is a determinant of health? How do I treat race and racism as variables in conceptualization and analysis? What is the narrative about race? Does this story medicalize race? Does it de-racialize medicine? Why is race used? Is its use discussed critically? Is there a more accurate measure we might use instead of race?

(continued)

Table 4.3 (continued)

Anti-racist research embraces intersectionality	Where am I positioned on social identity axes of race, gender, sexual orientation, ethnicity, nationality, (dis) ability, social class, education, or other positions of power? What is my positionality in relation to the research question and the community that I am doing research on/about/with? What are the broader systems of power and privilege that affect my research problem? How might this research measure and analyze those systems? How might sexism and other systems of oppression contribute to the observed effect? What sociodemographic characteristics am I measuring in this research? What am I NOT measuring? How might this create a hidden population in the data? Am I able to analyze the heterogeneity of groups? If not, what is the limiting factor? Is my measurement of race/ethnicity relevant to the community that I am doing research on/about/with? Is my measurement of other key sociodemographic factors equally relevant, such as socioeconomic class and gender?
Anti-racist research is participatory and emancipatory	Am I doing research *with* the community? Do I give power to the community as an essential part of the research team? How do I position myself as a facilitator rather than the host? Does the population want to be involved in research? Do I provide a structure and expectation of co-ownership of data and research outputs? Is the research *for* the community? What are the community's priorities? What is the community's research agenda? How can research be a tool to advance community priorities and align with the community's purpose? Do I engage with the community's ways of knowing? Do I equally balance "academic" knowledge with that of the community? What are the risks of participation for the community? What are the risks of participation for the researcher? Are these risks and benefits balanced? How do I value the community as a part of my research process? How are community members financially compensated? Are there other ways I could compensate the community or community members? Do I give co-researchers titles that reflect their importance and expertise on the team? How will the research lead to concrete change? Do I aim for and measure outcomes such as increasing capacity, skill development, shifting power structures and policy making? How do I plan for outputs other than the research report? How do I plan to disseminate to those in power and those engaged in advocacy work?

(continued)

Table 4.3 (continued)

Anti-racist research is decolonial in its practice and impact	How might Eurowestern-centrism be present in this research? What is the history associated with this research problem/population? How might the study population be "othered" or pathologized? What does my study approach and methodology say about my power? What is my relationship to the data/land that I am doing research on/about/with? Where do I feel discomfort in doing this research? Where is that discomfort coming from? How can I work to normalize the discomfort among myself and my research team? How does this research center participant/community needs? How has the community dictated what data is collected and how? Who owns the data? How is this research intrusive to the community? How can I mitigate that? Has the community determined the usefulness or impact of my research? Who am I responsible to? Have I invited the community to hold me accountable? Have I thoroughly explained the outcomes and benefits associated with the research for both the researcher and the participant/community? What opportunities are there for the community to determine the usefulness or impact of my research? What is the impact of my research? How might my research help unveil systemic injustice? How can my research advocate for reparations and/or land/data sovereignty?

References

Abel, E. K. (2004). 'Only the best class of immigration': Public health policy toward Mexicans and Filipinos in Los Angeles, 1910–1940. *American Journal of Public Health, 94*(6), 932–939. https://doi.org/10.2105/AJPH.94.6.932

Abrams, J. A., Tabaac, A., Jung, S., & Else-Quest, N. M. (2020). Considerations for employing intersectionality in qualitative health research. *Social Science and Medicine, 258*(June), 113138. https://doi.org/10.1016/j.socscimed.2020.113138

Agénor, M. (2020). Future directions for incorporating intersectionality into quantitative population health research. *American Journal of Public Health, 110*(6), 803–806. https://doi.org/10.2105/AJPH.2020.305610

Alexander-Floyd, N. G. (2012). Disappearing acts: reclaiming intersectionality in the social sciences in a post-Black feminist era. *Feminist Formations, 24*(1), 1–25. https://doi.org/10.1353/ff.2012.0003

Alhasan, D. M., Gaston, S. A., Braxton Jackson, W., Williams, P. C., Kawachi, I., & Jackson, C. L. (2020). Neighborhood social cohesion and sleep health by age, sex/gender, and race/ethnicity in the United States. *International Journal of Environmental Research and Public Health, 17*(24), 1–23. https://doi.org/10.3390/ijerph17249475

Bailey, Z. D., Krieger, N., Agénor, M., Graves, J., Linos, N., & Bassett, M. T. (2017). Structural racism and health inequities in the USA: Evidence and interventions. *The Lancet, 389*(10077), 1453–1463. https://doi.org/10.1016/S0140-6736(17)30569-X

Balls-Berry, J. E., & Acosta-Pérez, E. (2017). The use of community engaged research principles to improve health: Community academic partnerships for research. *Puerto Rico Health Sciences Journal, 36*(2), 84–85.

Balsam, K. F., Molina, Y., Beadnell, B., Simoni, J., & Walters, K. (2011). Measuring multiple minority stress: The LGBT people of color microaggressions scale. *Cultural Diversity and Ethnic Minority Psychology, 17*(2), 163.

Bastos, J. L., Celeste, R. K., Faerstein, E., & Barros, A. J. D. (2010). Racial discrimination and health: A systematic review of scales with a focus on their psychometric properties. *Social Science and Medicine, 70*(7), 1091–1099. https://doi.org/10.1016/j.socscimed.2009.12.020

Bauer, G. R. (2014). Incorporating intersectionality theory into population health research methodology: Challenges and the potential to advance health equity. *Social Science and Medicine, 110*, 10–17. https://doi.org/10.1016/j.socscimed.2014.03.022

Boonzaier, F., & van Nieker, T. (eds). (2019). *Decolonial feminist community psychology*. Springer.

Bowleg, L. (2012). The problem with the phrase women and minorities: Intersectionality-an important theoretical framework for public health. *American Journal of Public Health, 102*(7), 1267–1273. https://doi.org/10.2105/AJPH.2012.300750

Bowleg, L., & Bauer, G. (2016). Invited reflection: Quantifying intersectionality. *Psychology of Women Quarterly, 40*(3), 337–341.

Boyd, R. W., Lindo, E. G., Weeks, L. D., & McLemore, M. R. (2020). On racism: A new standard for publishing on racial health inequities. *Health Affairs Blog, 10*. https://doi.org/10.1377/hblog20200630.939347

Brayboy, B. M., Gough, H. R., Leonard, B., Roehl, R. F., & Solyom, J. A. (2012). Reclaiming scholarship: Critical Indigenous research methodologies. *Qualitative research: An introduction to methods and designs* (pp. 423–450).

Brewer, R., & Heitzeg, N. (2008). The racialization of crime and punishment. *American Behavioral Scientist*. https://doi.org/10.4324/9781315697475-6

Brophy, A. L. (2016). *University, court, and slave: Pro-slavery thought in Southern colleges and courts and the coming of civil war*. Oxford University Press.

Brown, K. S., Kijakazi, K., Runes, C., & Turner, M. A. (2019). Confronting structural racism in research and policy analysis. *Urban Institute*, 1–16.

Buchanan, N. C. T., & Wiklund, L. O. (2021). Intersectionality research in psychological science: Resisting the tendency to disconnect, dilute, and depoliticize. *Research on Child and Adolescent Psychopathology, 49*(1), 25–31.

Buchanan, N. C. T., Rios, D., & Case, K. A. (2020). Intersectional cultural humility: Aligning critical inquiry with critical praxis in psychology. *Women & Therapy, 43*(3–4), 235–243.

Bullough, R. V., & Pinnegar, S. (2001). Guidelines for quality in autobiographical forms of self-study research. *Educational Researcher, 30*(3), 13–21. https://doi.org/10.3102/0013189X030003013

Case, A. D. (2017). Reflexivity in counterspaces fieldwork. *American Journal of Community Psychology, 60*(3–4), 398–405.

Chicago Beyond. (2019). *Why am I always being researched?*, 1–112.

Clarke, A. R., Goddu, A. P., Nocon, R. S., Stock, N. W., Chyr, L. C., Akuoko, J. A. S., & Chin, M. H. (2013). Thirty years of disparities intervention research. *Medical Care, 51*(11), 1020–1026. https://doi.org/10.1097/MLR.0b013e3182a97ba3

Cole, E. R. (2009). Intersectionality and research in psychology. *American Psychologist, 64*(3), 170–180. https://doi.org/10.1037/a0014564

Coleman, B. R., Bonam, C. M., & Yantis, C. (2019). I thought ghettos just happened: White Americans' responses to learning about place-based critical history. *History and collective memory from the margins: A global perspective* (pp. 207–228)..

Collins, P. H., & Bilge, S. (2020). *Intersectionality*. Wiley.

Collins, S. E., Clifasefi, S. L., Stanton, J., The LEAP Advisory Board, Straits, K. J. E., Gil-Kashiwabara, E., Espinosa, P. R., et al. (2018). Community-Based Participatory Research

(CBPR): Towards equitable involvement of community in psychology research. *American Psychologist, 73*(7), 884–898. https://doi.org/10.1037/amp0000167

Combahee River Collective. (1977). *A Black feminist statement.*

Corburn, J. (2007). Our roots American urban planning. *Urban Affairs Review*, 688–713.

Crenshaw, K. (1989). Demarginalizing the intersection of race and sex: A Black feminist critique of antidiscrimination doctrine, feminist theory and antiracist politics. *University of Chicago Legal Forum, 139.*

Crenshaw, K. (2016). *The urgency of intersectionality.* Ted conferences. https://www.ted.com/talks/kimberle_crenshaw_the_urgency_of_intersectionality?language=en

Crenshaw, K., Gotanda, N., Peller, G., & Thomas, K. (1995). Critical race theory. In *The key writings that formed the movement* (pp. 276–291).

Dancis, J., & Coleman, B. R. (2022). Transformative dissonant encounters: Opportunities for cultivating antiracism in White nursing students. *Nursing Inquiry, 29*(1), e12447.

Daza, S. L., & Tuck, E. (2014). De/colonizing, (Post)(Anti)colonial, and indigenous education, studies, and theories. *Educational Studies, 50*(4), 307–312. https://doi.org/10.1080/00131946.2014.929918

Decorby-Watson, K., Mensah, G., Bergeron, K., Abdi, S., Rempel, B., & Manson, H. (2018). Effectiveness of capacity building interventions relevant to public health practice: A systematic review. *BMC Public Health, 18*(1), 1–15. https://doi.org/10.1186/s12889-018-5591-6

Dei, G. J. S., & Lordan, M. (2016). *Anti-colonial theory and decolonial praxis.* Peter Lang Publishing, Inc.

Democracy Now. (n.d.). *Shackles and Ivy: The secret history of how slavery helped build America's elite colleges.*

Dill, B. T., & Kohlman, M. H. (2021). Intersectionality: A transformative paradigm in feminist theory and social justice. In S. N. Hesse-Biber (Ed.), *The handbook of feminist research: Theory and praxis* (pp. 154–174). Sage.

Doll, K. M., Snyder, C. R., & Ford, C. L. (2018). Endometrial cancer disparities: A race-conscious critique of the literature. *American Journal of Obstetrics and Gynecology, 218*(5), 474–482.

Dzidic, P., & Bishop, B. (2017). How do our values inform ethical research? A narrative of recognizing colonizing practices. *American Journal of Community Psychology, 60*(3–4), 346–352. https://doi.org/10.1002/ajcp.12197

Ellis, C., Adams, T. E., & Bochner, A. P. (2011). *Autoethnography: An overview.*

Else-Quest, N. M., & Hyde, J. S. (2016). Intersectionality in quantitative psychological research: I. Theoretical and epistemological issues. *Psychology of Women Quarterly, 40*(2), 155–170.

Fine, M. (2013). Echoes of bedford: A 20-year social psychology memoir on participatory action research hatched behind bars. *American Psychologist, 68*(8), 687.

Fine, M., & Ruglis, J. (2009). Circuits and consequences of dispossession: The racialized realignment of the public sphere for U.S. youth. *Transforming Anthropology, 17*(1), 20–33. https://doi.org/10.1111/j.1548-7466.2009.01037.x

Ford, C. L., & Airhihenbuwa, C. O. (2018). Commentary: Just what is critical race theory and what's it doing in a progressive field like public health? *Ethnicity and Disease, 28*, 223–230. https://doi.org/10.18865/ed.28.S1.223

Ford, C. L., & Harawa, N. T. (2010). A new conceptualization of ethnicity for social epidemiologic and health equity research. *Social Science & Medicine, 71*(2), 251–258. https://doi.org/10.1016/j.socscimed.2010.04.008

Galan, C. A., Bekele, B. M., Boness, C. L., Bowdring, M. A., Call, C. C., Hails, K., McPhee, J., et al. (2020). A call to action for an antiracist clinical science. *Journal of Clinical Child & Adolescent Psychology, 50*(1), 12–57. https://doi.org/10.1080/15374416.2020.1860066

Garcia, N. M., López, N., & Vélez, V. N. (2018). QuantCrit: Rectifying quantitative methods through critical race theory. *Race Ethnicity and Education, 21*(2), 149–157. https://doi.org/10.1080/13613324.2017.1377675

Gaudry, A. J. (2011). Insurgent research. *Wicazo Sa Review, 26*(1), 113–136.

Gilbert, K. L., & Ray, R. (2016). Why police kill Black males with impunity: Applying Public Health Critical Race Praxis (PHCRP) to address the determinants of policing behaviors and 'justifiable' homicides in the USA. *Journal of Urban Health, 93*(1), 122–140.

Gillborn, D., Warmington, P., & Demack, S. (2018). QuantCrit: Education, policy, 'big data' and principles for a critical race theory of statistics. *Race Ethnicity and Education, 21*(2), 158–179. https://doi.org/10.1080/13613324.2017.1377417

Gordon-Larsen, P. (2006). Inequality in the built environment underlies key health disparities in physical activity and obesity. *Pediatrics, 117*(2), 417–424. https://doi.org/10.1542/peds.2005-0058

Greenwood, D. J., & Levin, M. (1998). Action research, science, and the co-optation of social research. *Studies in Cultures, Organizations and Societies, 4*(2), 237–261. https://doi.org/10.1080/10245289808523514

Grzanka, P. R. (2020). *From buzzword to critical psychology: An invitation to take intersectionality seriously from buzzword to critical psychology* (p. 3149). https://doi.org/10.1080/02703149.2020.1729473

Hancock, A. M. (2007). When multiplication doesn't equal quick addition: Examining intersectionality as a research paradigm. *Perspectives on Politics, 5*(1), 63–79. https://doi.org/10.1017/S1537592707070065

Hankivsky, O. (2012). Women's health, men's health, and gender and health: Implications of intersectionality. *Social Science and Medicine, 74*(11), 1712–1720. https://doi.org/10.1016/j.socscimed.2011.11.029

Haozous, E. A., Strickland, C. J., Palacios, J. F., & Arambula Solomon, T. G. (2014). Blood politics, ethnic identity, and racial misclassification among American Indians and Alaska natives. *Journal of Environmental and Public Health, 2014*. https://doi.org/10.1155/2014/321604

Hardeman, R. R., & Karbeah, J.'. M. (2020). Examining racism in health services research: A disciplinary self-critique. *Health Services Research, 55*(S2), 777–780. https://doi.org/10.1111/1475-6773.13558

Hardeman, R. R., Medina, E. M., & Kozhimannil, K. B. (2016). Structural racism and supporting Black lives – The role of health profesesionals. *New England Journal of Medicine, 375*(22), 2113–2115.

Hartman, S. V. (1997). Innocent amusements: The stage of sufferance. In *Scenes of subjection: Terror, slavery, and self-making in nineteenth-century America* (pp. 17–48).

Helms, J. E., Jernigan, M., & Mascher, J. (2005). The meaning of race in psychology and how to change it: A methodological perspective. *American Psychologist, 60*(1), 27.

hooks, b. (1981). *Ain't I a woman: Black women and feminism*. Routledge.

Horne, G. (2020). *The dawning of the apocalypse: The roots of slavery, White supremacy, settler colonialism, and capitalism in the long sixteenth century*. Monthly Review Press.

Illinois, Unviersity of. (2018). *Office of the chancellor: Land acknowledgement statement*. https://chancellor.illinois.edu/land_acknowledgement.html

Janes, J. E. (2016). Democratic encounters? Epistemic privilege, power, and community-based participatory action research. *Action Research, 14*(1), 72–87. https://doi.org/10.1177/1476750315579129

Kagawa Singer, M., Dressler, W., George, S., Baquet, C. R., Bell, R. A., Burhansstipanov, L., Burke, N. J., et al. (2016). Culture: The missing link in health research. *Social Science and Medicine, 170*, 237–246. https://doi.org/10.1016/j.socscimed.2016.07.015

Kaufman, J. S. (2008). Epidemiologic analysis of racial/ethnic disparities: Some fundamental issues and a cautionary example. *Social Science and Medicine, 66*(8), 1659–1669. https://doi.org/10.1016/j.socscimed.2007.11.046

Kelley, A., Belcourt-Dittloff, A., Belcourt, C., & Belcourt, G. (2013). Research ethics and indigenous communities. *American Journal of Public Health, 103*(12), 2146–2152.

Kendall, E., Muenchberger, H., Sunderland, N., Harris, M., & Cowan, D. (2012). Collaborative capacity building in complex community-based health partnerships: A model for translating knowledge into action. *Journal of Public Health Management and Practice, 18*(5), 1–13. https://doi.org/10.1097/PHH.0b013e31823a815c

Kendi, I. X. (2019). *How to be an antiracist*. One world.

Koster, R., Baccar, K., & Lemelin, R. H. (2012). Moving from research on, to research with and for Indigenous communities: A critical reflection on community-based participatory research. *The Canadian Geographer/Le Géographe Canadien, 56*(2), 195–210.

Lensmire, T. J., McManimon, S. K., Tierney, J. D., Lee-Nichols, M. E., Casey, Z. A., Lensmire, A., & Davis, B. M. (2013). McIntosh as synecdoche: How teacher education's focus on white privilege undermines antiracism. *Harvard Educational Review, 83*(3), 410–432.

Lewontin, R. C. (2005). The fallacy of racial medicine: Confusions about human races. *Genewatch: A Bulletin of the Committee for Responsible Genetics, 18*(4), 5–7.

Loomba, A. (2015). *Colonialism/postcolonialism*. Routledge.

Lykes, M. B., Lloyd, C. R., & Nicholson, K. M. (2018). Participatory and action research within and beyond the academy: Contesting racism through decolonial praxis and teaching 'against the grain. *American Journal of Community Psychology, 62*(3–4), 406–418. https://doi.org/10.1002/ajcp.12290

Marx, G. (1997, March 12). Opposition brewing to UIC expansion. *Chicago Tribune*.

Matsui, E. C., Perry, T. T., & Adamson, A. S. (2020). An antiracist framework for racial and ethnic health disparities research. *Pediatrics, 146*(6), e2020018572. https://doi.org/10.1542/peds.2020-018572

McClure, E. S., Vasudevan, P., Bailey, Z., Patel, S., & Robinson, W. R. (2020). Racial capitalism within public health-how occupational settings drive Covid-19 disparities. *American Journal of Epidemiology, 189*(11), 1244–1253. https://doi.org/10.1093/aje/kwaa126

McKnight, J. L., & Kretzmann, J. P. (2012). Mapping community capacity. In M. Minkler (Ed.), *Community organizing and community building for health & welfare* (pp. 171–186). Rutgers University Press. https://doi.org/10.1007/978-94-007-0753-5_102372

Memmi, A. (2013). *The colonizer and the colonized*. Routledge.

Merriam-Webster. (2021). *Emancipate*. https://www.merriam-webster.com/dictionary/emancipate

Minkler, M. (2012). *Community organizing and community building for health and welfare*. Rutgers University Press.

Moradi, B., & Grzanka, P. R. (2017). Using intersectionality responsibly: Toward critical epistemology, structural analysis, and social justice activism. *Journal of Counseling Psychology, 64*(5), 500.

Morgan, M. A. (2006). *Community engagement in public health*.

Morton Ninomiya, M. E., & Pollock, N. J. (2017). Reconciling community-based indigenous research and academic practices: Knowing principles is not always enough. *Social Science and Medicine, 172*, 28–36. https://doi.org/10.1016/j.socscimed.2016.11.007

Neblett, E. W. (2019). Racism and health: Challenges and future directions in behavioral and psychological research. *Cultural Diversity and Ethnic Minority Psychology, 25*(1), 12–20. https://doi.org/10.1037/cdp0000253

Nowell, B., & Harrison, L. M. O. (2011). Leading change through collaborative partnerships: A profile of leadership and capacity among local public health leaders. *Journal of Prevention & Intervention in the Community*. https://doi.org/10.1080/10852352.2011.530162

Obasogie, O. K. (2013). Foreword; critical race theory and empirical methods. *UC Irvine Law Review, 3*(2), 183–186.

Office of Extramural Research. (2001). *NIH policy on reporting race and ethnicity data: Subjects in clinical research*. National Institutes of Health.

Patel, L. (Leigh). (2014). Countering coloniality in educational research: From ownership to answerability. *Educational Studies, 50*(4), 357–377. https://doi.org/10.1080/00131946.2014.924942

Paul-Emile, K. (2014). Critical race theory and empirical methods conference. *Fordham Law Review, 83*, 2953.

Perez-Rodriguez, J., & de la Fuente, A. (2017). Now is the time for a postracial medicine: Biomedical research, the National Institutes of Health, and the perpetuation of scientific racism. *American Journal of Bioethics, 17*(9), 36–47. https://doi.org/10.1080/15265161.2017.1353165

Public Science Project. 2021. *Youth Justice Research Collaborative*. https://publicscienceproject.org/youth-justice-research-collabortaive/

Ratele, K., & Malherbe, N. (2020). What antiracist psychology does and does not (do). *South Africa Journal of Psychology, 50*(3), 296–300. https://doi.org/10.1177/0081246320947361

Riddell, J. K., Salamanca, A., Pepler, D. J., Cardinal, S., & McIvor, O. (2017). Laying the groundwork: A practical guide for ethical research with Indigenous communities. *The International Indigenous Policy Journal, 8*(2).

Rosenberg, M., Ranapurwala, S. I., Townes, A., & Bengtson, A. M. (2017). Do black lives matter in public health research and training? *Plos one, 12*(10), e0185957.

Sabati, S. (2019). Upholding 'colonial unknowing' through the IRB: Reframing institutional research ethics. *Qualitative Inquiry, 25*(9–10), 1056–1064. https://doi.org/10.1177/1077800418787214

Silva, D. F. D. (2007). *Toward a global idea of race* (Vol. 27). University of Minnesota Press.

Singh, S., Granski, M., del Pilar Victoria, M., & Javdani, S. (2018). The praxis of decoloniality in researcher training and community-based data collection. *American Journal of Community Psychology, 62*(3–4), 385–395. https://doi.org/10.1002/ajcp.12294

Smith, L.T. (2018). Indigenous insight on valuing complexity, sustaining relationships, being accountable. In *Tackling wicked problems in complex ecologies: The role of evaluation* (pp.45-66). Stanford University Press.

Stern, J. A., Barbarin, O., Cassidy, J., & Stern, J. A. (2021). Attachment & human development working toward anti-racist perspectives in attachment theory, research, and practice. *Attachment & Human Development, 00*(00), 1–31. https://doi.org/10.1080/14616734.2021.1976933

Stolley, P. D. (1999). Race in epidemiology. *International Journal of Health Services, 29*(4), 905–909.

Suzuki, S., Morris, S. L., & Johnson, S. K. (2021). *Using QuantCrit to advance an anti-racist developmental science: applications to mixture modeling*. https://doi.org/10.1177/07435584211028229

Taylor, K. Y. (Ed.). (2017). *How we get free: Black feminism and the Combahee River Collective*. Haymarket Books.

Tuck, E., & Yang, K. W. (2012). Decolonization is not a metaphor. *Decolonization: Indigeneity, Education and Society, 1*(1), 1–40.

University of Illinois Chicago. (2016). *Permanent campus site selection, 1958–1963. UIC History Exhibition*.

Wallerstein, N., Duran, B., Oetzel, J. G., & Minkler, M. (2017). *Community-based participatory research for health: Advancing social and health equity*. Wiley.

Ward, J. B., Gartner, D. R., Keyes, K. M., Fliss, M. D., McClure, E. S., & Robinson, W. R. (2019). How do we assess a racial disparity in health? Distribution, interaction, and interpretation in epidemiological studies. *Annals of Epidemiology, 29*, 1–7. https://doi.org/10.1016/j.annepidem.2018.09.007

Washington, H. A. (2006). *Medical apartheid: The dark history of medical experimentation on Black Americans from colonial times to the present*. Doubleday Books.

Wilder, C. S. (2014). *Ebony & Ivy: Race, slavery, and the troubled history of America's universities*. Bloomsbury Publishing.

Williams, D. R., & Mohammed, S. A. (2013). Racism and health I: Pathways and scientific evidence. *American Behavioral Scientist, 57*(8), 1152–1173.

Zakocs, R. C., & Edwards, E. M. (2006). What explains community coalition effectiveness? A review of the literature. *American Journal of Preventive Medicine, 30*(4), 351–361. https://doi.org/10.1016/j.amepre.2005.12.004

Alexis Grant is a scholar-activist and participatory researcher and evaluator. She is an African American, Jamaican, and Native American and is a cisgender woman, and the first in her family to earn a PhD. Her research focuses on cross-sector implementation of community health interventions, collaboration for community health, and power-sharing to dismantle systemic racism in public health systems, including those within academic institutions. She received her PhD in Community Health Sciences from University of Illinois Chicago.

Andrea L. DaViera is a scholar-activist and doctoral candidate in Community and Prevention Research. Andrea is a first-generation college student from Chicago who identifies as a cisgender white woman. She has broad interests in intersectionality, power, oppression, and participatory action research. The goal of Andrea's research is to actively disrupt systems of violence and inequity while understanding and bolstering what promotes thriving, resiliency, and resistance. As a student organizer at University of Illinois Chicago, Andrea challenges the university administration to strive for equity rather than simply diversity.

Chapter 5
Demystifying How Academic-Community Partnerships Use Reflexivity and Praxis to Promote Participatory Research Principles of Equity and Justice

Jeni Hebert-Beirne, Sylvia Gonzalez, Melissa Chrusfield, Adlaide Holloway, Jennifer Plascencia Lopez, and Dolores Castañeda

5.1 Introduction

There is widespread agreement among public health advocates that community-led, participatory action research is needed to name structural roots of health inequities experienced at the neighborhood level, understand the mechanisms at play, and identify solutions that enhance community strengths and assets (Bowleg, 2017, 679, 2019, 240; Wallerstein et al., 2018, 4; Thomas et al., 2011, 408.). Community organizers and advocates suggest that a healthy community is only possible when community members are the co-developers of their futures (Minkler, 2012, 38; Ledwith, 2020). However, most research remains disengaged from community assets and

J. Hebert-Beirne (✉)
School of Public Health, University of Illinois Chicago, Chicago, IL, USA
e-mail: jheber1@uic.edu

S. Gonzalez
Center for Healthy Work, School of Public Health, University of Illinois Chicago, Chicago, IL, USA
e-mail: sgonza43@uic.edu

M. Chrusfield · A. Holloway
Greater Lawndale Healthy Work Council, Chicago, IL, USA
e-mail: mcmosley78@gmail.com; adlaide.holloway@sinai.org

J. P. Lopez
Community Health Sciences, School of Public Health, University of Illinois Chicago, Chicago, IL, USA
e-mail: jplasc3@uic.edu

D. Castañeda
Center for Healthy Work. School of Public Health, University of Illinois Chicago, Chicago, IL, USA
e-mail: dcasta20@uic.edu

E. E. Anderson (ed.), *Ethical Issues in Community and Patient Stakeholder–Engaged Health Research*, Philosophy and Medicine 146,
https://doi.org/10.1007/978-3-031-40379-8_5

leadership due to layers of research-related inequities (Chicago Beyond, 2019, 7), influenced by a priori assumptions (Ford & Airhihenbuwa, 2010 S30) and researchers helicoptering in and out of communities in the name of solving communities' problems never to be seen again (Wallerstein et al., 2018, 4). There are signs of progress in naming the ways in which the academy has been complicit in the processes of structural violence (including in our own institution; Botterman et al., 2022) and in naming the need for decolonization of research processes (Smith, 2012). There are also recent concerns relating to new risks of greater colonization of research (see Chap. 4, in this volume), evidenced by the increased interest by academics who were made aware of the racialized, social production of health inequities due to the global consciousness raising with the murder of George Floyd (New York Times, 2020) but who are not trained in, nor committed to long-term community-engaged research (Lett et al., 2022, 2).

There are core reasons for the renewed emphasis on the need for authentic community stakeholder-engaged research. First, participatory research produces better, more "truthful" science (Wallerstein et al., 2018, 17), and second, participatory research processes build the capacity of community and academic partners to collaborate (Coombe et al., 2020). Yet, the power of the critical discourse that can emerge from having diverse stakeholders reflect on the injustices at the core of health inequities under investigation is underappreciated.

Authentic community stakeholder-engaged research can contribute to higher quality, more valid science by improving the degree to which each stage of the research process is rooted in community priorities, from research question identification to the dissemination of the findings (Israel et al., 1998, 180). Research hypotheses that are informed by people with lived experience on the phenomenon are more likely to provide the critical knowledge needed to best understand the inequities and identify solutions to the injustices at play (Ledwith, 2016, 139). The findings that emerge from community-engaged research are less likely to produce partial truths (Chicago Beyond, 2019, 7) and more likely to produce findings that present a counter-narrative to the hegemonic dominant discourse (Ledwith, 2020 170).

Authentic community stakeholder-engaged research is meant to be capacity building. Research processes build community capacity by centering and building on community assets. Authentic research can transform academia by repositioning academics to follow the lead of community experts (Hebert-Beirne et al., 2018). Perhaps least understood is the degree to which authentic community stakeholder-engaged research allows for the praxis required for real change on the injustices at the core of health inequities. When public health researchers and people who have lived experience with systems of oppression strategically, authentically, and reciprocally engage, the intentional discourse and reflexivity build critical consciousness on the role of power in the socio-political production of the unjust conditions that produce health inequities. The praxis, reflecting on the unjust contradictions at play, informs the intentional actions needed to address the injustice (Ledwith, 2016, 35). Through strategic engagement, we can begin to recognize diverse types of truths and identify how academia is complicit in producing research data that maintain a single, hegemonic narrative of everyday life that perpetuates inequalities (Minkler, 2012). Antonio Gramsci suggests this critical consciousness is produced by centering organic intellectuals and their lived experience in academic-research partnerships; this is the praxis, the basis of action for change (Ledwith, 2016, 74). Freire further suggests that dialogue and praxis are the basis of humanization (Ledwith, 2016, 24). Maintaining productive academic-community partnerships is key to sustaining the dialogue that fuels praxis. Freire, in fact, calls us to focus on the everyday contradictions and conflicts at the root of our research (Ledwith, 2016). By questioning what is happening in everyday life, we expose the contradictions of injustice that lead to and sustain oppression. When we listen, we question what is at the roots of injustice and oppression. This forces us to reject downstream changes that make life temporarily better, instead of insisting on radical change. We recognize the layers of inequities held in place by power that threaten the production of trust in research: access, information, validity, ownership, value, accountability, and authorship (Chicago Beyond, 2019). Transformative Communication Spaces – "the intellectual and social spaces that partners create and provide to each other for shared learning and trust-building" – are necessary structures for participatory inquiry that promotes and allows for shared learning, trust-building, and establishing a shared identity among partners as co-leaders of collaborative research (Hebert-Beirne et al., 2018, 417). Transformative Communication Spaces are needed to engage in critical dialogue and critical consciousness-raising to address the contradictions and conflicts that emerge in our research processes.

Below, we describe how our academic-community partnerships use reflexivity and practices to identify solutions to the everyday contradictions and conflicts to continually ground our partnership in principles of equity and inclusion.

Community Grounding

This story, from one of our authors, Dolores Castañeda, provides context for the research being done by the Greater Lawndale Healthy Work (GLHW) Project.

When I was a young child, I helped my mother sell eggs and vegetables at the local market in Guanajuato, Mexico. She worked all day at the market, went home in the evening to prepare cooked foods to sell, and returned to the local market to sell some more. Despite working all day long, she was still unable to support us economically. Due to the economic and political uncertainties in Mexico, my family and I immigrated to the U.S. We arrived in Little Village, a predominantly Mexican neighborhood on the southwest side of Chicago, which I have called home for the past 50 years.

While in the U.S., my family and I continued working long hours to make ends meet. Working in the factories was a dehumanizing experience; we were overworked and threatened if we did not work fast. When I spoke out, the supervisor fired me. As Paolo Freire states in *Pedagogy of the Oppressed*,

(continued)

"Dehumanization, which marks not only those whose humanity has been stolen, but also (though in a different way) those who have stolen it, is a distortion of the vocation of becoming more fully human" (Freire et al., 2018, 44). Put in other words, my supervisor and I were both stripped of our humanity. With my faith as my compass, I said enough was enough and have since dedicated my life to various social justice causes, such as immigrant rights, homelessness, workers' rights, and violence.

Recently, the father of my children suffered a work-related death, and as of yet, neither the U.S. Occupational Safety and Health Administration (OSHA) nor the company have provided answers or taken responsibility for his death. This tremendous loss in our family has been a source of pain and also a point of connection with others who share similar stories. In these moments of reflection with others, I have been troubled by a culture of overwork that has been deeply internalized by the worker, leaving no time to seek medical care or even rest. Workers are dying for their paycheck, and the system is at fault for perpetuating these precarious conditions.

Despite the collective pain and loss, I still remain hopeful and dedicated to working for reform. The words of Mariame Kaba deeply resonate with me and give me the words to describe the kind of world I want to build—a society where "we have everything we need: food, shelter, education, health, art, beauty, clean water, and more things that are foundational to our personal and community safety" (Kaba et al., 2021, 25). This world includes opportunities for work that are fair and just. When we have those right conditions in place for everyone to access their basic needs as well as healthy work, the need for policing, prisons, and surveillance will be obsolete.

5.2 Greater Lawndale Healthy Work (GLHW) Project Background

The GLHW project is a research project of the University of Illinois Chicago (UIC), School of Public Health Center for Healthy Work, a National Institutes of Occupational Safety and Health (NIOSH) Center for Excellence for *Total Worker Health*®. The GLHW project is a CBPR project that works in partnership with community residents and representatives of community-based organizations in two contiguous community areas in Chicago, North Lawndale and Little Village, which together form the Greater Lawndale area. The project aims to explore the role of work as a social determinant of health and to identify community solutions to promote worker health at the neighborhood level.

The GLHW project grew from an organic academic-community collaboration for community health inquiry and action. Our goal was to describe, in an ongoing capacity, the health needs and assets of the community, from an emic, grounded perspective, with attention to structural and social determinants of health, using iterative research methods, and producing new knowledge that is shared and disseminated in the community toward action. We use a community health assessment approach aligned with CBPR principles, including centering community priorities, leveraging the strengths of academic and community partners, and collaborating at each stage of the research, from research question identification to instrument development, data collection, and dissemination of findings (Israel et al., 1998). Work and occupation, as a social determinant of health, emerged as a central community concern as part of our iterative mixed methods research. This led to the current focus on the impacts of increasing precarity in work opportunities at the neighborhood level on community health. Precarious work is defined as that which is unstable, insecure, uncertain, and lacking control over hours and schedule, and that has limited social benefits (health insurance, retirement), few options for advancement, low wages, exposure to dangerous or hazardous conditions, and little protection from discrimination or exploitation (Tompa et al., 2007). We seek to identify evidenced-based, community-led community capacity-building efforts to promote healthy work opportunities (stable jobs with adequate pay, benefits, and opportunities for protection and advancement) at the neighborhood level.

Our structure for collaborative leadership has shifted over the years, adapting to our research and capacity-building needs. Our current academic-community partnership leadership structure is the GLHW Council, comprised of community members, representatives of community-based organizations in Greater Lawndale, and university faculty, staff, and students. The Council determines the vision and guiding principles and oversees the implementation of evidence-based interventions identified on our theoretically- and community-grounded GLHW Action Roadmap (manuscript in development). The Community Co-Chairs of the Council (the third and fourth authors of this chapter) and the faculty, staff, and student academic leads (the first, second, fifth, and sixth authors) meet regularly to reflect on contradictions and conflicts that emerge in our research partnership and our processes and to identify solutions.

5.2.1 GLHW Council Mission, Values, and Principles

The GLHW Council works collaboratively with community members and organizations to change the narrative on work, challenge traditional power structures, and demonstrate the social impact of precarious work. The GLHW Council envisions a community where we affirm the value and humanity of community members in Greater Lawndale by working to ensure healthy work options are within reach for all residents. The purpose of the GLHW Council is to identify, develop, and implement sustainable interventions/initiatives to promote healthy work in Greater Lawndale. This includes: leveraging the GLHW Action Roadmap to identify potential points of intervention; assessing community readiness for change; identifying partners within and outside the community; and assisting in developing and implementing sustainable, community-driven interventions. The GLHW project adheres to several principles:

1. We co-develop community-led interventions that build community capacity.
2. We are asset-oriented. We avoid "at risk," "vulnerable," or "target" language.
3. We commit to language justice, which allows everybody's voices to be heard, and deepening our commitment to equalizing power dynamics.
4. We use ecological thinking. Our interventions are at the systems, community level, not putting onus on workers to make social change.
5. Students are equal research partners.
6. We commit to equitable dissemination of our findings, giving credit where it is due.
7. We prioritize the development of the counter-narrative; worker testimonies and stories are valuable sources of data.
8. Our research should be healing; the healing component should come from the people in the community.
9. We commit to praxis (theory, action, reflection). Being in the community informs theory; being on the ground informs our thinking. Being present is the only way to identify solutions. Decisions remain in the community so we must be more present in the community.
10. We commit to ongoing co-learning. CBPR needs to be fully understood to be transformative.

5.3 Methods: Academic-Community Research Partnership Praxis

The administrative community-academic team (the authors of this chapter) is responsible for assuring that the GLHW activities align with our CBPR principles and our Council values, mission, vision, and principles. To hold ourselves accountable, our administrative team co-developed a process for reflexivity that aligns with our shared theoretical framework. We use an adaptive public health critical race praxis (Ford & Airhihenbuwa, 2010) and feminist frame (hooks, 1989) that suggests that for our research partnership to be productive, we need to:

1. Identify and work to transform research hierarchies
2. Maintain attention to equity and social justice as we do our research
3. Commit to the recognition that the dismantling of racism is central to health equity
4. Expand vocabulary used to discuss complex racial, class, gender, and sexuality concepts
5. Challenge racial and white supremacist hierarchies
6. Use methods that go beyond *unmuting marginalized voices* to rather center the research at the margins, recognizing the margins as a place of resistance and power (hooks, 1989, 203–209).

This critical framing is essential for our research as "critical perspectives interrogate, expose, and challenge assumptions about policies, institutions, and practices that obscure power relations that foster inequality and oppression and conceal how dominant groups construct knowledge, facts, and problems" (Bowleg, 2019, 15). Bowleg and others suggest critical frameworks are needed to challenge "epistemologies of ignorance," theories of knowledge production that ignore the role of systems of oppression such as white supremacy, racism, sexism, and classism. Uncritical research produces dominant narratives that maintain the status quo by manipulating people into not seeing the contradictions in the injustices underlying the phenomenon (Ledwith, 2016).

Our team co-developed guidelines for our reflexivity. We set aside time and space for reflexivity. We asked each other to read passages that inspired us from the work of Paulo Freire, bell hooks, Mariame Kaba and/or shared our own experiences with issues of injustice as fuel for praxis. We agreed to co-develop our shared language. When we introduced a new concept or term, we agreed to teach the group the concept. We agreed to hold each other accountable to the work by establishing and keeping deadlines for the review of material and group discussion. We discussed the contradictions and conflicts emerging in our work and brainstormed how to address these issues while staying true to our CBPR principles and GLHW Values. To do this, we borrowed the Being and Problematising and Conscientisation stages from the Rowan model to name an everyday contradiction, engage in critical discourse about the contradiction, and reflect on the socio-political context of the contradiction, respectively (Rowan, 1981). We recorded our discussion and decisions.

5.4 Results

5.4.1 Naming the Contradictions in our Research to Co-Develop Solutions

In order to engage in critical discourse and elevate our shared critical consciousness—a level of insight at which people recognize oppression as a structural problem rather than an individual failing (Freire in Ledwith, 2016)—we named the primary contradictions and conflicts in our research focus area.

> **Those whose ancestors were exploited to build our country experience the greatest number of structural barriers to healthy work.** The ancestors of those slaves and migrants whose exploited labor built this country continue to be systematically left out of healthy work and benefits that are tied to formal work (e.g., health insurance, social security, union participation).
>
> **The dominant narrative that "hard work pays off" does not hold true for those who work the hardest**. The dominant, mainstream narrative about work suggests that the poor are in the situation because they do not work hard, and those who work hard are deserving of health care, time off, profit, etc. Yet, those who work the hardest in terms of number of jobs, hours, and labor often have none of these benefits.

While transformative praxis is rooted in stories of everyday life experiences (Ledwith, 2016), internalized self-blame makes truth elusive. Community members internalize blame for their situation, in which they are trying to make ends meet. This is compounded at the interpersonal level where members in a social network blame each other. Individual and interpersonal blame allows for systems to remain unaccountable and for employers to exploit workers. Critical consciousness about structural injustices underlying work is necessary for developing a sense of agency and ultimately collective action for liberation (Freire et al., 2018).

The social justice framing that "Healthy work is a human right" does not match reality. The human rights and legal framing of our research do not reflect reality. In reality, "unhealthy employers" are not held accountable because legal systems value profit over people. People are not able to speak their truth to power. We need to create conditions that foster healthy work.

5.4.2 Praxis Adaptations across the Research Cycle

Our reflexivity allows us to calibrate our research process, such that it stays grounded in the GLHW vision and CBPR principles. Reflectivity around these four contradictions using our theoretical critical framework and GLHW principles to guide us led to adaptations of our research process across the research cycle. See Table 5.1 for how research process adaptions align with principles.

5.4.3 Conflicts with our GLHW Principles and Action Steps

In addition to engaging in reflexivity in light of inherent contradictions in our research focus, we experience regular conflicts in adhering to our GLHW Principles and theoretical underpinnings of our research. Table 5.2 depicts Action Steps taken in light of conflicts to assure alignment with our values.

5.5 Discussion

5.5.1 Impact on Our Academic-Community Partnership

The reflexivity we engage in through our research partnership not only produces iterative adaptation to our research processes, but it strengthens our partnership and commitment to the work. We have recognized through our praxis that this shared understanding of the theoretical underpinnings of our research that we develop takes a long time (this speaks to the rootedness of racial and academic hierarchies in research) and requires an ongoing commitment to learning. Our commitment to adoption of an equity lens and elimination of racism in our work requires regular

Table 5.1 Crosswalk of solutions to identified contradictions by GLHW theoretical underpinnings

	Research question identification	Research design	Instrument development/ training	Recruitment	Data collection	Data analysis	Dissemination of findings for action
Reflexivity outcomes	Center lived experience with the phenomena under investigation [1,5,6] Do not replicate harmful stereotypes by comparing neighborhoods to each other but rather build solidarity across [3,5]	Commit to research methods (storytelling, focus group, concept mapping) that inform nuanced understanding of well-known gaps toward solution identification to address community needs [1,2,4]	Co-develop instruments using language that is accessible rather than pre-validated items[1,6] Humanize our research by bringing a personal touch to every activity by having community researcher-facilitated data collection [2,6]	Be present in the community, raising awareness of work as a social determinant of health before during and after recruiting for research [2,4]	Bring a trauma-informed approach to data collection [2,4,6] Offer healing resources to research participants [2] Give research participants time they need[2,5,7] Provide resources after research participation [2,6]	Use an interpretive lens that recognizes historical systems of oppression to shift the mental frame of workers regarding deservedness, worthiness [1,3,6]	Commit to humanizing the issues; assure stories are heard broadly [1,6] Respect ownership of the research products including equity in copyrighting [1,6] Commit to doing things differently and teaching others [2,6]
GLHW theoretical underpinnings	1. Identify and work to transform research hierarchies 2. Maintain attention to equity and social justice as we do our research 3. Commit to the recognition that the dismantling of racism is central to health equity 4. Expand vocabulary used to discuss complex racial, class, gender and sexuality concepts 5. Challenge racial and white supremacist hierarchies 6. Use methods that go beyond unmuting marginalized voices to rather center the research at the margins recognizing the margins as a place of resistance and power						

Table 5.2 Crosswalk of action steps to adhere to our GLHW Principles

	GLHW principles	Conflicts	Actions/steps
1	We co-develop community-led interventions that build community capacity	NIOSH grant sits within the university IRB questioned using young people as interviewers in our COVID stories project	Community council co-chairs lead intervention mapping, development, and implementation We explained to the IRB our intentions to build community capacity
2	We are asset oriented. We avoid "at risk," "vulnerable" or "target" language	North Lawndale and Little Village neighborhoods have long been pitted against each other	We analyze the data as Greater Lawndale avoiding replicating deficit orientation
3	We commit to language justice	While almost all of our printed material is in English and Spanish, there were different ideas of what approaches would be best to accommodate the monolingual English and Spanish speakers in meetings	We began by holding meetings in both languages using small group discussion in one language or the other to serve as the equity approach. However, this resulted in segregated rather than collaborative conversations. We now use a simultaneous translator for all meetings
4	We use ecological thinking. Our interventions are at the systems, community level; we do not put onus on workers to make social change	Workers have long been called upon to "speak up and stand up for rights," risking their jobs	We take a community-level approach to align interventions at contextual spaces to build power, equity, and wealth
5	Students are equal research partners	Students are often in administrative roles (e.g., note takers, data cleaners)	We hold each other accountable to share roles equitably
6	We commit to equitable dissemination of our findings, giving credit where it is due	Publishing our findings in academic journals alone does not influence social change PI typically gets recognition for collaborative effort. Our greater Lawndale Loteria educational card game copyright solely recognized the university	We disseminate findings through community meetings, infographics, podcasts, and research briefs We are working with university lawyers to establish multiple copyrights so that local artists get credit for their work
7	We prioritize the development of the counter narrative; worker testimonies and stories are valuable sources of data	Typical research methods produce partial truths (Chicago Beyond, 2019, 7). In peoples' stories we center the consequences of structural power and identify possibilities for change	Our methods and approach to interpretation are grounded and iterative: Stories, concept mapping, member checking, listening sessions

(continued)

Table 5.2 (continued)

	GLHW principles	Conflicts	Actions/steps
8	Our research should be healing; the healing component should come from the people in the community	NIOSH funds do not support healing initiatives. How can we bring a healing experience to the research participant and trauma informed approach to the research? The university needs to recognize when the community is hurting and that when the university does not say something, that is violence	We implemented trauma-informed research protocol training for focus groups, interviews, and surveys We support COVID testing and vaccination efforts We use methods such as photovoice that can be uplifting Be present when the community is hurting
9	We commit to praxis (the intersection of theory, action, reflection). Being in the community informs theory; being on the ground informs our thinking. Being present is the only way to identify solutions. Decisions remain in the community so we must be more present in the community	NIOSH funds do not fund "being present" in neighborhoods outside of the context of research	GLHW staff participate in ongoing community events and meetings and provide information, resources, and GLHW lunchboxes We are present and answer questions in spaces where we are not recruiting for research purposes
10	We commit to ongoing co-learning. CBPR needs to be fully understood to be transformative	Developing reciprocal partnership/mutually beneficial relationship between community and academic partners takes time and creativity. Power and knowledge are interrelated; we cannot be agents of change without being agents of knowledge (Ledwith, 2016)	We commit to ongoing reflexivity on contradictions and conflicts to strengthen our partnership We conduct internal evaluations with CBPR-based questions to measure strengths and weaknesses in our partnerships

Glossary
NIOSH National Institutes for Occupational Safety and health
IRB Institutional review board
Greater Lawndale Loteria – An evidence-informed, historically grounded and worker justice-themed card game to promote awareness of precarious work at the neighborhood level

check-ins about decisions: Who is making the decision? Who is impacted? Who benefits? Who is impacted but is not here? This last question forces us to think about what community issues are represented on the Council and what gaps exist.

The focus on the contradictions in our research opens doors for honest conversation. As we listened to stories emerging from our data, we were forced be more reflective of each other on a personal level (e.g., regarding child care responsibilities, differences in COVID-19 risk and impact). We were called to consider the degree to which we ourselves foster a healthy workspace. In committing to our diverse leadership model, we make decisions that address power inequities in our partnership and accommodate and make room for each other as humans with work-life balance needs and unpredictable stressors. We hold each other accountable for where we meet (community or university), how we meet (in person or virtual), and who plays what roles in the meeting. As we commit to this model we are "finding out what connects us, reveling in our differences, this is the process that brings us closer, that gives us a world of shared values of meaningful communities" (hooks, 2003).

Freire argued that it is not enough for people to study the world; they also have a responsibility to act to create a more just world. For Freire, praxis was "a central defining feature of human life and a necessary condition of freedom" and "human nature is expressed through intentional, reflective, meaningful activity situated within dynamic historical and cultural contexts that shape and set limits on that activity" (Freire et al., 2018). We need to ask ourselves, 'What is our position in the community as researchers. How does it relate to liberation, to freedom?'

5.6 Conclusions

In our reflexivity, we focus on new ways of knowing that allow us to see our identities and realities within systems of oppression and find solutions that involve humanization and healing. "When our lived experience of theorizing is fundamentally linked to processes of self-recovery, of collective liberation, no gap exists between theory and practice" (hooks, 1994, 61). That said, in the same way that workers cannot be solely held accountable for the systems change needed to foster healthy work, individual, local academic-community partnerships cannot control the systems and institutions that maintain power imbalance between the academy and communities. It is time for a new norm of stakeholder-engaged research that does not document inequities but rather prioritizes community-driven social change solutions for health inequities. This requires naming and dismantling long held power advantages maintained by internal university processes in order to allow for genuine equity and reciprocity within academic-community research partnerships.

Acknowledgements This research is made possible by the collaborative efforts of UIC faculty, staff, students and Greater Lawndale Community Researchers: Sandra Avelar (UIC Graduate Student), Teresa Berumen (Saint Anthony Hospital), Tessa Bonney (UIC Department of Environmental and Occupational Health Sciences), Gabriela Bustos (Sinai Urban Health Institute), Robert Calhoun (Saint Anthony Hospital), Rosi Carrasco (Chicago Community and Workers' Rights), Arturo Carrillo (Community Resident), Dolores and Yvette Castaneda (Community Residents), Aeysha Chaudhry (UIC Graduate Student), Melissa Chrusfield (Community Resident), Lorraine Conroy (UIC Environmental and Occupational Health Sciences), Rolando Favela (UIC SPH Staff), Jennifer Felner (UC San Diego Graduate Student), Linda Forst (UIC Environmental and Occupational Health Sciences), Sylvia Gonzalez (UIC SPH Staff), Renee Hatcher (UIC Law School), Jeni Hebert-Beirne (UIC Community Health Sciences) Virgilio Hernandez (Chicago

Community and Workers' Rights), Adlaide Holloway (Sinai Urban Health Institute), Rodney Johnson (UIC Graduate Student), Morgan Lawson (UIC Graduate Student), Marsha Love (UIC SPH Staff), Adriana Magana (Community Resident), Natalie Merrick (UIC Graduate Student), Amanda Mongtomery (UIC Graduate Student), David Mosley (Community Resident), Jackeline Ortiz (Telpochcalli Community Education Project), Maria Post (Community Resident), Jennifer Plascencia Lopez (UIC Graduate Student), Preethi Pratap (UIC Environmental and Occupational Health Sciences), Laura Romero (Telpochcalli Community Education Project), Angelica Rosales (Community Resident), Leonarda Rosendo (Telpochcalli Community Education Project), Kathleen Rospenda (UIC Department of Psychiatry), Patricia Pereda (Telpochcali Community Education Project), Rev. Bob Smith (Community Resident), Maria Velazquez (Telpochcali Community Education Project), Alisa Velonis (UIC Community Health Sciences), Richard Wallace (Equity and Transformation), Madeline Woodberry (Sinai Urban Health Institute), Suzanne Zoheri Chopra (Saint Anthony Hospital).

Funding Funding for this chapter was made possible by the Centers for Disease Control and Prevention National Institute of Occupational Safety and Health under grant number U19 OH011232. Total Worker Health® is a registered trademark of the U.S. Department of Health and Human Services (HHS). The views expressed in written materials or publications do not necessarily reflect the official policies of the Department of Health and Human Services, nor does the mention of trade names, commercial practices, or organizations imply endorsement by the U.S. Government. Participation by the UIC Center for Healthy Work does not imply endorsement by HHS, the Centers for Disease Control and Prevention, or the National Institute for Occupational Safety and Health.

References

Botterman, L., Carey, J., Giloth, S., Schroeder, R., & Smith, D. P. (2022). UIC partnerships for anti-racist campus transformation. In S. Giloth (Ed.), *Healthviews magazine*. Office of Advancement in the UIC School of Public Health. Accessed March 31, 2022. https://publichealth.uic.edu/alumni/healthviews-magazine/#fall-2021-edition

Bowleg, L. (2017). Towards a critical health equity research stance: Why epistemology and methodology matter more than qualitative methods. *Health Education & Behavior, 44*(5), 677–684. https://doi.org/10.1177/1090198117728760

Bowleg, L. (2019). Perspectives from the social sciences: Critically engage public health. *American Journal of Public Health, 109*(1), 15–16. https://doi.org/10.2105/AJPH.2018.304825

Chicago Beyond. (2019). *Why Am I always being researched?* Accessed September 7, 2021. https://chicagobeyond.org/researchequity/

Coombe, C. M., Schulz, A. J., Guluma, L., Allen, A. J., Gray, C., Wilma Brakefield-Caldwell, J., Guzman, R., et al. (2020). Enhancing capacity of community-- academic partnerships to achieve health equity: Results from the CBPR partnership academy. *Health Promotion Practice, 21*(4), 552–563. https://doi.org/10.1177/1524839918818830

Ford, C. L., & Airhihenbuwa, C. O. (2010). Critical race theory, race equity, and public health: Toward antiracism praxis. *American Journal of Public Health, 100*(S1), S30–S35. https://doi.org/10.2105/AJPH.2009.171058

Freire, P., Ramos, M. B., Macedo, D. P., & Shor, I. (2018). *Pedagogy of the oppressed* (50th ed.). Bloomsbury Academic.

Hebert-Beirne, J., Felner, J. K., Kennelly, J., Eldeirawi, K., Mayer, A., Alexander, S., Castañeda, Y. D., et al. (2018). Partner development praxis: The use of transformative communication spaces in a community-academic participatory action research effort in a Mexican ethnic enclave in Chicago. *Action Research, 16*(4), 414–436. https://doi.org/10.1177/1476750317695413

hooks, b. (1994). Teaching to transgress: Education as the practice of freedom. *Journal of Engineering Education, 1*, 126–138.

hooks, b. (1989). Choosing the margin as a space of radical openness. *Framework: The Journal of Cinema and Media, 36*(36), 15–23.

hooks, b. (2003). *Teaching community: A pedagogy of hope* (Vol. 36). Psychology Press.

Israel, B. A., Schulz, A. J., Parker, E. A., & Becker, A. B. (1998). Review of community-based research: Assessing partnership approaches to improve public health. *Annual Review of Public Health, 19*(1), 173–202. https://doi.org/10.1146/annurev.publhealth.19.1.173

Kaba, M., Murakawa, N., & Nopper, T. K. (2021). *We do this 'Til we free us: Abolitionist organizing and transforming justice*. Haymarket Books.

Ledwith, M. (2016). *Community development in action: Putting Freire into practice*. Policy Press.

Ledwith, M. (2020). *Community development: A critical approach*. Policy Press.

Lett, E., Adekunle, D., McMurray, P., Asabor, E. N., Irie, W., Simon, M. A., Hardeman, R., & McLemore, M. R. (2022). Health equity tourism: Ravaging the justice landscape. *Journal of Medical Systems, 46*(3), 1–6. https://doi.org/10.1007/s10916-022-01803-5

Minkler, M. (2012). *Community organizing and community building for health and welfare*. Rutgers University Press.

Rowan, J. (1981). A dialectical paradigm for research. In P. Reason & J. Rowan (Eds.), *Human Inquiry* (pp. 93–112). Wiley.

Smith, L. T. (2012). *Decolonizing methodologies: Research and indigenous peoples* (2nd ed.). Zed Books.

The New York Times. (2020). How George Floyd died, and what happened next. *The New York Times, 8*, 2020. https://www.nytimes.com/article/george-floyd.html

Thomas, S. B., Quinn, S. C., Butler, J., Fryer, C. S., & Garza, M. A. (2011). Toward a fourth generation of disparities research to achieve health equity. *Annual Review of Public Health, 32*(1), 399–416. https://doi.org/10.1146/annurev-publhealth-031210-101136

Tompa, E., Scott-Marshall, H., Dolinschi, R., Trevithick, S., & Bhattacharyya, S. (2007). Precarious employment experiences and their health consequences: Towards a theoretical framework. *Work, 28*(3), 209–224.

Wallerstein, N., Duran, B., Oetzel, J. G., & Minkler, M. (2018). *Community- based participatory research for health: Advancing social and health equity* (3rd ed., pp. 3–16). Wiley.

Jeni Hebert-Beirne, MPH, PhD is an Associate Professor of Community Health Sciences at the University of Illinois Chicago (UIC) School of Public Health. She is a community-based participatory researcher (CBPR) focused on unpacking the structural drivers and social determinants of community health inequities and identifying community-led solutions to health equity. She is a lead investigator for the Greater Lawndale Healthy Work Project in the Center for Healthy Work. In partnership with student and community collaborators she has co-founded the UIC SPH Collaboratory for Health Justice, a center to foster reciprocal community engagement in the academy; the UIC Partnership for AntiRacist Campus Transformation (PACT), focused on institutional change as an objective to promoting health equity within the academy; and Epidemics of Injustice, an academic course open to the community and co-led by the Radical Public Health (RPH) student group.

Sylvia Gonzalez, MPH, DACM has served as a staff member on the GLHW Project since 2017. Sylvia has a Master of Public Health from the University of Illinois Chicago and a Doctorate of Acupuncture and Chinese Medicine from the Pacific College of Health & Science. Sylvia is passionate about providing trauma-informed and healing-centered approaches in both her clinical acupuncture practice and public health work.

Melissa Chrusfield is a long-time resident of the West Side of Chicago, residing formerly in North Lawndale and currently in East Garfield Park, an advocate for her community, and a mother of three amazing children. She is the Events Director at Lawndale Christian Health Center, has served as a member of the Community Advisory Committee for the Sinai Urban Health Institute for five years, is a member of the Better Baby Zone Committee in East Garfield Park, and was a member of the planning committee for West Side United. She desires deeply that the beauty, potential and great value of every human be recognized and affirmed with both words and action. She is a GLHW Project co-chair.

Adlaide Holloway is a Senior Community Health Worker (CHW) Consultant and Trainer at Sinai Urban Health Institute (SUHI) of Sinai Chicago. As a CHW, Adlaide has worked on numerous programs to provide asthma and diabetes education and management support and is also a lifestyle coach for the CDC's National Diabetes Prevention Program. Adlaide recently transitioned into training and facilitation with SUHI's Center for CHW Research, Outcomes, and Workforce Development (CROWD) where CHWs are trained and supported to connect under invested communities with equitable access to holistic health care. Adlaide is a co-chair on the GLHW Project Council and the Illinois CHW Association.

Jennifer Plascencia Lopez is a graduate research assistant pursuing her Master in Public Health with a focus on Community Health Sciences. She received her Bachelor of Science in Neuroscience from the University of Michigan in 2019. As a Chicago native, Jennifer recognized the health and social inequities impacting her community, and her interest in learning about public health ensued. In addition to her interest in learning about community health, Jennifer is passionate about supporting youth in pursuing higher education, as level of education has significant implications on health. Jennifer aims to utilize her knowledge in public health to serve her community in bringing health equity and social justice.

Dolores Castañeda, MPH, is a passionate community organizer and long-time Little Village resident. She is the co-founder of Padres Angeles, board member at Jorge Prieto Family Health Center, active parishioner at Saint Agnes of Bohemia Church, and a mutual aid volunteer on efforts regarding asylum seekers, street vendors, and unhoused people. She is the Outreach Coordinator for the Greater Lawndale Healthy Work Project. She has a Master of Public Health degree from the University of Illinois at Chicago.

Chapter 6
Reflexivity: A Strategy for Ethics- and Values-Driven Community Partnerships in Mental Health

Tommy Chou and Stacy L. Frazier

6.1 Ethics- and Values-Oriented Community Partnership with Reflexivity

Current research estimates a 17-year timeline from development to adoption of health care technologies in clinical settings (Chambers, 2018; Morris et al., 2011). To close this gap, investigators have increasingly turned to collaboration with community stakeholders as a means to build, disseminate, and implement culturally robust and contextually valid services in partnership with their intended users (Frazier et al., 2007; González Castro et al., 2010). Data show that more psychology researchers and providers have also become engaged in advocacy and activism in response to the broader sociopolitical climate (Winerman, 2017). These shifts have brought researchers and providers in psychology into new roles and settings, raising ethical challenges that overextend traditional professional guidelines such as the American Psychological Association's (APA) Ethics Code (Campbell & Morris, 2017; Chou & Frazier, 2019). Accordingly, an emerging body of literature explores the ethics of community-engaged research (CEnR) through case examples that highlight relevant theory, concepts, and codes of conduct; however, pragmatic guidance translating procedural ethics into ethical decision-making for psychologists engaged in CEnR remains sparse. At the same time, clinical psychology represents—at its core—a patient- and person-centered field wherein research is

T. Chou (✉)
Department of Psychiatry and Human Behavior, Brown University, Providence, RI, USA

Weight Control and Diabetes Research Center, The Miriam Hospital, Providence, RI, USA
e-mail: po-hun_chou@brown.edu

S. L. Frazier
Department of Psychology, Florida International University, Miami, FL, USA

E. E. Anderson (ed.), *Ethical Issues in Community and Patient Stakeholder–Engaged Health Research*, Philosophy and Medicine 146,
https://doi.org/10.1007/978-3-031-40379-8_6

inextricably tied to clinical practice. Training and professional growth, in particular, incorporate learning towards the resolution of ethical issues traditionally associated with mental health service provision. As a result, clinical psychologists may be especially well positioned to make meaningful contributions to the growing literature on ethical practice in CEnR. This chapter aims to accomplish multiple goals: (1) introduce reflexivity and complementary compassion- and mindfulness-based skills as strategies to support ethical decision-making in CEnR; (2) use real-world and conceptual examples to prompt reflections on readers' own current and future stakeholder-engaged practice; and (3) present 4R, a structure for reflexivity that we have utilized in our own community-engaged consultation and research.

Reflexivity—the active and ongoing examination of one's work and the learning and outcomes of one's practice—may support community-engaged investigators in reflecting on, evaluating, and continually improving their CEnR processes and procedures. Guilleman and Gillam (2004, 274) contextualize reflexivity in research by defining science as "an enterprise of knowledge construction…that requires scrutiny, reflection, and interrogation of the data, the researcher, the participants, and the context that they inhabit." With this definition in mind, they describe reflexivity as a two-step process for investigators that involves first collecting and interpreting data (i.e., "What did we learn?"), then reflecting upon how they arrived at their interpretations and conclusions (i.e., "How did we learn it?"). They posit that academic and sociopolitical perspectives and experiences influence the mission, aims, and values central to each investigator's program and process of research; the research questions they choose to pursue; the communities and participant samples they select; their predominant theoretical frameworks and data collection methodologies; analytic strategies and interpretation of findings; and the presentation of their conclusions and the pathways by which they publish and disseminate their work. As such, Guilleman and Gillam (2004) present reflexivity as a necessary and active process that should be incorporated into all stages of research.

To the same (or perhaps even greater) degree, these considerations hold true for CEnR, and extend well beyond study procedures. Across the various formats and goals of community partnership, the perspectives, values, and past experiences of both academic and community stakeholders impact the initial direction of the partnership and its progress over time (e.g., Case, 2017; Chou & Frazier, 2019; Haarlammert et al., 2017). Ultimately, a complex and cascading set of individual and group factors determine collaborations' trajectories through individual interactions—and the interpretations of those involved in these interactions—that build and influence each other over time. Take, for example, a simple comment that we have received upon returning to a community partner, an afterschool program hosted at a local school, for a second consultation visit: "We didn't think we'd see you again after last week!" One's first interpretation may be that program staff perceived us as disinterested or incapable to sustained commitment; however, active use of reflexivity (e.g., asking "Is this an assumption or is this a fact proven by substantial objective evidence?") might inspire an alternative range of possibilities. Perhaps the staff member was excited about our return, acknowledging how challenging the previous visit was, or simply surprised, based on past experiences with researchers who never returned.

An investigator's interpretation will likely influence subsequent interactions, albeit in subtle ways. In the above example, the first interpretation may result in a defensive stance, discouraging future visits to the site, whereas the alternatives may generate empathy and inspire the investigator to listen and learn more. Accordingly, reflexivity may support compassionate and values-oriented practice in response to ethical challenges. Often, as in the preceding example, there is an ambiguous interaction with competing interpretations that requires an immediate response, as well as a later opportunity for retrospective consideration and learning (Chou & Frazier, 2019). As such, we leverage reflexivity as a core routine practice and propose an explicit and structured approach to guide CEnR investigators at different levels of training and career progression.

We have found that recording details of partnered activities and engaging in an active routine of reflexivity, both individually and as a research team, provide several benefits (Chou & Frazier, 2019). First, utilizing reflexive practices encourages a mindful awareness of our stakeholders' values and workforce dynamics, as well as the patterns and standard procedures of our partnership. Second, it fosters awareness of "blind spots" by highlighting dimensions of ethical considerations in partnership that individual team members might otherwise miss. Third, it creates a platform through which to identify common precursors of ethical conflicts. Finally, it contributes to an overall team culture that maintains and prioritizes dialogue about ethical conduct, supports the growth of insight as a part of professional development, and promotes disclosure and group problem-solving around challenges in fieldwork. Over time, we arrived at 4R, a four-stage sequence—*Respond, Record, Reflect, Revise*—to navigate specific incidents and address overarching processes related to ethical conduct. This sequence is presented below.

Respond Case examples of ethical dilemmas often describe what seems like a slow and methodical process for decision-making, whereas in reality, most challenges in the field require immediate response and action. In our stakeholder-engaged work, we have found that the discomfort and ambiguity, especially in high-stakes situations, can interfere with taking any action for fear of making mistakes. At the same time, non-response when our support and expertise are most needed is itself a risky option, especially when safety is at stake. Further, we often find that our goals and values—such as maintaining safety and building rapport—represent competing priorities. For example, when deciding whether disciplinary practices common in our stakeholders' community warrant a report to agencies meant to protect and support children and families, we understand that doing so may damage rapport and decrease the likelihood that community members will seek necessary mental health support in the future. In this first step, we urge our team members to respond immediately, in the moment, to the extent that they can do so safely and ethically. At minimum, we value transparency; if the appropriate solution remains unclear, we let partners know we need more information and/or time to consult with others in order to identify a way forward. For trainees (i.e., undergraduate research staff, graduate trainees, even junior investigators operating under senior researchers' supervision), *Responding* includes both immediate actions to mitigate harm within the confines of their training and subsequent consultation with supervisors.

Record Following initial action and after resolving any imminent safety concerns, we encourage our team members to document ethical concerns privately and confidentially in detailed field notes for retrospective consideration both independently and with their team. In addition to allowing for more accurate recall of information after the fact, documentation helps to build evidence that can contribute to the CEnR ethics literature. Though researchers may tailor records to their own needs, we suggest that *Recording* at minimum include (1) an objective narrative of the circumstances preceding the ethical challenge; (2) their subjective experience including thoughts, emotions, physical feelings, and reactions; (3) any decisions and immediate actions (i.e., how did they *Respond*); and (4) plans for next steps to continue mitigating harm in the specific situation, prevent similar situations from occurring, and/or process events with community partners and stakeholders. All research team members involved in an ethically challenging situation can record their experiences independently. This ultimately provides robust documentation allowing for cross-validation in reflection (Creswell & Miller, 2000).

Reflect We encourage independent reflection as a means to critically examine events and actions, internal experiences, and explicit or implicit motivations and biases that influence interpretations (e.g.,, of others' communication or the level of risk) and decision-making. Having recorded the details of ethical challenges enables us to reference previous documentation to evaluate patterns over time, particularly in our own emotional, physical, and behavioral reactions that may contribute to current and future challenges. Further reflection with team members who were present, as well as those who were not, provides space for validation, constructive feedback, education, and growth. In our experience, holding routine discussions around ethical issues within and across research teams has facilitated a culture of learning and openness by creating space for different perspectives, alternative solutions, and mutual peer support and understanding. Depending on the nature of community partnership, investigators may also invite stakeholders to review the details of an event, share their own experience, provide perspective and guidance, and reflect together on how to resolve current and future issues. Overall, we have found nonjudgmental reflection both challenging and productive in providing an appraisal of ethical issues, constructive suggestions toward alternative solutions, and necessary revisions to standard operating procedures.

Revise Insights that emerge during reflection highlight many ways in which learning from the present ethical dilemma may inform our future ethical decision-making. The ways in which we have changed our approach in CEnR include (but are not limited to) exploring new and relevant literatures to gain necessary expertise for future consultation; obtaining training in novel interventions; developing new resources for our stakeholders; adjusting how we communicate with community partners and stakeholders during challenging situations and subsequent debriefing; and broadening, narrowing, or altogether changing the focus of our partnered goals and activities in collaboration with stakeholders. In general, we *Revise* to solidify lessons learned, apply these lessons to our general approach to partnership as well as specific operating procedures, and deepen the cumulative value over time of our records as a self-generated body of data that lives and grows alongside our partnership and practice.

We have developed this 4R structure for reflexivity over years of community partnerships. It rests on the consolidation of experience from the first and second authors (trainee and mentor, respectively), and was shaped over time through the contributions of other members of our research team, our academic collaborators, and our community stakeholders. We acknowledge that academic-community partnership is complex and takes many forms, and we anticipate that these exact steps may not suit all CEnR investigators and teams or every situation encountered in the field. Despite these challenges, we hope that the 4R framework provides a *blueprint for individualized plans for active, ongoing reflexivity*. We recognize, too, that reflexivity itself may feel daunting. When reflecting on interactions with stakeholders and their ethical implications, an investigator seeks to understand (1) the influence of their own biases and perspectives; (2) their stakeholders' biases and perspectives; (3) the circumstances of a specific event in time; and (4) the broader context of their partnership. Reviewing one's experiences in partnership, from one's own perspective, with the express purpose of expanding and revising one's perspectives and practices, presents a complex and dynamic challenge. In short, this challenge is perhaps best illustrated by Zen master Seng-Ts'an's statement, "If you work on your mind with your mind, how can you avoid great confusion?" (as quoted by Hayes et al., 2016).

To advance readers' ability to effectively navigate this process, next we present strategies drawn from compassion- and mindfulness-based conceptual models to ground active reflexivity in evidence-based practice. We leverage concepts from these traditions for a number of reasons. First, compassion-based concepts align with current models of community partnership and stakeholder engagement, which emphasize openness and transparency, joint decision-making, and a mindful regard for current and historic power dynamics (Belone et al., 2016; Damschroder et al., 2009). Second, compassion-based therapies such as Acceptance and Commitment Therapy (ACT) explicitly aim to promote *cognitive flexibility* (also known as *psychological flexibility*), or the ability to consider a wide range of potential explanations for and responses to events and ideas (Hayes et al., 2006; Scott, 1962). Third, literature in experimental psychology, health care, and education has identified meditation and mindfulness practice as effective ways to reduce the impact of implicit bias toward marginalized groups (Burgess et al., 2017; Carson & Johnston, 2000; Kang et al., 2014). Lastly, mindfulness and self-compassion (described below) bear particular relevance to the nonjudgmental regard of *negative* thoughts, emotions, and experiences in a balanced and neutral manner (Neff & Dahm, 2015). This in turn may support objective and productive reflection of past interactions, particularly when an investigators' response to an ethical issue may require repair or revision.

6.2 Relational Frames and Cognitive Fusion

Though a comprehensive overview of ACT, its theory, and its primary mechanisms is beyond the scope of this chapter, several concepts are particularly helpful when engaging in reflexive practice. Notably, relational frame theory has enabled us to "take a step back" from our process of community partnership to more objectively evaluate and improve our approach (Chou & Frazier, 2020). *Relational frame theory* posits that individuals retain information about concepts largely in relation to other concepts, or relational frames, that form semantic networks that impact how we view and respond to the world (Hayes et al., 2006). For example, you know a quarter is physically larger than a nickel, and a nickel is larger than a dime. Thus, you know that a quarter is larger than a dime. In a clinical context, relational frame theory may explain the pathways by which a patient who has experienced a severe trauma (e.g., a life-threatening car accident) might then associate related stimuli (e.g., driving) with abstract concepts (e.g., danger) (Hayes, 2018). As these connections become stronger, they may persist even in the face of contradictory information, and lead to *cognitive fusion*. In other words, the intellectual or conceptual understanding becomes "fused" with reality—thoughts become facts. In contrast, *cognitive defusion* refers to the process of "loosening" these relational frames (e.g., through exposures whereby a patient might gradually approach an anxiety-provoking situation such as driving to weaken the connection between driving and danger).

Importantly, ethical decision-making relies on relational frames, and the concepts of cognitive fusion and defusion from relational frame theory can promote objective evaluation of one's conduct. In other words, individuals judge real-time behaviors (i.e., ethics in practice) by their connection to personal beliefs and professional guidelines such as the APA Ethics Code (i.e., procedural ethics). The ways in which an individual interprets these abstract rulesets and links them to their specific stakeholder-engaged situations may determine the range of responses available to them. For example, in our work with non-profit afterschool organizations serving traditionally underserved communities at a local public school, we provided workforce support and in vivo consultation. In one incident, afterschool staff were informed that one of their middle schoolers had been physically disciplined, and visible marks resulted in a call to the local Department of Children and Families. As evening approached and children began leaving, the student sat in a classroom with the school social worker and two police officers waiting for her mother to arrive. School administrators assumed responsibility, while non-profit leadership—our community partners—asked staff to leave; however, our role as consultants was unclear. We knew the student well, having spent time on site, and when we approached them to check in, they reported feeling confused. Although we are trained in children's mental health, this student was not our patient, we were not providing direct service, and we had no authority to provide care. Thus, despite wanting to assist the student further, we instead operated on our most salient semantic ties in the moment: our *role* as consultant to the afterschool program most closely resembled the role of staff, thus our ethical *responsibility* was to follow guidance by program leadership and, as a result, the ethical *behavior* would be to leave as directed. Here, we suggest pausing to reflect on how you might have addressed this situation in your own practice.

Though the team member on site (the first author, a doctoral trainee at the time) initially left the school, discomfort at this decision prompted a call to his mentor (second author) during his commute. Discussion addressed two questions: What was the source of discomfort, and what was a *values-oriented* response? We determined that while leaving the school was reasonable according to basic professional ethics (by adhering to our community partner's request to staff), it generated a feeling of unease in its misalignment with our higher-level values and priorities (to keep youth safe and supported). Deconstructing this example through the lens of concepts presented above, attending to uncomfortable internal reactions through reflexivity as an *active, ongoing* practice prompted the call between trainee and mentor. Further, the call created space for cognitive defusion, as we evaluated together the extent to which adherence to relevant relational frames was the values-oriented choice. We re-established that as a scientific partner and on-site consultant, we could follow partnered leadership's request that their staff leave the school. At the same time, we identified that our role as collaborators who were also familiar with the school staff afforded latitude to stay if we felt that was necessary to uphold our responsibility to the youth we serve. We ultimately decided to return to the site in the event we could provide further support, moving to align with our higher order values.

6.3 Self-as-Context

The previous example also illustrates *self-as-context*, or the idea that individuals can arrive at a sense of self that exists outside of the "labels we give ourselves and the stories we tell about who we are as a person" (Godbee & Kangas, 2020, 918). Under this notion, over-identification with our labels and roles can result in unproductive internal experiences such as rigid adherence to role expectations or defensiveness in situations where others hold perspectives that contradict our own views about our roles. In other words, self-as-context aims to *defuse* individuals from their internal stories about themselves—it views the self as the context within which thoughts and feelings occur, not the product of those thoughts and feelings. It encourages individuals to think and act more flexibly, and take others' perspectives more successfully, by viewing themselves as *a person in their roles* as opposed to *a person defined by their roles*. To illustrate, the ethical obligation of a consultant to an organization is, arguably, to embrace its mission and goals, support the capacity and wellbeing of its workforce, and "do no harm" by acting in a way that aligns with organizational expectations (or, at the very least, not to operate in a contradictory way). In contrast, a person serving as a consultant—while still bound in part by the ethical obligations of that role—holds higher-level values and codes of conduct in consideration. While these distinctions may at first appear straightforward, proactive reflection, consideration in-the-moment, and retroactive evaluation of the subtle differences between the two perspectives as they apply to ethical challenges may promote values-oriented decision-making in practice. Thus, recognizing self-as-concept may support ethical decision-making and reflexive evaluation, especially when investigators feel conflicted even over choices that appear consistent with role expectations.

Furthermore, investigators might better recognize potential areas of tension and understand stakeholders' perspectives by "taking a step back" with the view of self-as-context. Let us consider, for example, the role of "researcher in psychology." An investigator who identifies with this label would likely consider themselves to be an individual who works toward the common good by acquiring, analyzing, and disseminating scientific information that promotes mental health and wellbeing. Alternatively, stakeholders may consider other aspects of the role of research or the field of psychology more salient, such as past injustices perpetrated upon disenfranchised and/or ethnic and racial minority populations (Lee, 2012; Satcher, 2012); long-standing misrepresentation of cultural minority practices in scientific publication (Haarlammert et al., 2017); or recent and historic breaches of ethics in psychology (Risen, 2015; Youngpeter, 2008). If an investigator holds too tightly their own conceptualization of their role as "researcher in psychology," they may fail to acknowledge stakeholder impressions that may impact the quality and effectiveness of partnership. Worse—and perhaps more relevant to the question of ethical practice—an investigator may inadvertently perpetuate negative impressions regarding their role and field without fostering an awareness of these issues through the lens of self-as-context. To that end, we suggest that readers take time to consider their various roles, how stakeholders might perceive them, and what implications these may have on ethical conduct both in discrete situations and, more broadly, in how they approach and conceptualize the process of partnership and relationship building.

6.4 Self-Compassion and Mindfulness

While discussing ethical issues in CEnR, Campbell and Morris (2017) observed that "identifying an ethical path can be a difficult, uncomfortable, *and often quite a lonely journey*" (491, emphasis added). In fact, research has demonstrated that ethical decision-making can increase emotional exhaustion in settings such as intensive care (Teixeira et al., 2014). Furthermore, community-engaged investigators—particularly those working in areas with high rates of violence exposure—frequently receive trauma narratives from collaborating stakeholders or participants (van der Merwe & Hunt, 2019), or experience acute stressors themselves (Chou & Frazier, 2020), which in turn may elevate burnout and vicarious (or direct) trauma exposure. Importantly, evidence also demonstrates a positive correlation between burnout and both risk taking and avoidant decision-making (Michailidis & Banks, 2016), each of which holds high-stakes consequences during ethical dilemmas. For example, a consultant experiencing significant burnout may be more likely to underestimate the risk to safety posed by community partners' practices, or postpone essential but difficult conversations with management about challenges faced by frontline staff, insufficient resources, or ineffective leadership practices with downstream effects on the quality of programming provided to youth.

We urge readers to consider their own experience with burnout, as well as their coping and self-care strategies. Literature in mindfulness and compassion-based theory and intervention—which often parallel and draw from Eastern philosophies (Fung, 2015; Hayes, 2002; Shonin et al., 2014)—recall the Buddhist concept of "flows of compassion": (1) outward flow (compassion *for others*); (2) inward flow (compassion *received from others*); and (3) self-compassion (Gilbert, 2014). Though evidence regarding effective ways to address burnout remains scarce, emerging research suggests that self-compassion programs and skills to decrease anxiety, depression, and compassion fatigue and increase well-being are promising strategies (Beaumont & Hollins Martin, 2016; Boellinghaus et al., 2014; Neff & Dahm, 2015). In addition to potential indirect effects on ethical decision-making through the reduction of burnout, mindfulness and compassion-focused meditation practice may reduce the impact of implicit bias on health care provider behaviors (Burgess et al., 2017). Moreover, research has demonstrated the effectiveness of meditation for improving patient-centered care, reducing stress and overall cognitive load, and—particularly relevant to the practice of reflexivity—empowering providers to *detect* their own implicit bias.

Mindfulness-based interventions and techniques to promote self-compassion show promise in addressing burnout and enhancing an individual's ability to objectively regard their past and inner experiences (Boellinghaus et al., 2014; Neff & Dahm, 2015). Randomized controlled evaluation of eight-week mindfulness-based stress reduction programs demonstrate their ability to reduce stress among health care professionals and improve both quality of life and self compassion (Shapiro et al., 2005). In our practice, we have employed more specific, discrete strategies such as the Gestalt two-chair technique and loving kindness meditation. In the former, an individual pictures two "selves"—one who provides critical judgment and another who receives that judgment (Neff, 2004). The individual imagines a "conversation" between the two individuals with the goal of recognizing the effects of receiving their self-criticism and practicing to "defend themselves" from a compassionate stance. Loving kindness meditation—a component of mindfulness-based stress reduction intervention and a long standing Buddhist practice—involves repeating a set of phrases that generate a sense of goodwill for oneself, often while visualizing an emotionally difficult situation such as an ethical challenge (Neff & Dahm, 2015). At their core, these practices aim to promote individuals' capacity to view themselves in the context of a common humanity (i.e., everyone makes mistakes) and show themselves the same support and kindness they would offer to a friend. This stance, in turn, can help reduce the intensity of internal distress, self-judgment, doubt, and guilt that may arise during and after an ethically challenging situation and create more space for objective evaluation and problem solving through reflexivity.

6.5 Conclusion

Ultimately, building and maintaining a robust and ethical practice of CEnR poses a dynamic and complex challenge. Partnerships may span a variety of settings and stakeholders, each with their own unique strengths, goals, and needs. The ambiguity and lack of certainty—coupled with high stakes related to safety and rapport—add considerable stress to the process of decision making when faced with ethical issues in the field. Thus, we encourage readers to address their concerns with all of the tools at their disposal: a growing body of ethics literature that may provide guidance, validation, and normalization (e.g., Campbell & Morris, 2017); research team members and partnered stakeholders who may lend additional support and extended perspectives; and a compassionate self-regard that may allow for objective, non-judgmental consideration that views mistakes as a common human experience and opportunities for growth.

References

Beaumont, E., & Hollins Martin, C. J. (2016). A proposal to support student therapists to develop compassion for self and others through compassionate mind training. *Arts in Psychotherapy, 50*, 111–118. https://doi.org/10.1016/j.aip.2016.06.005

Belone, L., Lucero, J. E., Duran, B., Tafoya, G., Baker, E. A., Chan, D., Chang, C., Greene-Moton, E., Kelley, M. A., & Wallerstein, N. (2016). Community-based participatory research conceptual model. *Qualitative Health Research, 26*(1), 117–135. https://doi.org/10.1177/1049732314557084

Boellinghaus, I., Jones, F. W., & Hutton, J. (2014). The role of mindfulness and loving-kindness meditation in cultivating self-compassion and other-focused concern in health care professionals. *Mindfulness, 5*(2), 129–138. https://doi.org/10.1007/s12671-012-0158-6

Burgess, D. J., Beach, M. C., & Saha, S. (2017). Mindfulness practice: A promising approach to reducing the effects of clinician implicit bias on patients. *Patient Education and Counseling, 100*(2), 372–376. https://doi.org/10.1016/j.pec.2016.09.005

Campbell, R., & Morris, M. (2017). The stories we tell: Introduction to the special issue on ethical challenges in community psychology research and practice. *American Journal of Community Psychology, 60*, 299–301. https://doi.org/10.1002/ajcp.12178

Carson, T., & Johnston, I. (2000). The difficulty with difference in teacher education: Toward a pedagogy of compassion. *Alberta Journal of Educational Research, 46*(1), 75.

Case, A. D. (2017). Reflexivity in Counterspaces fieldwork. *American Journal of Community Psychology, 398–405*, 398–405. https://doi.org/10.1002/ajcp.12196

Chambers, C. T. (2018). From evidence to influence: Dissemination and implementation of scientific knowledge for improved pain research and management. *Pain, 159*, S56–S64.

Chou, T., & Frazier, S. L. (2019). Supporting ethical practice in community-engaged research with 4R : Respond, record, reflect, and revise. *Ethics & Behavior, 0*(0), 1–15. https://doi.org/10.1080/10508422.2019.1645665

Chou, T., & Frazier, S. L. (2020). CORE: Compassion oriented reflection and engagement to guide academic-community partnership. *Journal of participatory research. Methods, 1*(1), 10.35844/001c.13314.

Creswell, J. W., & Miller, D. L. (2000). Determining Validity in Qualitative Inquiry. *Determining validity in qualitative inquiry., 39*(3), 124–130.

Damschroder, L. J., Aron, D. C., Keith, R. E., Kirsh, S. R., Alexander, J. A., & Lowery, J. C. (2009). Fostering implementation of health services research findings into practice: A consolidated framework for advancing implementation science. *Implementation Science, 4*(1), 1–15. https://doi.org/10.1186/1748-5908-4-50

Frazier, S. L., Abdul-Adil, J., Atkins, M. S., Gathright, T., & Jackson, M. (2007). Can't have one without the other: Mental health providers and community parents reducing barriers to services for families in urban poverty. *Journal of Community Psychology, 35*(4), 435–446. https://doi.org/10.1002/jcop.20157

Fung, K. (2015). Acceptance and commitment therapy: WesterN adoption of Buddhist tenets? *Transcultural Psychiatry, 52*(4), 561–576. https://doi.org/10.1177/1363461514537544

Gilbert, P. (2014). The origins and nature of compassion focused therapy. *British Journal of Clinical Psychology, 53*(1), 6–41. https://doi.org/10.1111/bjc.12043

Godbee, M., & Kangas, M. (2020). The relationship between flexible perspective taking and emotional Well-being: A systematic review of the "self-as-context" component of acceptance and commitment therapy. *Behavior Therapy, 51*(6), 917–932. https://doi.org/10.1016/j.beth.2019.12.010

González Castro, F., Barrera, M., & Holleran Steiker, L. K. (2010). Issues and challenges in the Design of Culturally Adapted Evidence-Based Interventions. *Annual Review of Clinical Psychology, 6*(1), 213–239. https://doi.org/10.1146/annurev-clinpsy-033109-132032

Haarlammert, M., Birman, D., Oberoi, A., & Moore, W. J. (2017). Inside-out: Representational ethics and diverse communities. *American Journal of Community Psychology, 414–423*, 414–423. https://doi.org/10.1002/ajcp.12188

Hayes, S. C. (2002). Buddhism and acceptance and commitment therapy. *Cognitive and Behavioral Practice, 9*, 58–66. https://doi.org/10.4324/9781315745138

Hayes, S. C. (2018). Improving workplace experience and reducing burnout in integrated care environments: Mindfulness and psychological flexibility. https://integration.samhsa.gov/about-us/Webinar_mindfulnessandstress.pdf

Hayes, S. C., Luoma, J. B., Bond, F. W., Masuda, A., & Lillis, J. (2006). Acceptance and commitment therapy: Model, processes and outcomes. *Behaviour Research and Therapy, 44*(1), 1–25. https://doi.org/10.1016/j.brat.2005.06.006

Hayes, S. C., Strosahl, K. D., & Wilson, K. G. (2016). *Acceptance and commitment therapy: The process and practice of mindful change* (2nd ed.). Guildford Press.

Javdani, S., Singh, S., & Sichel, C. E. (2017). Negotiating ethical paradoxes in conducting a randomized controlled trial: Aligning intervention science with participatory values. *American Journal of Community Psychology, 439–449*, 439–449. https://doi.org/10.1002/ajcp.12185

Kang, Y., Gray, J. R., & Dovidio, J. F. (2014). The nondiscriminating heart: Lovingkindness meditation training decreases implicit intergroup bias. *Journal of Experimental Psychology: General, 143*(3), 1306–1313. https://doi.org/10.1037/a0034150

Kanov, J., Powley, E. H., & Walshe, N. D. (2017). Is it ok to care? How compassion falters and is courageously accomplished in the midst of uncertainty. *Human Relations, 70*(6), 751–777. https://doi.org/10.1177/0018726716673144

Lee, S. S. J. (2012). Lessons learned from the U.S. Public Health Service syphilis study at Tuskegee: Incorporating a discourse on relationships into the ethics of research participation among Asian Americans. *Ethics and Behavior, 22*(6), 489–492. https://doi.org/10.1080/10508422.2012.730002

Michailidis, E., & Banks, A. P. (2016). The relationship between burnout and risk-taking in workplace decision-making and decision-making style. *Work and Stress, 30*(3), 278–292. https://doi.org/10.1080/02678373.2016.1213773

Mikesell, L., Bromley, E., & Khodyakov, D. (2013). Ethical community-engaged research: A literature review. *American Journal of Public Health, 103*(12), 7–14. https://doi.org/10.2105/AJPH.2013.301605

Morris, Z. S., Wooding, S., & Grant, J. (2011). The answer is 17 years, what is the question: Understanding time lags in translational research. *Journal of the Royal Society of Medicine, 104*(12), 510–520. https://doi.org/10.1258/jrsm.2011.110180

Neff, K. D. (2004). Self-compassion and psychological Well-being. *Constructivism in the Human Sciences, 9*(2), 27–37.
Neff, K. D., & Dahm, K. A. (2015). Self-compassion: What it is, what it does, and how it relates to mindfulness. *Handbook of Mindfulness and Self-Regulation*, 121–140.
Risen, J. (2015). American Psychological Association bolstered C.I.a. torture program, report says. *New York Times, June, 2004*, 1–5.
Satcher, D. (2012). The legacy of the syphilis study at Tuskegee in African American men on health care reform fifteen years after President Clinton's apology. *Ethics and Behavior, 22*(6), 486–488. https://doi.org/10.1080/10508422.2012.730005
Scott, W. A. (1962). Cognitive complexity and cognitive flexibility. *Sociometry, 25*(4), 405–414.
Shapiro, S. L., Astin, J. A., Bishop, S. R., & Cordova, M. (2005). Mindfulness-based stress reduction for health care professionals: Results from a randomized trial. *International Journal of Stress Management, 12*(2), 164–176. https://doi.org/10.1037/1072-5245.12.2.164
Shonin, E., Van Gorder, W., & Griffiths, M. D. (2014). The emerging role of Buddhism in clinical psychology: Towards effective integration. *Psychology of Religion and Spirituality, 6*, 123–137. https://doi.org/10.1037/a0035859
Teixeira, C., Ribeiro, O., Fonseca, A. M., & Carvalho, A. S. (2014). Ethical decision making in intensive care units: A burnout risk factor? Results from a multicentre study conducted with physicians and nurses. *Journal of Medical Ethics, 40*(2), 97–103. https://doi.org/10.1136/medethics-2012-100619
van der Merwe, A., & Hunt, X. (2019). Secondary trauma among trauma researchers: Lessons from the field. *Psychological Trauma: Theory, Research, Practice, and Policy, 11*(1), 10–18. https://doi.org/10.1037/tra0000414
Winerman, L. (2017). Trends report: Psychologists are standing up for science. *Monitor on Psychology*.
Youngpeter, K. (2008). Controversial psychological research methods and their influence on the development of formal ethical guidelines. *Student Journal of Psychological Science, 1*(1), 4–12.

Tommy Chou Po-hun "Tommy" Chou is a community-engaged researcher whose program of work centers on advancing health equity for those impacted by poverty and other forms of socioeconomic disadvantage. By partnering with community-based organizations and the stakeholders they serve, Tommy aims to leverage existing science to design and disseminate programs that improve individuals' and organizations' overall wellbeing.

Stacy L. Frazier PhD, (she/her/hers) is a professor in the Department of Psychology at Florida International University. She directs a program of community-partnered and inter-agency children's mental health research to support schools and after-school programs serving youth in communities systemically underserved by inequities in care and underrepresented in psychological science. Her studies examine tiered and technology-facilitated models of workforce support for care extenders (e.g., afterschool staff, school personnel, home visitors), that are historically, culturally, and contextually informed, and focused on leveraging teachable moments during natural education, service, and recreation routines.

Part II
In the Field

Chapter 7
How Do You Define Community and Why Is it Important?

Laurene Tumiel-Berhalter and Linda Kahn

7.1 Introduction

Communities are the populations we study and the samples we recruit. Communities influence the way people think and behave, and they contribute to the complexity of the human condition. Culture, tradition, and beliefs are important aspects of all communities. Communities can be structured or unstructured, obvious or hidden, and defined or undefined. As researchers we must consider this complexity when designing studies, defining eligibility criteria, developing surveys, and most importantly interpreting results. This chapter discusses the complexity of defining a community and the importance of understanding these complexities to the research enterprise.

7.2 What Is a Community?

Communities can be compared to living organisms that grow, evolve, and fade over time. They are dynamic and perceived differently by their members. In brief, a community is defined by a key characteristic or set of characteristics that bring people together. Characteristics include social norms, needs and commitment, and emotional connection (Fremlin, 2015; Bradshaw, 2008; Smith, 2013).

Community is often associated with a place or geographic location that may include the neighborhoods where we live or a rural versus an urban center.

L. Tumiel-Berhalter (✉) · L. Kahn
Department of Family Medicine, Jacobs School of Medicine and Biomedical Science, University at Buffalo, Buffalo, NY, USA
e-mail: tumiel@buffalo.edu; lskahn@buffalo.edu

E. E. Anderson (ed.), *Ethical Issues in Community and Patient Stakeholder–Engaged Health Research*, Philosophy and Medicine 146,
https://doi.org/10.1007/978-3-031-40379-8_7

Communities may be defined by ZIP code, county line, municipality, parish, or other geographically defined boundary (see Chap. 19, this volume). For example, in communities with strong Roman Catholic backgrounds, community is defined by the parish a person belongs to. These parishes, based on location, are correlated with income level and social status. While geographic communities may be circumscribed by physical boundaries, invisible boundaries may co-exist, corresponding to subcontexts within the geography. The "other side of the tracks" infers shared sociodemographic characteristics corresponding to a specific place, while other designations can signify allegiance with a political faction or organization. In one community of Buffalo, NY, a major road divides a geographic community creating an invisible border. In conversations with two community centers, one on each side of the divide, we learned that few residents cross this boundary to attend community programs.

Other communities are defined by common interests—political or social, hobbies (e.g., Alliance Française, Garden club, Knights of Columbus, etc.), or life stage. Membership within these social groups can fluctuate over time. Communities are also connected to social institutions such as schools or churches or other organizations. Examples include student bodies of schools and universities, occupational groups, patients of a particular practice, or clients of a particular service agency. There may be a shared symbolism associated with the community such as sports paraphernalia or a uniform worn by those in the same occupation. National and international sports franchises have communities that can extend worldwide. The Buffalo Bills National Football Team are well-known for having a strong local fan base. This fan base extends across the country where one can be sure to watch a game at a recognized Buffalo Bills bar.

Communities are often defined by ethnicity or religion or founded on cultural values, belief systems, and customs. These traditions may include food, language, and health care practices. Immigrant communities in the US may vary in levels of acculturation or observance of specific traditional practices. Doula programs exist to help new Americans with prenatal care and delivery in the United States to navigate the health care system for the first time (LaMancuso et al., 2016). Doulas also educate health care providers on traditional birth practices, for example, birth prayers or consumption of the placenta.

A community can also be defined by health conditions such as diabetes, lupus, cancer survivorship, or specific rare conditions. These communities can be formal and self-defined by members who are participating in support groups, or informal such as bonding with other people with the same condition. On-line patient communities offer not only emotional support but share best practices for living with certain conditions. Some examples of patient and family communities include Myeloma Crowd (https://www.myelomacrowd.org/myeloma/community) and National Alliance on Mental Illness (https://nami.org/Home).

We can also define a community by life experiences that are often laced with stigma, e.g., people living with addictions and their loved ones or those involved in the criminal justice system. Some of these communities are not easy to identify. These are often referred to as "hidden populations" made up of people who are marginalized and vulnerable. They are subject to discrimination and often experience health inequalities (Krabbe et al., 2021). These communities may share social norms, needs, or emotional connections. They may be engaged in unconventional activities such as drug use or sex work, or they may be involved in the criminal justice system (Boeri & Shukla, 2019). They may suffer from mental health issues or homelessness. They may be stigmatized, disenfranchised, and concerned that divulging their experiences puts them at risk (Ellard-Gray et al., 2015). These identities may be intersecting or overlapping (e.g., justice-involved mothers who use drugs), heightening their feelings of stigma and perceived vulnerability (Ellard-Gray et al., 2015). Their circumstances and risks of privacy, legal exposure, or re-traumatization may compel them to remain "hidden" or "hard-to-reach" and harbor a mistrust of outsiders, especially researchers (Ellard-Gray et al., 2015).

The proliferation of social media has resulted in "virtual communities," connecting people across national boundaries around shared interests and activities. This has increased the opportunity for connectivity. Virtual communities on Facebook and other social media platforms have exploded in the last decade. Increased connectivity diminishes the importance on place as part of the definition of community and increases the fluidity by which people become members of various communities (Bradshaw, 2008; Fremlin, 2015).

The commonalities that characterize the concept of community are broad and complex (Chavis & Lee, 2015; Smith, 2013). We all belong to multiple, diverse, formal, and informal communities. Some communities are easily recognizable, other are not. Some communities are self-identified, while others are identified by outsiders. Connections with other communities can ignite co-learning, sharing strategies, and sharing stories and can be mutually beneficial to those receiving as well as giving support. Communities are not homogenous in terms of their belief systems and cultural practices; communities are experienced differently by different members (MacQueen et al., 2001). Consider, for example, a geographic community. Two people live in the east side of town A. One may feel a strong connection to that geographic community. Perhaps they have lived their whole life there, have friends and family there, and participate in community events. Another person may not feel like a member of the community. Perhaps they moved there because of proximity to their job, do not participate in community events, and have social ties to other geographic locations. We must remember that no community exists in isolation. The cross-sectionality of communities makes this concept even more complex. We may not be able to address all sub communities, but all types of communities need to be acknowledged.

7.3 Why Is Understanding Community Important for Research?

Researchers are required to define populations and the sampling strategies they use for recruitment. These definitions ultimately become eligibility criteria. However, researchers must remember that these eligibility criteria relate directly to complex human beings that belong to various communities and have multiple influences. Researchers frequently interpret findings without fully understanding the nuances of the communities from which they are recruiting. This impairs interpretation of the results, generalizability of the findings, and assessments of strengths and weaknesses of a study design.

A researcher may define their population as patients in a practice or those living in a certain ZIP code. But what does that really mean? How much do the researchers know about that community? What are the demographics of the community? Is that patient population racially/ethnically diverse? What proportion of patients have Medicaid? Does the patient population live within walking distance or are they coming from a variety of neighborhoods? Is there a prevalent religious background? What is the percent living in poverty? Are there senior housing facilities located there? Is there a predominant set of occupations? Every community is complex but the more researchers know about it, the easier it will be to reflect on the intersectionality of these characteristics and how it may influence the intended research sample.

There are other important considerations. Which nuances within the intended population are important to the research? Which ones can impact recruitment, data collection, and the interpretation of findings? Is it important to have both men and women in the study? Are people of color disproportionately affected by the condition under study? Are people of lower income disproportionately affected by the condition? How will the research team ensure that these important nuances are accounted for?

Since everyone is a member of multiple communities, it is impossible to understand all potential communities to which research participants may belong. In fact, if it were possible, research communities would be reduced to individual levels and thus researchers would not be able to consider community/population health at all. However, researchers would be remiss not to be aware of the intersectionality of communities and their impacts on health and health behavior. For example, we conducted an intervention to improve cancer screening in a safety-net practice that had a large proportion of refugees from over 70 countries. Due to language barriers, we were unable to include most of these refugees in the study. However, to truly make change in the practice we needed to learn more about them. Like the English-speaking patients, they were poor and not being screened according to recommended guidelines. But they also had different cultural backgrounds and language barriers. We conducted a separate qualitative study with two of the larger groups of refugees in Buffalo, Somali Bantu and Karen patients (indigenous to the Thailand-Burma border), to understand their experiences pre- and post-settlement. Themes identified in these interviews reflected the need to introduce cancer screening using a trauma-informed approach (Schuster et al., 2019). These findings were useful to the practice and resulted in an educational document that used imagery to introduce cancer screening for refugee patients. Understanding experiences of members of different communities can help researchers fine tune their questions, assesses disparities faced by these communities, refine recruitment strategies, and assess whether proposed interventions would be equally as effective in the broader patient population.

Importantly, researchers must consider whether exclusion criteria systematically exclude any particular group, either intentionally or unintentionally. Unintentional exclusions may limit researchers' ability to address health disparities in their work. This can also limit the generalizability of the findings and may offer content for an extremely robust limitations section. By understanding the community from which potential participants will be recruited, researchers can determine whether their sample represents the intended community to the best of their ability. By giving more thoughtful consideration to the communities that reflect study eligibility criteria, first and foremost, researchers will be able to conduct research that is truly respectful and meaningful to potential participants. In addition, the research will be better. Recruitment strategies will be more specific and meaningfully facilitate participation. The understanding of community can influence what data is collected, how it is collected, and, most importantly, how results are interpreted. It will provide context that will contribute to the generalizability of findings and the potential to assess health disparities.

Community partners can identify the most important characteristics of community members that a researcher needs to be aware of and that should drive decision making about inclusion and exclusion criteria (Green & Mercer, 2001). For example, a researcher studying diabetes might know that their sample will include people of different ages, races, income levels, and sexual orientations. After reviewing the literature on health disparities, the researcher may purposefully decide to aim to be representative as possible across gender and race. Recruitment materials can then be constructed with that decision in mind. The researcher might consider whether the same recruitment materials will be appealing and meaningful to all groups, asking: What language choices should be used? Are the study titles and descriptions understandable? What photos should be used?

Community partners can also provide tremendous insight on where to share recruitment materials. Where will people trust the information and think about responding? Should the information be at doctors' offices, at barber shops, or at community centers?

Community partners can shed light on the questions that different groups have about their health conditions or risk factors, what outcomes are meaningful to them, and how they view improvement in quality of life. This insight can guide the types of questions that are being asked. Most importantly, community members can help interpret results. For example, a community health needs assessment we conducted included the CAGE questionnaire (Ewing, 1984) to assess risk of alcohol dependence. We presented data that showed little risk of alcohol dependence in the sample. Our community partners questioned the data stating that alcohol dependency was more prevalent in the community than the data showed. They asked where the non-drinkers were? We had coded the non-drinkers as low-risk based on their CAGE scores. The community partners suggested separating out the non-drinkers. Creating three categories, non-drinkers, low risk, and high risk, was more reflective of the predominately Puerto Rican community with a larger proportion of religious non-drinkers. Those that did drink, however, were more likely to be at risk of dependency (Center for Urban Studies in Primary Care, 1994).

Researchers must recognize the influence that community nuances have on the research process in order to appropriately choose their words and the messaging about why a study is important. For example, does the eligibility criteria and protocol allow for local or distal participation? This can create the opportunity for social media as a possible recruitment strategy. It can also influence local and distal registries (whether for disease-specific or general research participation).

Hidden communities are particularly challenging to work with because there are uncertain parameters with no existing sampling frames (Krabbe et al., 2021; Benoit et al., 2005). Individuals may feel that acknowledging that they belong to a particular group or community is threatening (Benoit et al., 2005). There is also a high degree of mistrust of outsiders—especially researchers (Benoit et al., 2005). We maintain a long-standing collaboration and friendship with the Medical Care Administrator of the Erie County Department of Health who also directs the county's Opiate Epidemic Task Force. Over the years, we have worked with her on numerous initiatives spanning many different public health issues including diabetes, HIV-AIDS, teen pregnancy, asthma, and substance use. Recently, she played an instrumental role in the design and implementation of a community-based study of people who use opioids and were rescued from overdose with naloxone (Kahn et al., 2020). She helped us conceptualize the study and develop the interview questions and co-authored publications (Kahn et al., 2020). Among our preliminary findings was that people rescued with naloxone will often resume using drugs for a variety of reasons, including staving off withdrawal symptoms. First responders (e.g., paramedics, police, fire) become frustrated when they must rescue the same person more than once. Our Health Department colleague incorporated our preliminary finding into her naloxone training program for first responders. She compares naloxone rescue for opioid overdose to reviving a person with a heart attack. She asks the first responders, "How often have the heart attack victims you saved changed their diet and lifestyle the very next day?" (Kahn et al., 2020). This is an example of how collaboration with community partners can result in a "win-win." They facilitate the research while the findings can benefit their programs.

Community members from groups that are underrepresented in research may not trust researchers. Memories of unethical research practices, such as those exemplified by the Tuskegee Syphilis Trials (https://www.history.com/news/the-infamous-40-year-tuskegee-study) persist. It is not unusual for Black Americans to mention Tuskegee in conversations about research. These discussions can provide an opportunity to acknowledge injustices and discuss the protections that are currently in place to prevent such travesties from occurring. Learning about the community and the injustices they have experienced in research and health care promotes trust between researcher and the community (see Chap. 10, this volume).

7.4 Strategies for Learning More about a Community

Learning about a new community with whom you will be conducting research may seem like a daunting task. Depending on your research discipline, you may not know where to start. The following strategies can help researchers to effectively learn about their research community.

7.4.1 *Data-Based Strategies*

Data sources exist that provide some insight into various communities. It is important to note that this is a necessary step but insufficient without additional community engagement strategies. Before planning research with or in any community, it is important to explore what data have already been collected and publicly available. While numbers can only skim the surface, they can provide a foundation that will be enhanced through community engaged and collaborative strategies.

United States census data (https://www.census.gov/data.html) is available to obtain demographic characteristics on state, city, ZIP code and other types of geographies. Other national data sources exist, such as the Behavioral Risk Factor Surveillance System or the National Health Interview Survey available through the Centers for Disease Control and Prevention's National Center for Health Statistics (https://www.cdc.gov/nchs/index.htm), that can provide prevalence estimates of conditions and behavioral risk factors. These sources are publicly accessible and can provide researchers with a sense of who makes up their intended communities.

Local and State Public Health Departments often have data dashboards online that describe the demographics of various populations. These are often shared data sources as described above but in a localized manner. Administrative data from medical practices or community-based organizations can also be useful tools in describing the demographic distribution of corresponding communities. Public Health Departments and hospitals are often required to conduct regular community health needs assessments to set priorities and guide strategic planning. These reports are publicly available, often on respective websites.

7.4.2 *Community Engagement Strategies*

Any level of *community engagement* can help to improve research, if done appropriately. There are several strategies that span the spectrum of community engagement (Community Engagement Key Function Committee Task Force, 2011). Incorporating community voice can help frame research to be the most inclusive and therefore the most generalizable. Researchers may want to partner with a public health researcher or epidemiologist who does community-engaged research and can help identify community partners. Linking with researchers who have already developed trust in the community can provide some warm hand-offs to facilitate potential partnerships. Utilize expertise, connections, and resources available at your institution. If an institution is part of a Clinical and Translational Science Award (https://www.ctsacentral.org/institutions/), the community engagement core can help researchers to better understand the community and link them with appropriate community partners.

Participant observation is an approach developed by anthropologists that entails immersion in a culture or community (Bernard, 2006). The researcher becomes both an "insider," establishing trust and rapport with community members, while at the same time maintaining objectivity as an "outsider" conducting research. Traditionally, the anthropologist or researcher spends a year or more conducting fieldwork within a specific community or culture. For example, L.K. spent a year living in a working-class Francophone community in Montréal, spending time in schools, churches, and people's homes (Kahn, 1992). A practical approach to participant observation in the context of community-based research is to begin attending meetings, or "hanging out" and meeting people at venues related to your research. This could be a local health clinic, churches, school meetings, community centers. Joining a task force tied to a relevant community-based issue is another practical approach. The goal is to establish trust and rapport with community members by getting to know them on a personal level. This will accelerate one's ability to understand the needs and issues of the community and ability to recruit study participants.

Another strategy is to utilize *Community Engagement Studios* (Joosten et al., 2015; Joosten et al., 2018). Community Engagement Studios are organized by trained staff and provide a one-time interface with people who would meet eligibility criteria to respond to a specific question about your proposed research. The group of potential participants may offer guidance on recruitment materials, data collection strategies, or data collection elements. Studios can be conducted in-person or virtually.

Reaching out to community-based organizations, patients, and other community stakeholders to form a *community advisory board* can offer insight into the population and help reach hidden populations (Strauss et al., 2001; Quinn, 2004; Newman et al., 2011). These boards can help researchers understand the politics of the community, invisible boundaries, and nuances that are not easily Googled. Community advisory boards meet consistently but the frequency by which they meet may vary (i.e., annually, quarterly, monthly). Members provide continuous feedback over the course of the development and implementation of a project or series of projects.

Developing *partnerships and collaborations* not only helps researchers gain access to the community but can also inform the research design and interpretation of results (Boeri & Shukla, 2019; Wallerstein & Duran, 2010). Community partners enable the researcher to view the community through the lens of its members. Partners can take on all shapes and sizes. They might be institutional (i.e., hospital or health department), organizational (i.e., community-based organizations or practices), or more grassroots (i.e., coalitions or patients). All bring unique and perhaps different perspectives (Tumiel-Berhalter et al., 2005). We have worked extensively with a group of older patients in our community, the Patient Voices Network, who help design interventions to screen underserved patients for a variety of cancers (Reilly et al., 2018) and have active roles in the implementation of these interventions. Patient Voices are involved in writing grant and disseminating results.

Approaches to working with hidden populations include working with community partners or partner organizations that represent these specific populations (Ellard-Gray et al., 2015; Benoit et al., 2005). Researchers can engage partners in developing projects and defining parameters of the specific group. Working with a trusted "insider" or "key informant" can expedite building rapport (Boeri & Shukla, 2019). When working with hidden populations it is especially important to communicate in private or "safe spaces," provide transportation reimbursements or arrange for transportation, utilize "snowball sampling" techniques that draw on personal networks, and maintain honesty and awareness of our role as researchers and relationship to our community partners (Boeri & Shukla, 2019). We have also collaborated with peers in recovery who have helped engage people who have overdosed on opioids. These peer key informants have played an instrumental role in developing questions for qualitative interviews. In our study of opioid overdose survivors, several questions asked about the context of how people began using drugs, including one that asked, "what did it feel like" the first time a person used a drug to get high. The peer advised us to remove that question because asking people to recall "their first high" could be a trigger, causing a relapse. Had we not consulted the peer, our study could have caused harm. We are currently working with another peer "key informant" on a study of mothers with substance use disorder involved with the criminal justice system.

Community partners "vouch" for the trustworthiness of the researcher and can also introduce the researcher to other community members. This relationship is especially important when working with highly stigmatized and vulnerable populations. Using a trusted "insider" to help recruit participants is an established approach that improves rapport with the researcher and ensures respectful interactions (Arditti, 2015; Benoit et al., 2005; Easterling & Johnson, 2015; Moore & Miller, 1999; Ellard-Gray et al., 2015; Monograph, 1990). We have successfully worked with trusted insiders to help recruit participants in studies on people in the criminal justice system and those with substance use disorders (Kahn et al., 2019; Kahn et al., 2020).

Finally, researchers can and should develop long-standing relationships and friendships with their partners (Kahn et al., 2020). Researchers are often viewed as not trustworthy. Taking the time to build relationships can help to establish trustworthiness. This reciprocity not only helps researchers make sense of the data and conceptualize future studies, but the relationship may benefit the community partner by providing new opportunities including exposure to research and university resources. Our Patient Voices project has helped community members learn about the ethics of human subjects research, clinical trials, and medical education, and facilitated contacts with physicians at our medical school.

7.5 Conclusions

When researchers understand community, both parties benefit. This understanding can help recruitment and improve study outcomes (Green & Mercer, 2001). Through effort, researchers will build trust with the community and leave something sustainable in the community. Better understanding community can ensure that research aligns with community priorities and result in community level improvements. For example, a study undertaken to address the impacts of environmental exposures on the prevalence of lupus among African Americans included active engagement of the community. This team became advocates for their health and their community resulting in a toxic site clean-up (Terrell et al., 2008) and policy changes (Williams et al., 2016).

We know that many communities are underrepresented in research, so it is often unclear how generalizable findings are to the larger population. The lack of attention to potential differences may contribute to systemic bias that prevents equitable health and health care. Purposeful attention to community nuances and the intersectionality of communities allows for more accurate interpretation of research findings leading to quicker progression of research and integration of promising practices into the delivery of health and health care. This, in turn, will reduce systemic bias that is prevalent in health care and research, reduce health disparities, and improve the delivery of health care for all (Dankwa-Mullan et al., 2010).

Researchers have an ethical responsibility to understand the communities they invite to participate in their research and whom their research ultimately impacts. Learning about a community through exploring existing data and engagement strategies helps researchers understand behavior and decision making. It will help researchers understand, for example, which side effects are tolerable and which interventions are acceptable. It also helps researchers to recognize that one size does not fit all. This impacts research findings and how generalizable they are to the broader community, and it allows research to directly improve the health of the community.

Acknowledgements We are truly grateful to the many community partners that we have worked with over the years that have shared their stories, their insight, and their passion with us. We are honored to have been part of your lives and humbled by all you have taught us.

References

Arditti, J. A. (2015). Situating vulnerability in research: Implications for researcher transformation and methodological innovation. *The Qualitative Report, 20*(10), 1568–1575.

Benoit, C., Jansson, M., Millar, A., & Phillips, R. (2005). Community-academic research on hard-to-reach populations: Benefits and challenges. *Qualitative Health Research, 15*(2), 263–282.

Bernard, H. R. (2006). *Research methods in anthropology: Qualitative and quantitative approaches*. Altamira press.

Boeri, M., & Shukla, R. K. (2019). *Inside ethnography: Researchers reflect on the challenges of reaching hidden populations*. University of California Press.

Bradshaw, T. K. (2008). The post-place community: Contributions to the debate about the definition of community. *Community Development, 39*(1), 5–16.

Center for Urban Studies in Primary. (1994). The lower west side health needs survey, 1994.

Chavis, D. M., & Lee, K. (2015). *What is community anyway?*. https://doi.org/10.48558/EJJ2-JJ82

Community Engagement Key Function Committee Task Force. (2011). *Principles of community engagement*. In Clinical, Community Engagement Key Function Committee Task Force on the Principles of Community Engagement Translational Science Awards Consortium, Agency for Toxic Substances United States, Registry Disease, Control Centers for Disease and Prevention. Dept. of Health & Human Services, National Institutes of Health, Centers for Disease Control and Prevention, Agency for Toxic Substances and Disease Registry, Clinical and Translational Science Awards (Eds.), Report.

Dankwa-Mullan, I., Rhee, K. B., Williams, K., Sanchez, I., Sy, F. S., Stinson, N., Jr., & Ruffin, J. (2010). The science of eliminating health disparities: Summary and analysis of the NIH summit recommendations. *American Journal of Public Health, 100*, 12–18. https://doi.org/10.2105/AJPH.2010.191619

Easterling, B. A., & Johnson, E. I. (2015). Conducting qualitative research on parental incarceration: Personal reflections on challenges and contributions. *The Qualitative Report, 20*(10), 1568–1575.

Ellard-Gray, A., Jeffrey, N. K., Choubak, M., & Crann, S. E. (2015). Finding the hidden participant solutions for recruiting hidden, hard-to-reach, and vulnerable populations. *International Journal of Qualitative Methods, 14*(5), 1609406915621420.

Ewing, J. A. (1984). Detecting alcoholism. The CAGE questionnaire. *JAMA, 252*(14), 1905–1907. https://doi.org/10.1001/jama.252.14.1905

Fremlin, J. (2015). *Identifying concepts that build a sense of community*. Accessed 30 Apr 2022. Media/Community Psychologist.

Green, L. W., & Mercer, S. L. (2001). Can public health researchers and agencies reconcile the push from funding bodies and the pull from communities? *American Journal of Public Health, 91*(12), 1926–1929. https://doi.org/10.2105/ajph.91.12.1926

Joosten, Y. A., Israel, T. L., Williams, N. A., Boone, L. R., Schlundt, D. G., Mouton, C. P., Dittus, R. S., Bernard, G. R., & Wilkins, C. H. (2015). Community engagement studios: A structured approach to obtaining meaningful input from stakeholders to inform research. *Academic Medicine, 90*(12), 1646–1650. https://doi.org/10.1097/ACM.0000000000000794

Joosten, Y. A., Israel, T. L., Head, A., Vaughn, Y., Villalta Gil, V., Mouton, C., & Wilkins, C. H. (2018). Enhancing translational researchers' ability to collaborate with community stakeholders: Lessons from the community engagement studio. *Journal of Clinical and Translational Science, 2*(4), 201–207. https://doi.org/10.1017/cts.2018.323

Kahn, L. S. (1992). *Schooling, jobs, and cultural identity: Minority education in Quebec, Garland reference library of social science*. Garland Pub.

Kahn, L. S., Vest, B. M., Kulak, J. A., Berdine, D. E., & Granfield, R. (2019). Barriers and facilitators to recovery capital among justice-involved community members. *Journal of Offender Rehabilitation, 58*(6), 544–565. https://doi.org/10.1080/10509674.2019.1621414

Kahn, L. S., Wozniak, M., Vest, B. M., & Moore, C. (2020). "Narcan encounters:" overdose and naloxone rescue experiences among people who use opioids. *Substance Abuse*, 1–14. https://doi.org/10.1080/08897077.2020.1748165

Krabbe, J., Jiao, S., Guta, A., Slemon, A., Cameron, A. A., & Bungay, V. (2021). Exploring the operationalisation and implementation of outreach in community settings with hard-to-reach and hidden populations: Protocol for a scoping review. *BMJ Open, 11*(2), e039451–e039451. https://doi.org/10.1136/bmjopen-2020-039451

LaMancuso, K., Goldman, R. E., & Nothnagle, M. (2016). "Can I ask that?": Perspectives on perinatal care after resettlement among karen refugee women, medical providers, and community-based doulas. *Journal of Immigrant and Minority Health, 18*(2), 428–435. https://doi.org/10.1007/s10903-015-0172-6

MacQueen, K. M., McLellan, E., Metzger, D. S., Kegeles, S., Strauss, R. P., Scotti, R., Blanchard, L., & Trotter, R. T. (2001). What is community? An evidence-based definition for participatory public health. *American Journal of Public Health, 91*(12), 1929–1938. https://doi.org/10.2105/AJPH.91.12.1929

Monograph. (1990). *The collection and interpretation of data from hidden populations*. NIDA Research.

Moore, L. W., & Miller, M. (1999). Initiating research with doubly vulnerable populations. *Journal of Advanced Nursing, 30*(5), 1034–1040. https://doi.org/10.1046/j.1365-2648.1999.01205.x

Newman, S. D., Andrews, J. O., Magwood, G. S., Jenkins, C., Cox, M. J., & Williamson, D. C. (2011). Community advisory boards in community-based participatory research: A synthesis of best processes. *Preventing Chronic Disease, 8*(3), A70–A70.

Quinn, S. C. (2004). Ethics in public health research. *American Journal of Public Health, 94*(6), 918–922. https://doi.org/10.2105/AJPH.94.6.918

Reilly, S. M., Wilson Crowley, M., Harold, P., Hemphill, D., & Tumiel Berhalter, L. (2018). Patient voices network: Bringing breast cancer awareness and action into underserved communities. *Journal of the National Medical Association, 110*(5), 448–454. https://doi.org/10.1016/j.jnma.2017.10.008

Schuster, R. C., Rodriguez, E. M., Blosser, M., Mongo, A., Delvecchio-Hitchcock, N., Kahn, L., & Tumiel-Berhalter, L. (2019). "They were just waiting to die": Somali Bantu and Karen experiences with cancer screening pre- and post-resettlement in Buffalo, NY. *Journal of the National Medical Association, 111*(3), 234–245. https://doi.org/10.1016/j.jnma.2018.10.006

Smith, M. K. (2013). *'Community' in The encyclopedia of pedagogy and informal education*. Accessed 30 Apr. https://infed.org/mobi/community/

Strauss, R. P., Sengupta, S., Quinn, S. C., Goeppinger, J., Spaulding, C., Kegeles, S. M., & Millett, G. (2001). The role of community advisory boards: Involving communities in the informed consent process. *American Journal of Public Health, 91*(12), 1938–1943. https://doi.org/10.2105/ajph.91.12.1938

Terrell, J. A., Williams, E. M., Murekeyisoni, C. M., Watkins, R., & Tumiel-Berhalter, L. (2008). The community-driven approach to environmental exposures: How a community-based participatory research program analyzing impacts of environmental exposure on lupus led to a toxic site cleanup. *Environmental Justice, 1*(2), 87–92. https://doi.org/10.1089/env.2008.0517

Tumiel-Berhalter, L., Watkins, R., & Crespo, C. J. (2005). Community-based participatory research: Defining community stakeholders. *Metropolitan Universities, 16*(1), 93–106.

Wallerstein, N., & Duran, B. (2010). Community-based participatory research contributions to intervention research: The intersection of science and practice to improve health equity. *American Journal of Public Health, 100*(S1), S40–S46. https://doi.org/10.2105/ajph.2009.184036

Williams, E. M., Terrell, J., Anderson, J., & Tumiel-Berhalter, L. (2016). A case study of community involvement influence on policy decisions: Victories of a community-based participatory research partnership. *International Journal of Environmental Research and Public Health, 13*(5). https://doi.org/10.3390/ijerph13050515

Laurene Tumiel-Berhalter is associate professor and director of the Community Engagement Core for the University at Buffalo's Clinical and Translational Science Institute. She is an epidemiologist with extensive experience conducting community-based participatory research and health disparities research to improve chronic disease self-management and cancer prevention among underserved communities. She has worked with a variety of partners from both urban and rural communities.

Linda Kahn is research professor and associate vice chair of Research Scholarship. She is a medical anthropologist and health services researcher, and examines the social, cultural, economic and political factors that influence health and risk behavior among vulnerable and complex populations. For two decades, her "research laboratory" has consisted of the community setting, medical practices, and recently the drug treatment courts.

Chapter 8
Community Researchers and Ethical Considerations: Burdens in the Field

Maghboeba Mosavel and Briona Phillips

8.1 Introduction

Capacity building is an integral part of research that engages community and patient stakeholders. To build capacity and encourage the authentic engagement of community residents, individuals with personal experiences of the research phenomenon being studied are increasingly hired by academic researchers to join research teams (Mir et al., 2013). An in-depth exploration of the community researcher role is necessary to avoid undue burden and develop safeguards to ensure ethical challenges are adequately addressed. Health disparities research centers on communities that have been affected by multiple inequities and who continue to experience ongoing racism, exclusion, and discrimination (Baciu et al., 2017; Hostetter & Klein, 2018). Therefore, community researchers working in such settings will likely experience a range of challenges as they navigate this role that invariably links them to an academic institution, often with its own storied reputation. Within this context, research study protocols may superimpose a set of rigid expectations that are out of sync with the real-world dilemmas that community researchers must navigate as they perform research tasks such as recruitment, informed consent, data collection and data dissemination while still being a community member, friend, relative, or neighbor. In this chapter, we draw upon our experiences from research projects involving community residents with no prior research training. Our aim is to provide practical recommendations for

M. Mosavel (✉) · B. Phillips
Department of Health Behavior and Policy, School of Population Health, Virginia Commonwealth University, Richmond, VA, USA
e-mail: mmosavel@vcu.edu; phillipsbm@vcu.edu

E. E. Anderson (ed.), *Ethical Issues in Community and Patient Stakeholder–Engaged Health Research*, Philosophy and Medicine 146,
https://doi.org/10.1007/978-3-031-40379-8_8

academic researchers to operationalize policies and practices that can facilitate the credible representation of community members in this multidimensional frontline role as community researcher.

8.2 Ethical Challenges Experienced by Community Researchers

Three overarching ethical principles, also known as the *Belmont* principles – respect for persons, beneficence, and justice (National Commission for the Protection of Human Subjects of Biomedical and Behavioral Research, 1979) – serve as guideposts for academic researchers as they engage with communities, build capacity, and develop relationships with key stakeholders and community members to advocate and work toward the elimination of health disparities (Guillemin & Gillam, 2004; Shrader-Frechette, 1994; Pimple, 2002). In community-based participatory research (CBPR) specifically, social justice considerations are critical to the conduct and credibility of research.

Significant contextual factors including research mistrust, negative experiences with academic institutions, and concerns about lack of direct benefit to the community provide a backdrop for ethical challenges that arise in community-engaged research. Community members join research studies for a variety of reasons including personal commitment to the issue being studied, desire for employment, professional development opportunities, and other intrinsic motivations such as wanting to make a difference (Mosavel et al., 2011; Legood, 2005). Importantly, community researchers share characteristics, affiliations, and strong commitments to the well-being of their communities. However, these very qualities may result in tensions arising from their dual roles – one as a community researcher and the other as a community member.

Dual Roles Community members hired and trained to serve as community researchers are usually either physically located in the neighborhoods where the research occurs and/or share a set of experiences related to the condition being studied (e.g., chronic disease, poverty, substance use, violence). Therefore, they simultaneously occupy dual roles (e.g., church member and recruiter, data collector and friend, etc.) that require carefully balancing community and research needs (Salway et al., 2015). When community researchers' roles conflict, this may result in cognitive (Salway et al., 2015; Flicker et al., 2007) or ethical dissonance (Barkan et al., 2015). While the presence of community researchers has been shown to be beneficial to both the research team and community (Kelly et al., 2018; Berger, 2015; D'Cruz & Gillingham, 2017), navigating ethical challenges can place considerable burden on these community researchers (Attree et al., 2011) and potentially impact research outcomes. For example, community members may mistrust the community researcher based on their affiliation with, and perceived loyalty to, their new employer, the academic institution, and now, insider status (Flicker et al., 2007;

Mosher et al., 2015; Flicker, 2005; Jewkes & Murcott, 1998; Cornwall & Jewkes, 1995).

Recruitment may pose inherent dilemmas for the community researcher (Flicker et al., 2007; Mosher et al., 2015) or for the research protocol. For instance, despite general mistrust of the research or academic institution, community residents may be more amenable to participating in the research because they trust the community researcher. On the other hand, the community researcher may, at times, too enthusiastically recommend that a community member participate to receive study benefits. During the conduct of research, community researchers also may obtain private, confidential information about community members that they may not otherwise have known. Outside of the research, it may be challenging for the community researcher to navigate their previous relationships knowing this private information (Salway et al., 2015). Thus, unlike information sharing between the academic researcher and community participant, which is time-specific and transient, the ongoing presence of the community researcher in their community introduces nuanced dimensions associated with privacy and confidentiality. These ethical challenges of dual roles can inadvertently create stressors for the community researcher, which in turn have ethical implications for recruitment, informed consent, and community relationships.

Proximity Emerging dilemmas associated with the close physical and emotional proximity to the research topic and intended community, and its unintended burdens on the community researchers have been identified (Kai & Hedges, 1999; Rowe, 2006). Given mistrust in research institutions, community researchers may be able to gain access to individuals more easily than academic researchers (Salway et al., 2015; Cornwall & Jewkes, 1995). Inherent challenges based on proximity, such as being too close to the research issue, could present undue burden on the community researcher. They may also be perceived to be associated with any negative impacts or lack of impact of the research (Salway et al., 2015). Such dilemmas associated with "being too close to the community" and the intensely personal significance of the research (both topic and community) are not only burdensome, but may also affect community researchers' personal relationships with research participants and other community residents once the research concludes (Salway et al., 2015).

Emotional proximity to the issues being studied can present additional challenges. For example, when cancer survivors conduct research with other cancer survivors (Mosavel & Sanders, 2014), or when past substance users work with those currently using substances, this may trigger a range of emotions (Vaughn et al., 2018). Similar to experiences of other frontline workers who are in the helping professions, these triggers may lead to burnout, fatigue, and feeling emotionally overwhelmed (Vaughn et al., 2018; Zellmer, 2004; Grant & Kinman, 2014; Cocker & Joss, 2016).

There remains a dearth of information related to the unintended burden and dilemmas inadvertently created by community researchers' dual roles and shared identities

(Salway et al., 2015; Flicker et al., 2007; Vaughn et al., 2018). Research protocols tend to be based on the idealistic interactions of researchers and participants as strangers in a controlled, laboratory setting and do not always consider some of the common situations that community researchers encounter (Ogden, 1999; Flicker et al., 2007; Plunk, 2011; Puckett, 2017; Brown et al., 2010; van der Merwe & Hunt, 2019). Most protocols do not address how to manage the emotional burdens that may arise when community researchers work within their own community. We aim to contribute to a gap in the field by applying traditional research ethics guidance to these frontline dilemmas caused by community researcher proximity and dual roles.

8.3 Lessons from Our Work

Here, we draw upon various community-engaged research experiences addressing cervical cancer disparities in South Africa and Cleveland, Ohio, (Mosavel et al., 2011) and obesity in Petersburg, Virginia (LaRose et al., 2021). These research projects were conducted in low-income, under-resourced, primarily Black and Brown communities that historically have borne the brunt of the impacts of a range of social, economic and political inequities. These projects all included hiring and training local residents as community researchers (Mosavel et al., 2005; Simon & Mosavel, 2010). In the cervical cancer project in South Africa, we hired seven community residents to conduct semi-structured interviews with 157 women about cancer beliefs and knowledge, social support, and harnessing their relationship with their adolescent daughter to promote cancer preventive behaviors (Mosavel et al., 2005). We also draw upon experiences in a cancer survivor study conducted in Cleveland where we trained eight cancer survivors and two cancer caregivers as community researchers who conducted 32 interviews with cancer survivors, caregivers, and health care professionals (Mosavel & Sanders, 2014). Our research focusing on obesity, the Wellness Engagement (WE) project, involved an extensive needs assessment using various methodologies including asset mapping, key informant interviews, house chats (similar to focus groups but led by a community researcher in a home setting with members of their social network) (Mosavel et al., 2016), community surveys, (Mosavel et al., 2020) and a pilot intervention (LaRose et al., 2021).

In these projects, community researchers were residents of the city where the research was being conducted, and a concerted effort was made to recruit community researchers from distinct neighborhoods within the community. Community researchers were hired as part-time, hourly paid staff. In the US-based projects, as hourly university employees, they were required to undergo a background check.

Below, we examine specific real-world ethical dilemmas experienced when community residents serve as community researchers and provide recommendations to academic researchers and community partners to address these challenges through process, protocol, and systems changes.

8.4 Key Ethical Considerations

Dual Roles The community researcher is on the frontline of any research study while they simultaneously continue to function as a full member of their community. These dual roles can create considerable tension. In our studies, community researchers became familiar with research expectations, rigor, ethical accountabilities, and other insider knowledge about the research enterprise. This new knowledge informed and modified how they viewed research, and some experienced conflict integrating their initial and emerging perceptions. In the WE project, for example, several community researchers, reflecting community sentiment, started out being somewhat skeptical about research. During onboarding and training, their understanding of research requirements and study implementation expanded, and they learned about required protections for research participants. At weekly meetings, the team discussed recruitment, informed consent, and voluntariness. Some community researchers initially had to be reminded that their enthusiasm for the project should not intentionally influence the choices of others related to study participation, and that they need to be especially careful when potential participants were known to them. As they became more knowledgeable about regulatory efforts to respect individual autonomy, community researchers became frustrated regarding the limitations of the research project to create change at a community level. This frustration was especially evident in the South Africa study where community researchers indicated that while this role led to personal empowerment, it also served to highlight the community's needs, which subsequently exacerbated their own concerns related to those needs. This tension is evident in the following refrains often heard at research team meetings: "what can we do, how can we help the community, we should do more than just research."

Tensions caused by navigating dual roles can create unintended burdens for the community researcher as well as the research project. For example, in the WE project, a community researcher, also a community activist, would frequently and rightly so, speak up at the local city, often contentious, council meetings. However, their personal views were often wrongly attributed to the research project, resulting in negative perceptions about the research. Consequently, the research team had a transparent conversation reminding community researchers that whenever they spoke publicly in their personal capacity, they should clearly indicate their views were distinct from those of the research project.

Emotional Burden Community researchers are often selected because of their lived experiences in a particular community or because of personal association with the topic. However, these exact selection criteria can introduce unexpected emotional burdens. Academic and community researchers alike may wrongly assume that shared lived experiences of the community researcher somehow inoculate them from emotional impact of the research topic. Academic researchers may inadvertently hold these views due to their lack of cultural sensitivity or lack of knowledge about secondary trauma (Pelzang & Hutchinson, 2017; Stacciarini et al., 2011;

LaVeaux & Christopher, 2009). Despite being insider researchers, research with in-depth community knowledge, community researchers may not fully anticipate that their status and familiarity with the community will not protect them from emotional burdens in our work with community researchers, we found that they experienced two types of salient emotional burdens: personal identification and community worry.

Personal Identification Community researchers often strongly identify with the experiences of research participants, and at times, data collection can trigger an unexpected, deep emotional reaction. In South Africa, the community researchers shared similarities with research participants including age, sex, parenting, and economic status. While working with the South African community researchers and witnessing the effects of listening to traumatic experiences of participants, the research team began to comprehend the extent of this emotional burden. In team debriefings, the community researchers reported that their own pain and trauma were exposed when conducting the semi-structured interviews with mothers. This personal identification and experience across multiple shared identities, combined with the use of semi-structured interviews, elicited storytelling that caused them to recall similar traumatic experiences. Their personal identification with these mothers' stories resulted in an unexpected emotional burden. Similar experiences were reported by the cancer survivor community researchers who interviewed other cancer survivors (Mosavel & Sanders, 2014). Several indicated that they found it emotionally taxing to hear about the research participants' experiences as they would become quite invested. However, others reported that hearing about research participants experiences served to affirm their own cancer journey.

In the WE Project, the community researchers' demographic profiles were more varied, and while from the same city, not all of them could relate to the personal experiences of participants. In this context, community researchers who shared fewer similarities and were less familiar with the lived experiences of the research participants would often express surprise at the extent of violence, poverty, and community hardships. Regardless of shared experiences, working directly with individuals and communities experiencing personal and structurally-based hardships proved emotionally exhausting to all community researchers. However, this also resulted in several community researchers expressing increased commitment to addressing economic and social disparities.

Community Worry Learning community context has the potential to increase awareness of societal issues and can increase overall worry and concern for the community. Community researchers reported that, in this role, they obtained a first-hand perspective of how community and systems-level factors exacerbated personal conditions. Their direct interaction with research participants, which meant repeatedly hearing themes of poverty, unemployment, violence, and overall lack of resources, brought heightened awareness and created a sense of urgency regarding the outcomes of the research project. However, for several of the community researchers, this intimate access to participants' daily lives served as motivation to become advocates within and beyond the research project. They subsequently asked more specific questions about eligibility requirements, intervention design, and sustainability. They encouraged collaboration beyond the research with community organizations that could more comprehensively address social determinants of health and develop programming to address salient needs.

Proximity The physical proximity of community researchers to potential participants is a significant asset in community-engaged research. However, this proximity may create certain ethical dilemmas (Richman et al., 2012). Given the emotional and physical proximity of community researchers, transparency and vigilance during the informed consent process is especially crucial. Our experience with community researchers suggests that participants' comfort asking questions and mutual trust with the community researcher can strengthen the process. However, it is imperative that the research team directly address potential dilemmas during initial and continued booster training (True et al., 2011).

Bias due to physical proximity may be associated with increased personal identification, which could cause the community researcher to question the research protocol, particularly related to recruitment eligibility (Mosavel et al., 2006). In South Africa, community researchers would lament the restrictiveness of the eligibility criteria if they encountered someone they thought "should" be eligible but was excluded because of age, grade of daughters, or cancer screening status. These concerns were exacerbated by perceived community need for the research stipend, general discomfort with exclusion criteria, and perception that the research had limited community benefit. These discussions provided the opportunity for the academic researchers to reexamine, or provide additional rationale for, the criteria. Nevertheless, the scientific rationale did not always adequately address concerns about community benefit.

In the WE Project, the house chat methodology (Mosavel et al., 2016) required that community researchers recruit members of their social network and lead discussions on micro and macro barriers and solutions to living a healthy lifestyle. The methodology also aimed to reach community members, particularly friends and family, who would not ordinarily participate in research. To address potential bias in the recruitment of their social network members, the entire team collaboratively developed the protocol for recruitment. First, we created a shared understanding of the rigor and uniformity required for implementation. Next, we agreed on the importance of diverse representation across different generations and households. Based on these tenets, the house chat leaders agreed to invite only one person per family unit. Likewise, in the WE project, (Mosavel et al., 2020), the team collectively agreed that community researchers would first recruit for a community-wide survey of 1200 residents directly from their neighborhood thus benefitting from the knowledge about their geographic location and access. This recruitment approach, which started with the geolocated strengths of the community researchers, helped to address potential transportation barriers and allowed the researchers to recruit in their own communities. Concerns about recruitment bias can be addressed by applying specific eligibility criteria and partnering with community researchers to develop a shared understanding of fairness and importance of diverse representation, while at the same time, providing ongoing training and support bolstered by a robust quality control process.

Community-Level Considerations A perception that a potential research study lacks community-level benefits can cause considerable tension. At the start of the WE project, there was a high level of mistrust and concern about a lack of tangible research benefits to the community. It is imperative that community-level benefit be discussed with the community research co-lead, community organizations who are part of the research advisory board or council, and community researchers to ensure that community benefits are realized and sustained beyond the end of the research study. This dialogue should be transparent and include research project limitations in order to strengthen academic-community partnerships and maximize outcomes.

In the WE project, we operationalized community-level benefits in several ways. First, we established an independent, community-led coalition to address health disparities, including obesity and other salient health concerns, using a collaborative, partner-engaged approach (Mosavel et al., 2019a, b). This coalition has continued beyond the research project, serving as a tangible exemplar of community-level benefit. Second, capacity building was considered a key component of community benefit. The project made a commitment to workforce development and hired and trained more than 20 residents as community researchers. Several of the community researchers used these skills to secure other research-related positions, some pursued higher educational opportunities, and several became more active at the civic level. Community-level considerations are especially critical when working in historically marginalized Black and Brown communities.

Inclusion University systems, perhaps unintentionally, perpetuate the exclusion of grassroots community voices. As a result, universities must make intentional changes to be inclusive of community voice. At our institution, as at many others, community researchers who are hired as hourly employees are subject to a background check. However, Black and Brown communities are more likely to experience racially motivated arrests for misdemeanor crimes such as driving without a drivers' license and non-attendance at a court date (Williams, 2019). Therefore, recruiting community residents from such communities result in background checks which may disclose criminal records. In the WE project, background checks revealed arrest records for two potential community researchers, driving without a license and check forgery. These records made them ineligible for hire. However, cognizant of known racial inequities in the criminal justice system, the academic and community research leads met with each community researcher to determine the context of their arrest. It was critical that the academic and community research leads determine that the past documented crimes would not pose any risk to research protocol fidelity or research integrity. Once this was determined, we advocated with the university administration that they should be hired despite their records. Eventually, the viable option from an administrative aspect was to consider hiring them as independent contractors, for which no background check was needed. One community researcher agreed and the other decided not to work with the university bureaucracy.

Community-engaged research teams will be confronted by multiple ethical dilemmas. It is critical that the existing community-engaged infrastructure, which typically includes community partners, community coalitions, community advisory boards, and community researchers, be engaged as partners in deciding how to address these dilemmas. In our research, the community partner and the academic researcher jointly made decisions and engaged the rest of the team as appropriate based on specific concerns. Transparency, collaborative decision-making, and thoughtful deliberation are prerequisites for addressing ethical dilemmas emerging during fieldwork.

8.5 Recommendations

The Academic Researcher and Research Team Must be Proactive in Planning for Challenges At an individual level, academic researchers have an ethical responsibility to critically examine research procedures to identify and avoid certain ethical dilemmas when possible. For academic-based researchers, it is critical to ensure that research practices are inclusive of a wide range of community voices and capacities. Academic researchers should advocate for changes at the institutional level, including fair payment of community researchers; this may also include questioning hiring and other policies that exclude and unfairly disadvantage marginalized communities.

Furthermore, the academic researcher needs to examine their own privileges and how these may lead to assumptions about the community researcher's role and ability to manage challenging field experiences. There may be the implicit assumption that because someone is from a particular community, they may be able to manage turmoil due to similarities in their shared lived context. However, community researchers are not insulated from the traumatic effects of poverty, violence, and unemployment. Therefore, adequate training, resources, and ongoing support must be provided.

Establishing a community advisory board is fundamental to ensure a formal structure for learning from community experts and anticipating and brainstorming challenging situations (Cramer et al., 2018; D'Alonzo, 2010; Wallerstein et al., 2008). An advisory board can be instrumental in identifying community-level ethical concerns that arise related to data sharing, disseminating research findings that may perpetuate negative stereotypes, ensuring community representation, and minimizing community harms (see Chap. 16, this volume).

Community researchers may not be aware of or prepared for the various challenges they will encounter (Flicker et al., 2007; Boynton, 2002). For example, in the case of the South African community researchers, we provided them access to professional counseling to help them cope with the emotional reactions that emerged during data collection with mothers. To minimize emotional burden, community researchers need resources training, and ongoing support.

Academic Institutions Have a Critical Role in Addressing Systemic Issues that Could Lead to Ethical Dilemmas University hiring authorities need to be willing to examine systems and policies that continue to exclude employees from marginalized communities. For example, mandatory employment background checks can disproportionately exclude many individuals from low-income Black and Brown communities from obtaining paid university positions as community researchers due to their higher likelihood of experiencing stops and arrests compared to other groups. Academic-community research partnerships must have transparent conversations about restrictive hiring protocols to ensure inclusive environments for community members in this role.

8.6 Conclusion

Community researchers are frontline staff directly engaging with research participants and the community more broadly. Therefore, the academic researcher must consider and prepare for the unintentional barriers and ethical conundrums that may arise when hiring a community member in this role. Ethical concerns such as burdens of physical, social, and emotional proximities must be addressed, and appropriate training and support provided. The paradox is that the community researcher is often selected because of these various proximities; therefore, the research team must carefully anticipate and address burdens and ethical issues that could arise for the community researcher in this role. Academic researchers must continue to ask critical questions to facilitate institutional level changes, including the extent to which university expectations or aspects of the research protocol may contribute to community researcher burden, and ultimately, the exclusion of meaningful, community representation.

Acknowledgements We would like to sincerely thank the community researchers who have contributed their expertise and time to the various projects.

References

Attree, P., French, B., Milton, B., Povall, S., Whitehead, M., & Popay, J. (2011). The experience of community engagement for individuals: A rapid review of evidence. *Health & Social Care in the Community, 19*(3), 250–260.

Baciu, A., Negussie, Y., Geller, A., Weinstein, J. N., & National Academies of Sciences, Engineering, and Medicine. (2017). The root causes of health inequity. In *Communities in action: Pathways to health equity*. National Academies Press (US).

Barkan, R., Ayal, S., & Ariely, D. (2015). Ethical dissonance, justifications, and moral behavior. *Current Opinion in Psychology, 6*(Dec), 157–161.

Berger, R. (2015). Now I see it, now I don't: Researcher's position and reflexivity in qualitative research. *Qualitative Research, 15*(2), 219–234.

Boynton, P. M. (2002). Life on the streets: The experiences of community researchers in a study of prostitution. *Journal of Community & Applied Social Psychology, 12*(1), 1–12.

Brown, P., Morello-Frosch, R., Brody, J. G., Altman, R. G., Rudel, R. A., Senier, L., Pérez, C., & Simpson, R. (2010). Institutional review board challenges related to community-based participatory research on human exposure to environmental toxins: A case study. *Environmental Health: A Global Access Science Source, 9*, 39. https://doi.org/10.1186/1476-069X-9-39

Cocker, F., & Joss, N. (2016). Compassion fatigue among healthcare, emergency and community service workers: A systematic review. *International Journal of Environmental Research and Public Health, 13*(6), 618. https://doi.org/10.3390/ijerph13060618

Cornwall, A., & Jewkes, R. (1995). What is participatory research? *Social Science & Medicine, 41*(12), 1667–1676.

Cramer, M. E., Lazoritz, S., Shaffer, K., Palm, D., & Ford, A. L. (2018). Community advisory board members' perspectives regarding opportunities and challenges of research collaboration. *Western Journal of Nursing Research, 40*(7), 1032–1048.

D'Alonzo, K. T. (2010). Getting started in CBPR: Lessons in building community partnerships for new researchers. *Nursing Inquiry, 17*(4), 282–288.

D'Cruz, H., & Gillingham, P. (2017). Participatory research ideals and practice experience: Reflections and analysis. *Journal of Social Work, 17*(4), 434–452.

National Commission for the Protection of Human Subjects of Biomedical and Behavioral Research. (1979). *The Belmont Report: Ethical principles and guidelines for the protection of human subjects of research*. https://www.hhs.gov/ohrp/regulations-andpolicy/belmont-report/read-the-belmont-report/index.html#xethical.

Flicker, S. (2005). *Critical issues in community-based participatory research* (PhD thesis). University of Toronto.

Flicker, S., Travers, R., Guta, A., McDonald, S., & Meagher, A. (2007). Ethical dilemmas in community-based participatory research: Recommendations for institutional review boards. *Journal of Urban Health: Bulletin of the New York Academy of Medicine, 84*(4), 478–493. https://doi.org/10.1007/s11524-007-9165-7

Grant, L., & Kinman, G. (2014). Emotional resilience in the helping professions and how it can be enhanced. *Health and Social Care Education, 3*(1), 23–34.

Guillemin, M., & Gillam, L. (2004). Ethics, reflexivity, and "ethically important moments" in research. *Qualitative Inquiry, 10*(2), 261–280.

Hostetter, M., & Klein, S. (2018, September 20). *In focus: Reducing racial disparities in health care by confronting racism*. Commonwealth Fund. Retrieved September 7, 2021, from https://www.commonwealthfund.org/publications/2018/sep/focus-reducing-racial-disparities-health-care-confronting-racism

Jewkes, R., & Murcott, A. (1998). Community representatives: Representing the "community"? *Social Science & Medicine, 46*(7), 843–858.

Kai, J., & Hedges, C. (1999). Minority ethnic community participation in needs assessment and service development in primary care: Perceptions of Pakistani and Bangladeshi people about psychological distress. *Health Expectations, 2*(1), 7–20.

Kelly, B., Friel, S., McShane, T., Pinkerton, J., & Gilligan, E. (2018). "I haven't read it, I've lived it!": The benefits and challenges of peer research with young people leaving care. *Qualitative Social Work, 19*(1), 108. https://doi.org/10.1177/1473325018800370

LaRose, J. G., Lanoye, A., Ferrell, D., Lu, J., & Mosavel, M. (2021). Translating evidence-based behavioral weight loss into a multi-level, community intervention within a community-based participatory research framework: The Wellness Engagement (WE) Project. *Translational Behavioral Medicine, 11*(6), 1235–1243.

LaVeaux, D., & Christopher, S. (2009). Contextualizing CBPR: Key principles of CBPR meet the indigenous research context. *Pimatisiwin, 7*(1), 1.

Legood, G. (2005). The recruitment and role of lay members. *Research Ethics Review, 1*(4), 135–138. https://doi.org/10.1177/174701610500100407

Mir, G., Salway, S., Kai, J., Karlsen, S., Bhopal, R., Ellison, G. T., & Sheikh, A. (2013). Principles for research on ethnicity and health: The Leeds Consensus Statement. *The European Journal of Public Health, 23*(3), 504–510.

Mosavel, M., & Sanders, K. D. (2014). Community-engaged research: Cancer survivors as community researchers. *Journal of Empirical Research and Human Research Ethics, 9*(3), 74–78. https://doi.org/10.1177/1556264614540598

Mosavel, M., Simon, C., van Stade, D., & Buchbinder, M. (2005). Community-based participatory research (CBPR) in South Africa: Engaging multiple constituents to shape the research question. *Social Science & Medicine (1982), 61*(12), 2577–2587. https://doi.org/10.1016/j.socscimed.2005.04.041

Mosavel, M., Simon, C., & Van Stade, D. (2006). The mother-daughter relationship: What is its potential as a locus for health promotion? *Health Care for Women International, 27*(7), 646–664. https://doi.org/10.1080/07399330600803790

Mosavel, M., Ahmed, R., Daniels, D., & Simon, C. (2011). Community researchers conducting health disparities research: Ethical and other insights from fieldwork journaling. *Social Science & Medicine (1982), 73*(1), 145–152. https://doi.org/10.1016/j.socscimed.2011.04.029

Mosavel, M., Ferrell, D., & LaRose, J. G. (2016). House chats as a grassroots engagement methodology in community-basedparticipatory research: The WE Project, Petersburg. *Progress in Community Health Partnerships: Research, Education, and Action, 10*(3), 391–400. https://doi.org/10.1353/cpr.2016.0046

Mosavel, M., Winship, J., Ferrell, D., & LaRose, J. (2019a). Data dissemination in CBPR: Accountability and responsiveness. *Collaborations: A Journal of Community-Based Research and Practice, 2*(1), 1–11.

Mosavel, M., Winship, J., Liggins, V., Cox, T., Roberts, M., & Jones, D. S. (2019b). Community-based participatory research and sustainability: The Petersburg wellness consortium. *Journal of Community Engagement and Scholarship, 11*(2), 7.

Mosavel, M., Ferrell, D., LaRose, J. G., Lu, J., & Winship, J. (2020). Conducting a community "Street Survey" to inform an obesity intervention: The WE Project. *Family and Community Health, 44*, 117–125. https://doi.org/10.1097/fch.0000000000000271

Mosher, H. I., Moorthi, G., Li, J., & Weeks, M. R. (2015). A qualitative analysis of peer recruitment pressures in respondent driven sampling: Are risks above the ethical limit? *The International Journal on Drug Policy, 26*(9), 832–842. https://doi.org/10.1016/j.drugpo.2015.05.027

Ogden, R. (1999). Ethical review in community-based HIV/AIDS research. *Canadian HIV-AIDS Policy & Law Newsletter, 5*(1), 39–40.

Pelzang, R., & Hutchinson, A. M. (2017). Establishing cultural integrity in qualitative research: Reflections from a cross-cultural study. *International Journal of Qualitative Methods, 17*(1), 1609406917749702.

Pimple, K. D. (2002). Six domains of research ethics. *Science and Engineering Ethics, 8*(2), 191–205.

Plunk, A. (2011). Improving institutional review of community-based participatory research applications. *AMA Journal of Ethics, 13*(2), 102–104.

Puckett, Y. (2017). Bringing the IRB into the community: A new framework for the ethical regulation of CBPR. *MedCrave Online Journal of Public Health, 5*(5), 183–118.

Richman, K., et al. (2012). Proximity, ethical dilemmas and community research workers. *American Journal of Bioethics, 3*(4), 19–29.

Rowe, A. (2006). The effect of involvement in participatory research on parent researchers in a Sure Start programme. *Health & Social Care in the Community, 14*(6), 465–473.

Salway, S., Chowbey, P., Such, E., & Ferguson, B. (2015). Researching health inequalities with community researchers: Practical, methodological and ethical challenges of an 'inclusive'research approach. *Research Involvement and Engagement, 1*(1), 1–21.

Shrader-Frechette, K. S. (1994). *Ethics of scientific research*. Rowman & Littlefield.

Simon, C., & Mosavel, M. (2010). Community members as recruiters of human subjects: Ethical considerations. *American Journal of Bioethics, 10*(3), 3–11.

Stacciarini, J. M. R., Wiens, B., Coady, M., Schwait, A. B., Pérez, A., Locke, B., et al. (2011). CBPR: Building partnerships with Latinos in a rural area for a wellness approach to mental health. *Issues in Mental Health Nursing, 32*(8), 486–492.

True, G., et al. (2011). Misbehaviors of front-line research personnel and the integrity of community-based research. *Journal of Empirical Research and Human Research Ethics, 6*(2), 3–12.

van der Merwe, A., & Hunt, X. (2019). Secondary trauma among trauma researchers: Lessons from the field. *Psychological Trauma: Theory, Research, Practice and Policy, 11*(1), 10–18. https://doi.org/10.1037/tra0000414

Vaughn, L. M., Jacquez, F., & Zhen-Duan, J. (2018). Perspectives of community co-researchers about group dynamics and equitable partnership within a community–academic research team. *Health Education & Behavior, 45*(5), 682–689.

Wallerstein, N., Oetzel, J., Duran, B., Tafoya, G., Belone, L., & Rae, R. (2008). What predicts outcomes in CBPR. *Community-Based Participatory Research for Health: From Process to Outcomes, 2*, 371–392.

Williams, T. (2019). Black people are charged at a higher rate than whites. What if prosecutors didn't know their race? *New York Times*, June 12.

Zellmer, D. D. (2004). Teaching to prevent burnout in the helping professions. *Analytic Teaching, 24*(1).

Maghboeba Mosavel is a Professor in the Department of Health Behavior and Policy. Her research focuses on cancer prevention and control, healthy lifestyle interventions, oral health disparities, and deceased tissue donation.

Briona Phillips is a PhD candidate in the Department of Health Behavior and Policy. Her research agenda focuses on racial implicit bias in oral health and its impact to Black patients' psychosocial wellbeing and engagement with oral health care service delivery.

Chapter 9
Community-Engaged Research with People with Developmental Disabilities: A Conversation with Community Researchers about their Ethical Inclusion

Brendan Durkin, Micah Fialka-Feldman, Jacob Myers, Ariel Schwartz, and Katherine McDonald

9.1 Introduction

People with developmental disabilities experience many injustices—including long-standing practices to segregate them and deny their rights to community living, education, sexuality, parenting, and decision-making. Disability rights and self-advocacy movements have achieved important social and legal changes including the promotion of models of disability that account for individual and environmental factors and their interactions that emphasize the impact of disabling environments. These movements also call for believing in all peoples' abilities and skills, rather than thinking about what they cannot do. Disability is increasingly understood as a social factor and people with disabilities represent a large and diverse population experiencing health disparities. Community-engaged research is a promising

B. Durkin
Boston College, Boston, MA, USA

M. Fialka-Feldman
Taishoff Center, School of Education, Syracuse University, Syracuse, NY, USA
e-mail: mfialkaf@syr.edu

J. Myers
Boston University, Boston, MA, USA

A. Schwartz
Institute on Disability, University of New Hampshire, Durham, NH, USA
e-mail: ariel.schwartz@unh.edu

K. McDonald (✉)
Falk College of Sport and Human Dynamics, Syracuse University, Syracuse, NY, USA
e-mail: kemcdona@syr.edu

E. E. Anderson (ed.), *Ethical Issues in Community and Patient Stakeholder–Engaged Health Research*, Philosophy and Medicine 146,
https://doi.org/10.1007/978-3-031-40379-8_9

practice to increase the representation of people with developmental disabilities in research and address disparities in health outcomes, the social determinants of health, how people are treated when they seek healthcare, access to healthcare, and health outcomes.

We are community (Brendan, Micah, Jacob) and academic (Ariel, Katie) researchers who have worked together for many years on several community-engaged research projects with communities of people with developmental disabilities. We share here a conversation about how academic researchers can help community researchers feel respected and meaningfully included as research partners. Neither of these experiences—respect and meaningful inclusion—are common experiences for people with developmental disabilities. The presence of people with developmental disabilities is critical in community-engaged research projects and relies on interpersonal interactions that integrate disability-related accommodations and uphold commitments to the community. We believe these actions improve accountability to populations experiencing health disparities and are building blocks to ethical community-engaged research with communities of people with developmental disabilities.

9.2 Creating a Sense of Belonging

In our conversation, we talked about the importance of the positive relationships that community researchers develop on research teams. For example, Jacob shared feeling a sense of belonging: "*I think it's important that someone with a disability is on a research team. They can be included, they can feel part of a family.*" Brendan and Micah also felt it was important to be included and, like Jacob, they have experiences of developing strong relationships with other research team members. However, such positive experiences do not happen all the time for people with developmental disabilities who are frequently seen as incapable and less worthy. Brendan, Micah, and Jacob all shared that having long-term relationships with people who took the time to understand and know them individually, understand their strengths, and provide disability-related accommodations strengthened relationships and promoted a sense of belonging.

For example, Micah shared, "*I think having good people to help me. Katie's very good at understanding, and [asks me] good questions.*"

When community researchers feel a sense of belonging, they feel comfortable and confident to speak up and share their ideas for the project. When Ariel asked Jacob what helped him speak up or connect with others, he said, "*The other research team members. It felt like a family, it felt really connected. It felt like you fit in if you wanted to.*" Katie asked, "*What are the things that people did or said that helped you get that family feeling and feel connected and accepted?*" and Jacob responded, "*They were just welcoming. You could just see in their-in their faces, their facial expressions, their body language. It just felt like we're part of something special. You were making a difference, helping people. You're not alone.*" Jacob's comments demonstrate the importance of having all research team members embrace the inherit dignity, worth, and abilities of people with developmental disabilities.

Providing needed and desired disability accommodations reflects these views and, as such, are an essential ethical responsibility of academic researchers doing community-engaged research with communities of people with developmental disabilities. Accommodations can come in the form of research materials, providing multiple forms of communication, and personal support. Brendan emphasized the importance of having a go-to person and one-on-one support so that he knew who to go to when he had questions or was confused. Having a go-to person to provide the support he needed helped him work on challenging tasks; together, these experiences of support helped him feel he belonged. A conversation between Brendan and Ariel highlighted the benefits of personal support.

Brendan: *You know, actually, I love that question. I really do…I think it's the research staff, really the staff that's mostly important, the individual. I think what helped me to be more processing of my life as a [part of research] is definitely having you guys around… I think about what the [knowledge I have from the] community brings to that research.*

Ariel: *I know that having the one-on-one can be a way to connect with people. Is there anything with big groups that made you feel welcome or like you could speak up?*

Brendan: *Even when welcomed to any group, I just feel like having that special person would just take that, uh, out of a scenario and be with a bigger group…[A bigger group] that can be a bad situation, where you don't know the [answer to the question]. That was my hard problem over time…I love how you connect, bonding wise to have one-on-one, so that will help you to be yourself. It's amazing to be with people like you [Ariel] and others [for such a long time].*

We also talked about the importance of meeting and working with other people with disabilities. Having peers on the same project team strengthened relationships and abilities to complete the work. Brendan's and Jacob's reflections on being a part of a group of people with disabilities highlighted how tokenistic inclusion of just *one* community researcher is ethically problematic and ineffective for fostering meaningful inclusion and contributions.

Brendan: *I want to see us working together. I want to see us, like, bonding together. We should have groups of two or four groups. I think it's fun, also, to be with others.*

Jacob: *I think Brendan and Micah really, really said what I was going to say about being with a group of people with a disability helping in research is to maybe relate to them and see that they might have the same similarities as me, and I feel comfortable in that environment.*

We talked about how social time—whether as part of research project meetings or spending time together outside research project meetings—can also help build strong relationships.

Brendan: *If I were part of the group...I would...have some ice breakers and something. Have a lunch break because that break would actually help and get to know others that way.*

However, not all dynamics are easy or positive. Sometimes teamwork can present challenges to teams and create ethical dilemmas. Our research projects share a core belief that disability is not inherently negative, and that disability rights and pride are valued and beneficial. Yet these beliefs are not universally shared. Micah shared an experience of having a different view than a teammate:

Micah: *In one of our meetings, I was saying that I was proud to have a disability and, and somebody in the group was very, like, disappointed that I said that. It was just surprising that somebody was very upset that I said I was very happy and proud to have a disability.*

In this case, team members were able to have private meetings to discuss the situation, their feelings about it, and plan for how to move forward. Ultimately, trusting and respectful relationships helped team members have these difficult discussions and agree on how to move forward as a team.

9.3 Fostering Respect and Meaningful Inclusion and Collaboration through Disability-Accommodations

While all community-engaged research teams need to foster respectful relationships and build trust among team members, accommodations play a unique role in community-engaged research with communities of people with developmental disabilities. In addition to the above discussion of one-on-one support, we talked about the importance of cognitive accessibility. For all research team members, it is difficult to understand and contribute when meetings are disorganized or there is too much information. Brendan, Micah, and Jacob shared how academic researchers can foster meaningful inclusion and collaboration by providing visually-supported structure, breaking down information into smaller parts, and being responsive to requests for accommodations. Of note, these types of accommodations may also benefit community researchers from other communities, especially those with lower levels of literacy and education. We also note that these accommodations can require a lot of time and resources, but their need and significant positive impacts make these investments necessary and worthwhile.

Micah: *[Academic researchers should] meet with [community researchers] and talk to them and ask them how they would be helpful when they do research...making sure that you ask the person with the disability how they're feeling in research.*

Jacob: *I would say stay organized...I think one way to help people with disabilities in research is to organize into, maybe, set each topic in one page, one line, or...in one sentence...Let's say, [number 1]..."tools for the researcher". Number 2 is, "techniques", number 3, so, then researchers don't have to go back and forth... it will be more helpful and not overwhelming.*

Brendan agreed with Jacob about the importance of breaking down tasks and added the importance of having clear goals.

Brendan: *You have to have a step-by-step, you have to have kind of like, a super category....how can you get step-by-step goals...I can't set goals if I don't know what to do. Well, that should be part of research.*

9.4 Meeting Expectations

Co-creating and disseminating products that can positively impact the lives of community members are important ethical responsibilities in community-engaged research. Brendan, Micah, and Jacob all talked about enjoying being a part of making sense of research data and sharing it with others.

Brendan: *You invited me to my school in the transition fair, [I] talked about what I've done at my school. That was very, very cool for me to learn.*

Micah, however, talked about how difficult it would be if a project team lead does not fully meet their responsibility of widely sharing co-created materials.

Micah: *I would say other projects that, sometimes, if you do so much work and then you don't see the final project...it would be kind of sad. It would just make me sad if we did all this work, but we didn't show it out in the public. Like, some of the people in Boston, probably, would like to, probably, learn about or see the stuff that we have done. It's sad that all the work, would just be sitting somewhere, and it could be being used at conferences or at things to help people. It's hard to think about something like that happening.*

Micah emphasized how important it is that academic researchers meet expectations for the outcomes and potential impact of community engaged work. To prevent such experiences, Micah stressed the importance of understanding and agreeing on outcomes up front:

Micah: *If you're going to do research projects, maybe explain what the hope is that you will get out of it. You do all the work and then it's sits in the corner? Then nothing comes from it? Explain if you do it, you're hoping that you can share with other people than having it sit in a back-on a computer and, and you can't share with anyone. Maybe, making sure that people sign a contract or sign something to make sure that you know what you're doing.*

9.5 Conclusions

Meeting ethical responsibilities to community researchers and their communities is necessary in community-engaged research and may require academic researchers to adjust the ways they meet this responsibility for different communities. In working with communities of people with developmental disabilities, community researchers Brendan, Micah, and Jacob emphasize the importance of creating a team dynamic that creates a genuine sense of belonging and fosters respect and meaningful inclusion. They shared how building strong personal relationships, providing disability accommodations, and following through on promises to co-create products that can positively impact people with developmental disabilities are some ways to foster this positive environment. In our conversation, Brendan, Micah, and Jacob shared that their long-term involvement in community-engaged research and relationships with research team members has helped them grow; they have learned new things and now feel more confident in sharing their views and expertise. Through their involvement in community-engaged research they have also developed new relationships and experienced new opportunities within and beyond research projects.

People with developmental disabilities are part of a large population experiencing health disparities *and* are also members of other populations (e.g., gender, ethnic, religious, and sexual minorities, people living in poverty, etc.) that experience health disparities. Given the power of community-engaged research, we hope more community-engaged research teams worldwide will create a space at their table for communities of people with developmental disabilities.

Acknowledgements Thank you to all of our research partners on the following teams: Project ETHICS, Research Ethics for All: Research Ethics Training for Patient Stakeholders with Intellectual and Developmental Disabilities, and the Inclusive Cool Cats (Developing the Pediatric Evaluation of Disability Inventory-Patient Reported Outcome, PEDI-PRO).

Funding and Conflicts of Interest This work was supported in part by the Eunice Kennedy Shriver National Institute of Child Health & Human Development of the National Institutes of Health under Award Number R21HD075078 (PI McDonald), the Patient-Centered Outcomes Research Institute (PCORI; EASC-IDD-00301 Co-Leads McDonald and Schwartz), National Center Medical Rehabilitation Research, National Institute of Child Health and Human Development/National Institute Neurological Disorders and Stroke, National Institutes of Health K12 HD055931 (PI Kramer), and Eunice Kennedy Shriver National Institute of Child Health and Human Development of the National Institutes of Health R41HD090772, 2R42HD090772-03A1 (PI Kramer).

The content is solely ours and does not necessarily represent the official views of the National Institutes of Health.

The authors have no conflicts of interest to report.

Bibliography

Academic Publications

Bigby, C., Frawley, P., & Ramcharan, P. (2014). Conceptualizing inclusive research with people with intellectual disability. *Journal of Applied Research in Intellectual Disabilities, 27*(1), 3–12.

Garcia-Iriarte, E., Kramer, J. C., Kramer, J. M., & Hammel, J. (2009). "Who did what?": A participatory action research project to increase group capacity for advocacy. *Journal of Applied Research in Intellectual Disabilities, 22*, 10–22.

McDonald, K. E., & Stack, E. (2016). You say you want a revolution. An empirical study of community-based participatory research with people with developmental disabilities. *Disability and Health, 9*(2), 201–207.

Nicolaidis, C., Raymaker, D., Kapp, S. K., Baggs, A., Ashkenazy, E., McDonald, K., et al. (2019). The AASPIRE practice-based guidelines for the inclusion of autistic adults in research as co-researchers and study participants. *Autism, 23*(8), 2007–2019.

Raymaker, D. M. (2017). Reflections of a community-based participatory researcher from the intersection of disability advocacy, engineering, and the academy. *Action Research, 15*(3), 258–275.

Schwartz, A. E., & Durkin, B. (2020). "Team is everything": Reflections on trust, logistics and methodological choices in collaborative interviewing. *British Journal of Learning Disabilities, 48*(2), 115–123.

Schwartz, A. E., Kramer, J. M., Cohn, E. S., & McDonald, K. E. (2019). "That felt like real engagement": Fostering and maintaining inclusive research collaborations with individuals with intellectual disability. *Qualitative Health Research, 30*(2), 236–249.

Web-Based Resources

Inclusive Research Network: https://www.inclusiveresearch.net/

The Academic Autistic Spectrum Partnership in Research and Education (AASPIRE): https://aaspire.org/

Toolkit for Remote Inclusive Research: https://yell.ot.phhp.ufl.edu/research/engaging-in-research-during-emergencies/toolkit-for-remote-inclusive-research/

Brendan Durkin lives in Newton, MA, and has been doing research for 9 years at Boston University. Brendan is well-known in the Boston area for his public speaking at universities and various organizations such as the Massachusetts Down Syndrome Congress.

Micah Fialka-Feldman holds a Certificate in Disability Studies from Syracuse University and is an Outreach Coordinator at the Taishoff Center and a Teaching Assistant in the School of Education. He is also a national speaker, self-advocate and pioneer who fights for disability justice and inclusion. Micah previously served on the President's Committee for People with Intellectual Disabilities.

Jacob Myers lives in Massachusetts and works at Whole Foods. He has been involved in research for 10 years at Boston University and MGH Institute of Health Professions. He is an EPIC Service Leader for the Boston Chapter of Empowering People for Inclusive Communities (EPIC). In this role, he gives back to his community, advocates for disability rights, and helps lead other young adults with disabilities in community service projects.

Ariel Schwartz is a Research Assistant Professor committed to advancing knowledge about the use of inclusive/participatory research approaches with individuals with intellectual and developmental disabilities. She actively partners with young adults with intellectual and developmental disabilities to study participation and wellness for transition age young adults.

Katherine McDonald is an Associate Dean of Research and Professor of Public Health. Katie uses socio-ecological theory and community-engaged research to understand and promote the inclusion of individuals with disabilities with an emphasis on ethical, legal, and social issues in research with adults with developmental disabilities and disability-based disparities. Katie is a Fellow of the American Association on Intellectual and Developmental Disabilities (AAIDD), Chair of Syracuse University's Institutional Review Board, and a member of the Editorial Board for Autism in Adulthood.

Chapter 10
Community Conversations about Culturally Responsive Health Research for African American Communities

Adina Black, Millicent Robinson, Paige Castro-Reyes, Al Richmond, Latajah Lassus, and Nancy Shore

10.1 Introduction

As we witness persistent health disparities in the United States (US), the need for cultural responsiveness in health research and policies is increasingly recognized. Cultural responsiveness is one of many terms used to highlight the importance of being sensitive, appropriate, safe, competent, and respectful of the behavior, norms, knowledge, beliefs, arts, laws, customs, capabilities, and practices of individuals belonging to a shared group. Cultural responsiveness in action requires acknowledging that these aspects influence delivery, navigation, and acceptance of services, interactions, and outcomes (Federation of Saskatchewan Indian Nations, 2013; Sasakamoose et al., 2017). Research on health disparities demonstrates that cultural diversity, inclusion, competency, and acknowledgement of individuals and their cultural frameworks are required for improved health outcomes (Purnell & Fenkl, 2019). In marginalized communities that have historically been harmed by powerful institutions, the implementation of culturally responsive approaches is pivotal.

A. Black · P. Castro-Reyes · A. Richmond
Community-Campus Partnerships for Health (CCPH), Raleigh, NC, USA

M. Robinson
School of Social Work, University of North Carolina, Chapel Hill, NC, USA

L. Lassus
Clark Atlanta University, Atlanta, GA, USA

N. Shore (✉)
Community-Campus Partnerships for Health (CCPH), Raleigh, NC, USA

Social Work, University of New England, Portland, ME, USA
e-mail: nshore@une.edu

E. E. Anderson (ed.), *Ethical Issues in Community and Patient Stakeholder–Engaged Health Research*, Philosophy and Medicine 146,
https://doi.org/10.1007/978-3-031-40379-8_10

Racism is a determinant of health status; it impacts behaviors, attitudes, and access to healthcare. Racism against African Americans in the US has been a persistent contributor to health disparities and inequities, resulting in a disproportionate burden of cardiovascular disease, HIV, and kidney disease and other illnesses in African Americans (Chinn et al., 2021). For example, African Americans have the highest rates of diabetes and cardiovascular disease mortality (Erves et al., 2016; Wright & Merritt, 2020). These persistent health inequities are also costly for the US economy. According to a recent report from the Joint Center for Political and Economic Studies, health disparities cost an estimated $400 billion annually. Anderson (2012) suggests that doing nothing comes with a human and financial cost that we as a society cannot continue to bear. This requires further research.

Policies such as the federal regulations for the protection of human participants in research (45 CFR 46) do not fully account for cultural considerations, nor do they provide the necessary guidance to ensure culturally responsive practices (Shore et al., 2015). While guidelines and recommendations from professional organizations exist to supplement federal guidance, effective approaches require a deeper understanding of community and a commitment to action to address persistent disparities and poor outcomes (Ihara, 2019).

For over a decade, Community-Campus Partnerships for Health (CCPH) has listened to diverse communities across the US to better understand what culturally responsive research and health care looks like. Lessons learned underscore the importance of trust, transparency, and equitable partnership approaches (CCPH, 2017). Building on previous work and through a community-academic partnership with the University of New England, CCPH engaged representatives of four ethnic communities—Black/African Americans, Native Hawaiians, Latino/a/x, and Hmong in a series of listening sessions and a community forum to develop recommendations for strategies to enhance culturally responsive research. This chapter reports lessons learned from CCPH-facilitated listening sessions with members of the African American community in North Carolina.

10.2 Methods

The team constructed an interview guide informed by a review of the literature and from the team's previous work. This included interview questions based upon core concepts of the Research Partnership Checklist, the Healing by Heart Model for Culturally Responsive Health Care, and the National Collaborative Study Team's proposed core competencies for researchers (Shore et al., 2015; University of Minnesota, 2021; Vawter et al., 2003). Topics covered included (1) experiences with research, both positive and negative, (2) reasons for participating or not in research, (3) benefits and risks of research, and (4) strategies to enhance cultural responsiveness of research.

The project team created an email invitation for the listening sessions to include individuals who had experience as a researcher, study participant, and/or observer of research within one's ethnic community. The invite underscored how participation was voluntary and that the project was part of a community engagement award intended to enhance the cultural responsiveness of research. CCPH recruited individuals based upon existing relationships enhanced by snowball recruitment. University of New England's institutional review board (IRB) determined the research to be exempt. The full report from all listening sessions and community forums is available on CCPH's website (ccphealth.org).

CCPH facilitated two listening sessions in North Carolina, inviting former and current research partners who were also asked to identify additional participants. A total of 15 individuals participated across the two listening sessions. Attendees included experienced community researchers, case managers, consultants, health educators, and college students. Participants were asked to consider their experiences as study participants, members of research teams, and/or their observations of research within their communities.

Members of the project team facilitated conversations, which ranged from 60–90 minutes. The conversations were recorded with participants' permission and transcribed. Members of the project team conducted thematic analysis by independently coding transcripts line by line using Dedoose, a cross-platform app for qualitative data analysis (Salmona et al., 2020). The team members discussed the coding decisions and one member took the lead in drafting a report of the findings. This draft was then reviewed by other team members and discussions occurred to finalize the report.

10.3 Findings

The select findings from the listening sessions are organized around four overarching themes associated with researchers learning from and relating respectfully to people from African American cultures: reasons for not wanting to be involved in research, community benefits of research, community risks of research, and culturally responsive research. These themes inform recommendations presented in the conclusion for developing and sustaining culturally responsive approaches.

10.3.1 Reasons for Not Wanting to Be Involved in Research

Participants voiced many reasons why they do not want to get involved in research, primarily focusing on reasons they would not want to be a study participant. These reasons were framed both in terms of potential individual-level harm as well as concerns about lack of community benefit. Participants acknowledged historical trauma that has fostered a multigenerational distrust between members of the African American community and researchers. Participants discussed that members of their communities are hesitant to get involved with research because of this distrust. Key reasons for not wanting to be involved in research include past harms, inadequate explanation of research, and the absence of African Americans on the research team.

Listening session participants cited the US Public Health Service-sponsored Syphilis Study in Tuskegee and other ethical violations as specific factors contributing to distrust in research and hesitation to participate in research. Historically, research involving African Americans has benefited other communities without concern for African Americans and has caused significant harm to individual research participants and African American communities.

Distrust is further exacerbated when researchers are not transparent and do not clearly communicate relevance and purpose of the research. Participants described experiences of being recruited for research where they did not receive sufficient information regarding what the research would include, what it was for, and who would benefit. As one participant shared:

> I think people always think back to the Tuskegee experiment and not having all of the information. So the trust factor is definitely, I would think is probably the highest ranking reason why people don't wanna do it. Um and also because when you think of the word "research" alone, a lot of us look at it as us being guinea pigs as if we're being tested um for the benefit of somebody else. So …we don't think about it necessarily benefiting us. We think about it benefiting other people. You know whether that be another culture or whether that's our culture but later on down the line. So, we won't see it. And so those are some of the things that I've heard about research.

Additionally, research team composition influences participants' willingness to be involved in research. Participants noted that most individuals and groups conducting research within their community and providing the funding to do so do not look like them, which diminishes their trust. This exacerbates participants' fears that the information they provide to researchers could be used against them and members of their communities:

> Depending on who is presenting the research project—if it's someone that looks like me, I trust you a whole lot more than our counterparts so and generally you know from what I've seen, those are people who are in charge of the research project.

10.3.2 Community Benefits of Research

Participants spoke about not only the importance of addressing potential community concerns but also the importance of ensuring community benefits such as building community capacity. This included research that creates jobs for community members and boosts the local economy as well as increases access to needed resources.

As part of building community capacity, participants identified raising community awareness about research as a collective benefit that could result from research involvement. Several participants expressed that their respective communities did not have a lot of knowledge regarding research in general, why it is important, and how findings are used. In considering health research, participants believed that raising awareness of health issues prevalent within the African American community would help improve outcomes for their communities. For example, one participant shared her story of being diagnosed with diabetes. She firmly believes that if she had been provided education earlier regarding diabetes, things may have been different for her:

> I just feel like for things like sickle cell and diabetes, it's so prevalent in the African American community. Don't nobody tell us about it till we get it. So, and like then that's when the research comes. The research needs to happen before so we can know how to prevent it. Like pre-diabetes is a thing. Like somebody needs to tell them "oh you're ten, maybe you should be looking up what this means" or how to live an active life. Like they tell you you should be active, they don't tell you why. They just say to be healthy. Okay, what's healthy? It's just like "What is that?". Okay I guess I'll go outside for 60 minutes.

The potential for research to help future generations was also considered a community benefit that may increase the likelihood of people choosing to participate in a given research project. As one person shared:

> Because they're hoping that it'll help the next generation in terms of whatever the health disparity is that you're focusing on, the research is focusing on. Hoping that it'll help you know come up with an answer or cure for things like cancer or HIV or something like that. So, I think that is what compels people to do it.

Another participant spoke to how increased awareness can result in improved health outcomes as well as fostering a sense of community empowerment:

> I think that for our community, participating in research could empower us to empower other people in our community to be part of it...oftentimes we are under-represented in clinical trials in the forms of research anyway. So, if we aren't there, then they are doing research on what looks like most of America, until a few years from now. And so what treatment might work for them might not work for us.

10.3.3 Community Risks of Research

Several community risks were noted during the listening sessions. Exploitation of African American communities was a key concern. Participants expressed that they already know what is wrong with their communities and that too often research is not providing new information for them. These individuals provided examples of how researchers have entered their communities and extracted information from the community that does not help the community. At times this comes from the research not being applicable to the community or the researchers not sharing findings and following up with the community:

> Biggest risk is being exploited. Someone comes out and does all this wonderful research but the product is nothing that you can use as a community member but they made money through that process of doing that research. So, it's just like where's the equitability there...so some community members will lose trust in the research process especially when researchers are constantly coming out and saying issues that they already knew were there.

> Like saying there's hog waste in my well so now you are telling me I have health problems because of it. I already have asthma, I already have all these problems. I already knew this. And nothing comes of that research as well. So, it's just like why are you doing this.

Additionally, stigmatization surfaced as a potential risk of research involvement. Simply targeting a community for research can create stigma as can the framing of findings. Participants discussed instances of research overly focused on deficits that too often resulted in researchers further stereotyping their community:

> I know for our community because we have a very high prevalence of chronic diseases, some of the people feel like we are forever stigmatized or we are always being looked at as a community that has so many issues in a negative way. And so we want to be perceived as a positive community or something...when will we have research that magnifies some of the good qualities that we have?

Researchers' lack of cultural understanding was identified as a factor increasing community-level risks. Participants felt that researchers who are not themselves African American lack insight into the culture and do not truly understand the African American community. Compounding the issue, participants believed that once information is obtained from African Americans, it can be misinterpreted due to willful negligence stemming from structural racism where researchers impose a dominant cultural perspective and fail to understand community experiences and beliefs:

> So with looking the same, say you were Caucasian, and you were to ask me about the African American community, you're not going to understand what I'm saying because you're not from that community. You can get the gist of it and be like 'oh okay, I see what you mean.' But you're not going to understand.
>
> Getting the information back to us. It's like if you not African American or someone of our skin tone, it's hard for us to get the information, like the right information back to us cause somebody done watered it down, mixed it up then put something else in there. It's like if I tell her a secret, and it gets back to me, it ain't gone be the same. Just need to be informed.

10.3.4 Culturally Responsive Research

Participants identified research-related factors that made them feel that researchers respect their culture. In part, this requires researchers listening to the community and addressing the identified community risks and benefits cited above. Responsive research also requires being respectful and transparent. Participants want researchers to be honest about their purpose, goals, and who they are, or as one participant shared, "Don't put up a façade. Just be you." Participants also felt that honesty in the beginning of the project is necessary to establish a relationship of trust. Researchers should be honest about who will benefit from the research and what form those benefits will take. By establishing transparency in the beginning, researchers enable community members to participate how they choose, and this may help to recruit others:

> People lose trust. But, to build trust is to be respectful to our gender, culture, and religion. Be respectful of everything. Be forthcoming with information. Be open in presenting to what the research is. How will it benefit the individual, the community, or whoever it is that you are working with? That way, not only do they get the research done, but they get the participants helping to bring in other people into the study. They can help with the recruitment. You can turn your study subjects into really owning the research.

Respectful communication requires that researchers resist making assumptions. For example, statistics that say that all African Americans are at high risk of a chronic disease should not have more weight than community-identified research priorities. As one person shared:

> I think also finding out what their needs are. You may have statistics saying there is a higher rate of whatever, but the folks in the community, that may not be a concern of theirs. Like diabetes. We may say, if we have more fresh fruit, fresh food available, and have more education, this may decrease diabetes. But if you came up in an environment where everybody in your family had it, you are just assuming that you are going to have it, that's not a real concern of yours.

Participants also expressed that they wanted verification that research was properly vetted by an IRB and that researchers working in their community are properly trained to ensure effective, ethical, and sound research. Such assurances provide comfort and ease of mind in engaging with the research team. Researcher training also shows respect for the fact that African American participants have valid reasons for mistrusting researchers due to historical abuses and exploitation:

> Finding some way to show the participants that you are credible is needed. It's a checks and balances system. You can't just come up to the school and be like, "hey, I'm here to do research." For what? Who are you? Where did you come from? You can't just pop up. It's a thing of credibility.

Participants also discussed the importance of recognizing the humanity of African Americans across the continuum of care. Researchers can demonstrate respect for African American culture by acknowledging that the community is made up of people with human rights and dignity. As African Americans, when they seek out assistance, they do not want to feel disrespected or stereotyped. They want researchers to understand and be mindful and considerate of cultural and lived experiences. This also includes acknowledging within the Black community that culture varies by beliefs, religion, and location. This acknowledgement highlights cultural differences across the diaspora:

> Just realize that people, researchers, doctors, whomever, you have to realize that people are human, regardless of who they are, what culture they come from, what color they are. They are human beings and they should be treated as such. You would not like nobody coming to your office and disrespecting you when you're trying to help them. Well they are coming for help, and they don't want you disrespecting them, belittling them, because of who they are or whatever culture they come from.

> Understand the culture for yourself in the area in which you plan to research...know we are different pockets...culture will differ from pocket to pocket (area) and going out and embracing that.

For research to be truly culturally responsive research, participants also spoke to the need for researchers to understand African American culture, for example, African American intergenerational cultural norms. When researchers enter the community with their own ideas and priorities, they should be mindful and respectful of cultural beliefs and practices that may conflict with these ideas and priorities. Participants cautioned that cultural practices will not change just because researchers believe they should. Researchers can make suggestions but cannot force change in the community. As one participant shared:

> "There are cultural norms that have been around forever. So, making sure that we don't go in telling people what to do but advising what we feel are some of the best practices because you will get resistance real quick from the older people."

10.4 Discussion

Based upon the listening sessions, key strategies recommended to enhance the cultural responsiveness of research are outlined here:

1. *Do not approach the Black community as a monolith.* Researchers must acknowledge the cultural differences across the diaspora and not assume all Black people identify as African American. Researchers should instead recognize how culture varies across generations and regions, among other factors. This requires researchers to recognize what culture means to the engaged community and how it is expressed.
2. *Develop researcher competencies.* Listening session participants identified numerous researcher competencies to increase culturally responsive practices. These included being honest, transparent, respectful, and authentic. Associated with these competencies is the need for researchers to resist making assumptions, become more culturally aware, and recognize reasons for why African Americans may want, or not, to participate in research.
3. *Diversify research teams.* Participants spoke at length about the value of diversifying research teams and ensuring members identify with the community in order to increase the likelihood of cultural understanding and to facilitate trust building. Several listening session participants spoke to the connection between enhancing culturally responsive research practices, trust building and improved research approaches. As one participant shared, ensuring researcher competencies does not necessarily translate to culturally responsive practices, underscoring the importance of diverse research teams.
4. *Spend time in the community to build rapport.* This requires taking time to develop a relationship and build trust. For some of the participants, this best occurs within equitable community-academic partnerships. To build trust, researchers should establish deep and lasting ties with the community, community members should be included on the research team, and the research approach should be comprehensive of African American cultural norms and preferences.

These factors are central to enhancing culturally responsive research and thus critical to protecting research participants.

5. *Ensure community benefits.* As participants pointed out, too often research is not community driven nor does it benefit the community. Across both listening sessions, participants instead spoke to how historically, research done on African Americans is experienced as exploitative, is overly deficit focused, and fails to address community identified priorities.
6. *Engage the community beyond research participation.* Participants spoke to how their communities want to help and have the experiences and wisdom to do so. The community knows their needs and can present the best practices to help their own community in a collaborative effort. Engagement also honors how communities want ownership of the research.

These recommendations echo prior research regarding engaging African American communities and resonate with what we (the authors) continue to witness (Braithwaite & Warren, 2020; Cooks et al., 2015; Erves et al., 2016; Lima et al., 2020; Nuriddin et al., 2020; Stein, 2017). African American communities are vulnerable and still reeling from historical trauma and abuse from research and healthcare institutions. Researchers need to acknowledge exploitation and mistrust that has developed from past treatment and honor the voices, the wisdom, the individualism within, and the priorities of the communities with whom they conduct their research. For example, listening session participants emphasized how culturally responsive research requires a critical understanding of the geo-political context, including the existence of structural inequities that have become even more apparent during COVID-19. Community-based research review processes may be one means of effectively vetting research proposals for cultural considerations. Though cultural considerations may fall outside the scope of routine institution-based IRB practices, community review processes can provide a "regulatory plus" review that better accounts for cultural and regulatory considerations in the review of research proposals (Shore et al., 2011, 2015). (See Chaps. 19 and 20, in this volume.)

Another important finding was the need to highlight experiences of members across the Black diaspora, which includes African descendants not identifying as African American. According to the U.S. Census Bureau (2021), millions of people who identify as being of African descent live in the US, with an ever-increasing number being foreign-born individuals from African or Caribbean nations. The experiences of Black individuals can be dramatically different depending on their national and racial heritage. It is dangerous, harmful, and disrespectful not to acknowledge these differing experiences across the diaspora. It is important to recognize the obstacles faced by those identifying as Black are not the same as that of the African American community, and that these individuals should not be forced to fit their story and experiences within the narratives shared by the African American community (Wallerstein & Duran, 2010). This finding was presented in the listening sessions as participants expressed differences within African American culture depending on other cultural factors such as location and religion.

10.5 Conclusion

While this chapter reports findings from just two listening sessions held in North Carolina, findings align with many of the values and principles of community-based participatory research (CBPR) (Israel et al., 1998). The listening session participants' recommendations echo CBPR principles that building and sustaining trustworthy relationships between communities and institutions is central to conducting culturally responsive research. A sense of distrust and concern, however, should not be seen as opposing research but rather highlighting the critical need for responsive research that addresses community priorities and concerns. The listening session participants' recommendations, stemming from their concerns about and desires for research, align with the study team's recommendation for core capacities that researchers should demonstrate as they engage with communities: humility, relational integrity, and accountability (Castro-Reyes et al., 2015). The ideas expressed by participants further align with other values and principles of CBPR, including translating findings into action that results in community benefits (Israel et al., 1998; Livingston & Pierce, 2013).

Regarding the understanding of cultural differences across Black communities, a need for similar processes that identify how to increase engagement of these other ethnic groups through culturally responsive approaches is highlighted. After all, these communities are often included in data that highlights Blacks as having disparate health outcomes, yet there is no distinction between African Americans and other communities across the diaspora. The COVID-19 pandemic, for example, did not create, but further exacerbated pre-existing structural inequities within the United States. Yet health data continue to problematically lump all of these communities under one category called "Black."

As the public health sector continues to mobilize against the COVID-19 pandemic, we must listen to communities and center their experiences to ensure culturally responsive approaches that address community identified priorities and concerns and attempt to resolve persistent inequities. We see this work that breaks down active structures that continue to result in poor health outcomes in Black and African American communities, and that also utilizes voices and stories from these communities to reconstruct systems that will yield effective and sustainable outcomes, as ongoing and simultaneous. We must rebuild the house as we dismantle it.

Acknowledgements This chapter would not have been possible without our entire study team and partners, Ahahui Malama I Ka Lokahi, SoLaHmo Partnership for Health and Wellness, and the University of New England. We thank the Native Hawaiian participants in Hawaii, African-American participants in North Carolina, Latino/a/x and Hmong communities in Minnesota for sharing their expertise and wisdom, and CCPH staff for their invaluable and informational insight.

Funding CCPH received a Patient-Centered Outcomes Research Institute Eugene Washington Community Engagement Award *(Patient Engagement: Enhancing Culturally Appropriate Research, Project Leads Alan Richmond & Nancy Shore, EA #6177)* to fund this work.

References

Anderson, K. M. (2012). Progress since 2000: Workshop summary. *How Far Have We Come in Reducing Health Disparities?* https://doi.org/10.17226/13383

Braithwaite, R., & Warren, R. (2020). The African American petri dish. *Journal of Health Care for the Poor and Underserved, 31*(2), 491–502. https://doi.org/10.1353/hpu.0.0026

Bureau, US Census. (2021). American Community Survey (ACS). *The United States Census Bureau*. Accessed 19 September https://www.census.gov/programs-surveys/acs/

Castro-Reyes, P., Cooks, J., Drew, E., Edwards, K., Freeman, E., Isaacs, M. L., & Wat, E. (2015). Research Ethics Reconsidered in the Context of Community-Engaged Research. Accessed September 20.

Chinn, J. J., Martin, I. K., & Redmond, N. (2021). Health equity among black women in the United States. *Journal of Women's Health, 30*(2), 212–219. https://doi.org/10.1089/jwh.2020.8868

Community-Campus Partnerships for Health. (2017). The convening journey: Facilitating patient & stakeholder engagement through partnerships. https://ccphealth.org/wp-content/uploads/2019/06/PCORI-Combined-Report-LKG.pdf

Cooks, J., Shore, N., Park, A., & Seifer, S. D. (2015). Galveston Island Community Research Advisory Committee: Gatekeepers for health and well-being for African-Americans in Galveston, TX. *CES4Health*. Accessed 19 September: http://www.ces4health.info

Erves, J. C., Mayo-Gamble, T. L., Malin-Fair, A., Boyer, A., Joosten, Y., Vaughn, Y. C., Sherden, L., Luther, P., Miller, S., & Wilkins, C. H. (2016). Needs, priorities, and recommendations for engaging underrepresented populations in clinical research: A community perspective. *Journal of Community Health, 42*(3), 472–480. https://doi.org/10.1007/s10900-016-0279-2

Federation of Saskatchewan Indian Nations. (2013). "Cultural Responsiveness Framework". Accessed on 19 September: http://allnationshope.ca/userdata/files/187/CRF%20-%20Final%20Copy.pdf

Ihara, E. (2019). Cultural competence in health care: Is it important for people with chronic conditions? *Health Policy Institute*. https://hpi.georgetown.edu/cultural/

Israel, B. A., Schulz, A. J., Parker, E. A., & Becker, A. B. (1998). Review of community-based research: Assessing partnership approaches to improve public health. *Annual Review of Public Health, 19*(1), 173–202. https://doi.org/10.1146/annurev.publhealth.19.1.173

Lima, K., Phillip, C. R., Williams, J., Peterson, J., Feldman, C. H., & Ramsey-Goldman, R. (2020). Factors Associated with Participation in Rheumatic Disease–Related Research among Underrepresented Populations: A Qualitative Systematic Review. *Arthritis Care & Research, 72*(10), 1481–1489. https://doi.org/10.1002/acr.24036

Livingston, M., & Pierce, L. (2013). Not all blacks are African American: The importance of viewing advisees as individuals in a culturally mosaic context. *The Mentor: Innovative Scholarship on Academic Advising., 15*. https://doi.org/10.26209/MJ1561284

Nuriddin, A., Mooney, G., & White, A. I. (2020). Reckoning with histories of medical racism and violence in the USA. *The Lancet, 396*(10256), 949–951. https://doi.org/10.1016/s0140-6736(20)32032-8

Purnell, L. D., & Fenkl, E. A. (2019). Transcultural diversity and health care. In *Handbook for culturally competent care* (pp. 1–6). Springer.

Salmona, M., Lieberman, E., & Kaczynski, D. (2020). *Qualitative and mixed methods data analysis using Dedoose: A practical approach for research across the social sciences*. SAGE Publications.

Sasakamoose, J. L., Bellegarde, T., Sutherland, W., Pete, S., & McKay-McNabb, K. (2017). Miýo-Pimātisiwin developing indigenous cultural responsiveness theory (ICRT): Improving indigenous health and Well-being. *International Indigenous Policy Journal, 8*(4). https://doi.org/10.18584/iipj.2017.8.4.1

Shore, N., Brazauskas, R., Drew, E., Wong, K. A., Moy, L., Baden, A. C., Cyr, K., Ulevicus, J., & Seifer, S. D. (2011). Understanding community-based processes for research ethics review: A National Study. *American Journal of Public Health, 101*(S1). https://doi.org/10.2105/ajph.2010.194340

Shore, N., Park, A., Castro, P., Cooks, J., Freeman, E., Isaacs, M. L., Sablan-Santos, L., Wat, E., Drew, E., & Seifer, S. D. (2015). A National Collaborative Study of Community-Based Processes for Research Ethics Review. *Community Engaged Scholarship for* Health. Accessed 19 September. http://www.ces4health.info/find-products/view-product.aspx?code=YGTTLYZH

Stein, R. (2017). Troubling history in medical research still fresh for Black Americans. *NPR*. Accessed 19 September. https://www.npr.org/sections/health-shots/2017/10/25/556673640/scientists-work-to-overcome-legacy-of-tuskegee-study-henrietta-lacks

University of Minnesota. (2021). Tools & Resources. *Clinical and Translational Science Institute.* Accessed 19 September https://ctsi.umn.edu/services/community-engagement/tools-resources

Vawter, D. E., Culhane-Pera, K. A., Babbitt, B., Xiong, P., & Solberg, M. M. (2003). A model for culturally responsive health care. *Healing by Heart*, 297–356. https://doi.org/10.2307/j.ctv16h2nfv.23

Wallerstein, N., & Duran, B. (2010). Community-based participatory research contributions to intervention research: The intersection of science and practice to improve health equity. *American Journal of Public Health, 100*(S1), S40–S46. https://doi.org/10.2105/ajph.2009.184036

Wright, J. E., & Merritt, C. C. (2020). Social equity and Covid −19: The case of African Americans. *Public Administration Review, 80*(5), 820–826. https://doi.org/10.1111/puar.13251

Adina Black has years of experience in community engagement work collaborating with organizations and key stakeholders to build relationships with academic, clinical, and professional partners in their journeys to become more responsive to their communities' needs. She serves as a consultant with non-profits, academic institutions, and researchers to develop and execute strategies related to engaging community leaders, building community capacity, and improving community outcomes.

Millicent Robinson is a postdoctoral research fellow through the Carolina Postdoctoral Program for Faculty Diversity. She earned her PhD in Community Health Sciences from the Jonathan and Karin Fielding School of Public Health at UCLA, and her BA, MSW, and MPH from UNC-Chapel Hill. Millicent's research agenda integrates theories and perspectives from Social Work, Public Health, African, African American, and Diaspora Studies, and Medical Sociology to address four key issues: (1) interconnections between mental and physical health, (2) culturally-relevant forms of coping, (3) complementary and alternative medicine, and (4) ethnic heterogeneity among Black women.

Paige Castro-Reyes joined CCPH in 2013 upon graduating from the University of Washington and now serves as deputy director. She completed a BS in Biology and a BA in International Studies: Comparative Religion. Paige served as project coordinator for multiple multi-partner projects focused on community engagement, ethics of research, and culturally responsive research practices. These projects included planning and facilitating virtual and in-person convenings centered on patient and community engagement and were funded by the National Institute of Environmental Health Sciences, the Robert Wood Johnson Foundation, the Patient Centered Outcomes Research Institute, and the Greenwall Foundation. Paige brings her unique lived and learned experience as a mestisa CHamoru woman to her work.

Al Richmond is executive director of CCPH and is a global thought leader advocating for the increased role of communities in research and public health. Al is advancing CCPH's commitment to social justice and health equity. His work includes creating guidelines for the conduct of community engaged research and serving as principal investigator on projects focused on patient engagement, community-engaged research ethics and health disparities. He has harnessed the organization's network to provide leadership at the national level in response to the COVID19 pandemic.

Latajah Lassus recently graduated from Clark Atlanta University with her Bachelor of Arts in Psychology. She is a scholar, creative, and social advocate. Her work in psychology aims to serve underrepresented and underserved communities such as African Americans, immigrants and LGBTQ+ individuals. She is using creative outlets like poetry, dance, music and visual arts to cultivate safe spaces for these communities to express themselves and cope with their spiritual, mental, and physical health challenges.

Nancy Shore is a professor and senior consultant for CCPH. In partnership with community groups and organizations, Nancy works toward strengthening community-engaged research ethics, enhancing culturally responsive research practices, reducing educational disparities, and fostering equitable philanthropic practices.

Chapter 11
The Power of Personal Narrative: My Experience with SACHRP, the FDA, and Bioethics

Gianna McMillan

"How important is this invitation?" I asked the administrator of my institutional review board (IRB). She had recruited me 3 years previously to serve as a community member on the UCLA committee and had become my mentor in the new (to me) world of research ethics. "I mean, in the context of the field, is this a big deal?"

"This is a very big deal, Gigi," she said. "An invitation to SACHRP is the best invitation anyone can get."

I learned that SACHRP—the Secretary's Advisory Committee for Human Research Protection—advises the Secretary of Health and Human Services (HHS) on issues related to the protection of human research participants (SACHRP Committee, 2016). This Secretary was a cabinet member—an advisor to the President of the United States—so my friend was right, this opportunity was a big deal. I was intrigued but nervous.

Two months earlier, I had spoken at a conference about the research participant's perspective of an informed consent process. The lights on the stage had been blinding and my "Ps" popped into the microphone. I told the story of my then five-year-old son, his brain cancer, and the clinical trial that would test a lower-than-standard dose of radiation while adding a chemotherapy drug never before used in children. I remember sharing how difficult that decision was and choking up at the end when I thanked the research community for their efforts to save children like mine. It had been emotionally exhausting to relive my personal experiences, but the enthusiastic audience response kindled something in me, a whisper that grew louder in passing days, telling me I had a meaningful message that could help future research participants. This feeling was confirmed by subsequent invitations to speak, and now an

G. McMillan (✉)
Bioethics Institute, Loyola Marymount University, Los Angeles, CA, USA
e-mail: gianna.mcmillan@lmu.edu

E. E. Anderson (ed.), *Ethical Issues in Community and Patient Stakeholder–Engaged Health Research*, Philosophy and Medicine 146,
https://doi.org/10.1007/978-3-031-40379-8_11

invitation to serve on a new SACHRP subcommittee. It felt like I was hovering at the edge of river rapids—and I could jump in or retreat. I jumped.

11.1 Secretary's Advisory Committee for Human Research Protection

A new SACHRP subcommittee was formed in 2005. The charge was to examine Subpart A of 45 CFR 46 (also known as the Common Rule), which is the section of federal regulations about biomedical research with humans. We were to evaluate each phrase, and determine where modification might be required, new interpretation appropriate, or additional guidance offered. Quarterly meetings in Washington, DC, would be supplemented by conference calls in between.

My first meeting was in the Office for Human Research Protections (OHRP) in Rockville, Maryland. I remember how quiet it was and that the conference room smelled like a new car. The leadership was excellent, and the people gathered in the room were experts from all over the country—very smart people. I couldn't help but wonder, "What am I doing in a room with *these* people?" Imposter syndrome is when a person doubts their abilities, when they feel like a secret fraud despite their valid qualifications. Businesswomen talk about this when they break into male-dominated professions, and famous entertainers often admit their inner certainty that their lack of talent will be revealed at any moment. It is not surprising that lay people who are invited to advise scientists or other well-trained groups of practitioners also feel this way. We are the nobody-outsiders talking to the important-insiders, and despite our internal fist-pumping that, "Finally! I get to share my hard-won knowledge that will help other people," we secretly wonder what the experts could possibly learn from us. I felt this when I first joined the UCLA IRB but had grown into my role. This time I understood that SACHRP wanted my non-academic, non-scientific perspective, my insight as the caregiver of a research participant, and my experience as the parent of a child who had cancer. I knew my value but was still awe-struck.

There was no time to be self-conscious because there was immediate heavy lifting. The Subpart A subcommittee identified key topics to address, drafted a tentative schedule, and agreed on methods for communication, record keeping, and final work product. We had the luxury of as much time as needed to do a good job, something I did not appreciate as much as I should have. Those meetings—and that work—are among the most satisfying in my career. Many of the other members had collaborated before, so there was an easy, collegial atmosphere. I never felt like an outsider or "token" non-scientist member, but it took hard work to pull my own weight. This meant extra research on technical agenda items and finding the courage to request real-time explanations during discussions. My questions were welcomed because an issue that seems obvious to professionals but murky to a patient advocate indicated that there was a problem to be addressed. Some of the thoughtful explanations prompted by my questions inspired content for future recommendations.

The subcommittee painstakingly crafted guidance based on ethical practice, like the definitions of minimal risk and reasonable (and enforceable) parameters for consent forms. We also considered whether new segments of law needed to be written. The over-riding challenge was that 45 CFR 46 was known as the "Common Rule" because other federal agencies (now numbering 20) had agreed to honor the stipulations, making it law "in common" to all of them, so any changes in the text of the regulations required unanimous agreement from each of those agencies—a herculean proposal. This meant our subcommittee leaned heavily toward reinterpretation of existing wording (when needed) and proposing the development of new guidance documents. These constraints were frustrating, but we created a body of work to be proud of—more than 80 recommendations in my tenure. (Note: In 2011, there was an "Advanced Notice of Proposed Rule Making" regarding the Common Rule, which led to actual revision of regulatory text in 2018, which went into effect in 2019.)

I served 6 years on this committee, rotating off when family circumstances no longer accommodated the travel. I saw, first-hand, that when people from different fields and mindsets are brought together to untangle a problem or create a novel strategy, it is the interaction of distinct points of view that ultimately reveals the best answer. The perspectives of patients and the general population are crucial. Rules and guidance must logically address the lived reality of the people. Do the laws make sense? Are they explained in a way understandable to the people? Do they address the priorities of the population? With the SACHRP subcommittee, as with the IRB, I saw that well-intentioned experts sometimes operated at an altitude far above the normal citizen on the street, and usually appreciated reminders that theoretical conversations must have practical application. My self-confidence grew and I learned when to insist on my point. Consensus was not always easy, but it was always worth the energy and hugely satisfying.

11.2 U.S. Food and Drug Administration

Toward the end of my time on the SACHRP Subpart A subcommittee, I was invited to be a Patient Representative for the U.S. Food and Drug Administration (FDA). This program trains patients and caregivers about FDA mission and procedures and invites them to provide advice, based on their personal knowledge, to the agency as it regulates drugs and devices (About the FDA, 2018). A Patient Representative is called to service, on average, about once a year. On the SACHRP subcommittee, I was supposed to be objective but use my personal experience to identify themes for discussion and then create or evaluate public-friendly documents. As an FDA Patient Representative, specific events in my life were used like case studies. My personal experience was intended to influence the actual process of drug development. I was not supposed to present generalizable knowledge or be objective. I was just supposed to share my own narrow experience. It was an interesting switch to make.

I had grown accustomed to the easy (albeit focused) conference room atmosphere of SACHRP subcommittee deliberation, which sometimes included homemade baklava from good-hearted OHRP staff. FDA meetings were something else entirely. Imagine airport security in the lobby of FDA headquarters, and then walking through a concrete and glass campus to a cavernous room. The front was roped off and featured a huge horseshoe table, draped in black cloth and sporting microphones and name cards at each seat. There were huge television screens on all the walls and large video cameras pointed at various sections of the table. Transcribers and audio-visual technicians discretely worked from around the room. Those of us sitting at the large table faced the other half of the auditorium, which was lined with chairs for the visiting public, lobbyists, or other federal employees assigned to the proceedings. There were lots of people in uniform, and we were warned to avoid the press.

Each meeting included pharmaceutical company presentations, PowerPoint slides with FDA analysis, and public commentary. The committee asked questions after each stage, and then had lengthy public discussions before agreeing to vote or offer advice. I experienced cognitive dissonance. Asked to share my personal experience, I again struggled to feel worthy of the invitation. After a couple meetings, I realized that no matter how well-prepared I was, I was going to be nervous when it came time for me to speak. I learned to write down my comments so that jittery words fell from my mouth in the correct sequence. My contributions were best received when accompanied by an anecdote relating to my child's experience or what I knew others had experienced. This created pragmatic connections between the reality of patient life and the science under discussion. FDA staff, industry representatives, and other experts valued this perspective, and while I had to maneuver for airtime in the deliberation, this was not due to indifference but because *every* person at the meeting had something important to say.

An obvious theme from my time on IRBs, the SACHRP subcommittee, and as a Patient Representative at the FDA, is my insecurity about the value of my perspective, and my growing realization that my story needed to be framed correctly to be effective. From years as a patient advocate and parent support group leader, I knew that there were *healing* stories that tumbled into the world from trembling lips and that by being voiced, empowered and comforted the teller. This kind of personal narrative comes easily to most people and is a crucial part of processing life trauma. These stories can inspire empathy in others and an awareness of a common human element. Then there are *representative* stories where the speaker is the voice for a community, an example offered to the public of a citizen who has experienced a particular set of circumstances. These stories inspire conversation and problem-solving. Finally, there are *teaching* stories, where the experienced narrator weaves their plot points into an educational thrust, intended to initiate action. While no personal story is ever *wrong*, the intent and the context in which it is offered affects how listeners will respond. The experienced community representative in the research arena should strategize about how their input can be presented for maximum effect.

11.3 Bioethics

The public presentation I mentioned at the beginning of this essay showed me the usefulness of my own experiences. This was at a conference sponsored by PRIM&R (Public Responsibility in Medicine & Research). PRIM&R is a nonprofit organization whose mission is to ensure the highest ethical standards in research by providing education and other professional resources to the research and research oversight community (PRIM&R, 2022). Every year after that first presentation, even as I worked with SACHRP and the FDA, I was a PRIM&R panelist or session contributor. I became fascinated by the history of research ethics and began working on an oral history project about early leaders in the field of research ethics. I filmed, edited, and curated these videos on the PRIM&R website. In the space of 5 years, the project created over 500 video clips, and I was privy to more than 100 personal accounts of career paths and ethical reflection, spanning from the early days of the *Belmont Report* to present day challenges with genomic sequencing and biobanking. The journey of each research ethics professional was unique, but I saw patterns in thought, personal development, academic perspective, professional behavior, regulatory oversight, hospital policy, public response, and scientific advancement. Ethical issues related to risk, consent, sharing of results, resource allocation, and patient-engagement rang familiar with my own experience. My small-scale, real-life experiences of caring for a child with cancer, enrolling him in a clinical trial, leading parent support groups, becoming an IRB member, and advising regulatory committees were manifest, large-scale, in the timeline of the field. I got a real sense of how individual contributions of hundreds of thousands of research participants added to the momentum of scientific advancement, and in this way, we were partners with the researchers. It was gratifying to know that the hardships my child and family had undergone had been of tangible help.

I wanted to know more. What were the ethical theories that guided research ethics policies? Who created these? How did they affect the general population? Why, after so long, was I only beginning to learn about this side of an important event I had lived through? After 20 years as a civilian patient advocate, and with my youngest child grown, I went back to school for a Master of Arts degree in Bioethics and then continued for a Doctorate. It was challenging to be a student again, in my 50s, but I was uniquely positioned to absorb the theoretical and historical context of the subject matter, given my "in the trenches" understanding. In many ways, I was doing double the work of the other students, because I was learning new concepts and then reprocessing my life milestones according to this knowledge. When I was finally introduced to the academic journal *Narrative Inquiry in Bioethics*, I felt as though I had found the final piece to my puzzle.

Narrative Inquiry in Bioethics collects the personal stories of patients, caretakers, clinicians, and researchers about a health issue, and then invites relevant experts to read the collection and comment on the bioethical themes that are woven through the narratives (NIB, 2019). The typical reader is a healthcare provider, researcher, academic, or policymaker involved in health professional education, bioethics guidance, and clinical decision making. I was a guest editor for an issue of parent stories about caring for children with brain tumors and I saw, firsthand, how empowering it was for these families to share their life lessons in a way designed to help other caregivers, instruct healthcare professionals, educate the public, and promote key patient issues. For more than 20 years, patients and caregivers had been telling me that they were experts about their own experience with their disease, but they did not feel that doctors wanted to learn from them. In this academic journal, these voices are collected in a credible way, and experts analyze these narratives for knowledge. These collections can then be used by patient communities for education, advocacy, and fundraising. I had come, full circle, back to the power of storytelling—so I returned to the classroom one more time, for a Master's in Fine Arts in Creative Nonfiction.

11.4 The Power of Narrative

These days I teach Research Ethics at Loyola Marymount University in Los Angeles, serve on the FDA's Pediatric Advisory Committee and the board of PRIM&R, and am the Director of Community Engagement for *Narrative Inquiry in Bioethics*. I look back 27 years to when my child was first diagnosed with brain cancer and I see a life-upending event that set me on the path to family support programs, IRB work, regulatory committees, research ethics, and academic bioethical reflection. In each instance, my primary identity is that of patient advocate—but my understanding of how *to be* this, and what *to do with* it has expanded as the parameters of my participation grew larger. My community-voice on IRBs and government committees is enhanced by my understanding of bioethical principles and my ability to draw direct connection between the abstract theories and real-life events. By the same token, my scholarly reflection is grounded by vivid memories of struggling to communicate with healthcare providers and investigators. I see that success at each milestone hinged on communication, and this was based on storytelling.

Time and again, I have seen a well-told story bridge gaps in factual understanding, forge empathetic bonds, and inspire meaningful collaboration between parties who didn't, before, speak the same language. The best thing that community and patient research partners can do in *any* arena, is to tell their story, but the telling should be well-considered, appropriate, and carefully crafted. What is the message? Who is the audience? Is the intent to heal, represent, or teach? There is a craft to storytelling; it is a skillset that can be learned—and because the stories we offer have value, we should not be shy about the planning or strategies needed for the physical act of delivering our message. By honoring and respecting our own narrative with thoughtful preparation, we invite others to do likewise, creating opportunity for the best of ethical reflections.

References

About the FDA Patient Representative Program. (2018). U.S. Food & Drug Administration. https://www.fda.gov/patients/learn-about-fda-patient-engagement/about-fda-patient-representative-program

Narrative Inquiry in Bioethics (NIB). (2019). https://nibjournal.org/

Public Responsibility in Medicine and Research (PRIM&R). (2022). https://primr.org/

SACHRP Committee. (2016). U.S. Department of Health & Human Services. https://www.hhs.gov/ohrp/sachrp-committee/index.html

Gianna McMillan is the Associate Director of the Bioethics Institute. She is on the Board of Directors for PRIM&R (Public Responsibility in Medicine & Research) and a member of the FDA's Pediatric Advisory Committee. She is the Director of Community Engagement for *Narrative Inquiry in Bioethics.*

Part III
Unique Ethical Considerations

Chapter 12
Patient Advocacy Organizations and Conflicts of Interest in Research

Lisa Parker and Barbara Mintzes

12.1 Introduction

Patient advocacy organizations are non-profit groups, often with a charitable status, with important roles in advocacy for patient interests, support for patients and carers, and education for patients, carers, clinicians, and the wider public. Many patient organizations are also involved in research (Rose et al., 2017). Organizations may be local, regional, or national in scope, and umbrella groups exist at a regional or international level. Most patient organizations focus on specific conditions or body systems, such as diabetes or heart disease, while others have a broader patient rights perspective. Some groups aim to represent specific populations that have faced discrimination in health service provision, for example: women, older people, or those with mental health issues. In this chapter we use the term 'patient organization' to mean any and all of these groups.

Patient organization roles in research include: funding of research grants; supporting and informing academic and/or industry research; carrying out their own studies; recruiting participants for clinical trials and registries; advocacy for public funding and/or changes in research regulations; and informing members about research findings (Pinto et al., 2016; O'Donovan, 2007; Parker et al., 2021). Rose et al. (2017) surveyed over 200 US patient organizations and found that 80% reported participating in research and 40% provided funding for biomedical and clinical research. Some organizations position themselves solely as medical research charities (O'Donovan, 2007).

L. Parker (✉) · B. Mintzes
School of Pharmacy and Charles Perkins Centre, Faculty of Medicine and Health, The University of Sydney, Sydney, NSW, Australia
e-mail: lisa.parker@sydney.edu.au; barbara.mintzes@sydney.edu.au

E. E. Anderson (ed.), *Ethical Issues in Community and Patient Stakeholder–Engaged Health Research*, Philosophy and Medicine 146,
https://doi.org/10.1007/978-3-031-40379-8_12

Around the world there is enthusiasm for the inclusion of patients in research, with strong encouragement from governments and other research funding bodies (Patient-Centered Outcomes Research Institute (PCORI), 2022; National Health and Medical Research Council and Australia, 2016; National Institute for Health Research, 2020; Hoddinott et al., 2018; den Oudendammer et al., 2019). There are many reasons why biomedical research should include patient organizations (Epstein, 2008; Pinto et al., 2016; Terry et al., 2007). For example, people with lived experience of illness can usefully shape the direction of research, prompting researchers to focus on questions and treatment outcomes that are important to patients. Patient organizations can prompt a more person-focused research design, informing patients about their rights as study participants and striving for participant safety in a way that, historically, some researchers have neglected. They can also disseminate findings quickly to public audiences that might otherwise struggle to get access. At a philosophical level, involving patient organizations can be seen as the right thing to do simply because people are worthy of respect, and so the study of particular population groups should arguably involve representatives of those people.

Patient organizations have traditionally had grassroots origins, arising out of the needs and interests of patients and carers, and aimed at providing patient support, promoting targeted research, and upskilling members in consumer rights activism for patient and health services advocacy. Recently, however, patient organizations have become more dependent on commercial funding, leading to concerns that these financial ties could undermine their independence and ability to represent the interests of their members in research as well as other activities (O'Donovan, 2007; Parker et al., 2019a, b; Mulinari et al., 2020; McCoy et al., 2017; Batt, 2017; Moynihan & Bero, 2017).

12.2 What Are Conflicts of Interest?

Patient organizations that accept funding from companies with marketed products used within healthcare services, such as pharmaceutical and medical device companies, are at risk of altering their public views or behaviour in a way that aligns with their funders rather than their own institutional agenda. This may occur for a range of reasons, including unconscious biases, reliance on information materials provided by sponsors, and deliberate avoidance of positions that might alienate current or future funders. According to the widely used definition of conflict of interest in medicine, these organizations *at risk* are thus regarded as having a conflict of interest. The U.S. Institute of Medicine has defined conflicts of interest broadly as "circumstances that create a risk that professional judgments or actions regarding a primary interest will be unduly influenced by a secondary interest" (Institute of Medicine, 2009). For patient groups, the primary interest is to represent the membership; a potential secondary interest is to be aligned with commercial entities providing funding. Pharmaceutical and medical device companies have a duty to pursue profit and returns for shareholders, achieved through developing and marketing health care products and recouping costs in research investments via sales. These are important societal aims but are not necessarily always consistent with the aims of patients and healthcare users. The language we use here is precise. It perhaps differs from how a conflict of interest involving a politician is often reported in the press, where the story may be about wrongdoing or corruption, such as providing public funding for a project that flows to a family member. In this chapter, we are using conflict of interest to represent a situation *of risk*, and we acknowledge that not all of those risky situations will necessarily result in bias or in corrupt behaviour.

Patient organization and industry agendas do sometimes align. For example, patient groups may be interested in achieving regulatory approval or subsidy for new medicines or devices that they believe are important for their members (Parker et al., 2019a; Jones, 2008). However, interests may not always align, including in the context of product safety, pricing, global access, and restricting excessive marketing (Mulinari, 2016; O'Donovan, 2007; Parker et al., 2019a). As noted above, patient organization activities may be skewed towards industry interests for a number of reasons, including a need to secure funding. At an extreme, some patient organizations are called 'astroturf' groups, because instead of having 'grassroots' origins they were created directly or indirectly by a pharmaceutical company for the purpose of furthering industry interests (O'Donovan, 2007; Angell, 2004, 151). For example, the group 'Patients Rising' has been called an astroturf organization because it was founded by a corporate communications consultant, receives funding from major pharmaceutical companies, and has attacked critics of the high prices of newer cancer drugs (Perry, 2016).

A broader concern is that in most countries limited public funding is available to support the activities of patient organizations. This constrains the scope and size of organizations that do not have commercial funding. Organizations may have internal policies not to accept industry funding, or they may represent a health condition without drug or device treatments and are therefore of limited interest to commercial sponsors (Jones, 2008). In contrast, organizations that are of interest to companies can be offered substantial sums of money, and if a company's support for a patient organization both provides a tax break and a means to support increased sales, the company can afford to be quite generous. This imbalance in funding sources has created a patient organization sector dominated by the louder voices of larger, well-funded industry sponsored groups. This has implications for the sector as a whole; it fosters a slant towards industry-friendly advocacy, education, and research, with less of a focus on key issues that conflict with sponsors' interests, such as affordability of medicines or ensuring high regulatory standards for effectiveness and safety (Parker et al., 2019a).

What does this all mean for the involvement of industry-funded patient organizations in research? To explore this issue, we discuss the literature around pharmaceutical and medical device funding of patient organizations, and the evidence around industry funder influence over patient organization activities, including research, and over the sector as a whole. We conclude by discussing strategies to remove or reduce the influence of industry funders.

12.3 How Common Is Industry Funding of Patient Organizations?

Pharmaceutical and medical device companies commonly seek to fund patient organizations. These companies have a lot to gain or lose from what patient organizations say and do. Patient organizations have increasing power to affect sales of medicines and devices in many ways (Lofgren, 2004). This might include advocacy for government approval or subsidy (Edwards, 2017; Abola & Prasad, 2016; Applebaum, 2009); communication with patients and health providers about product benefits (or safety concerns); disease awareness (or disease mongering) campaigns (Moynihan & Henry, 2006; Jorgensen & Gotzsche, 2004; Applebaum, 2009); and support for particular research agendas and methodologies.

A systematic review of industry funding of patient organizations identified 15 studies that measured how often patient groups are funded by industry within a population or a systematic sample (Fabbri et al., 2020). Eight of these studies looked at funding rates for all patient groups within a country or other defined population in nine mostly high-income countries: the United States (US), United Kingdom (UK), Canada, Australia, South Africa, Finland, Spain, Ireland, and the Netherlands. Funding rates ranged from 43% to 83%. Another three studies focused on funding of patient groups representing a specific condition. They found a broader range of rates, from 20% for rare diseases to 30% for cancer, and 75% for breast cancer. Given the small number of studies and varied conditions and settings (US, Australia, and Italy), reasons for these differences remain unclear. The remaining four studies looked at industry funding rates among patient organizations that responded to specific public consultations or participated in an advisory group to a regulatory agency. Rates of industry funding ranged from 34% to 75% of these patient organizations. Overall, this systematic review found that the amount of industry funding varied greatly per patient organization, from a small proportion to almost the entire group's budget.

Public transparency about industry funding of patient organizations is poor. In Australia, the national pharmaceutical industry association, Medicines Australia (MA), has required its member companies to publish information on the MA website documenting all company funding to patient organizations since 2013. Using this data, Lau et al. (2018) examined a random sample of 130 patient organizations that were industry funded between 2013 and 2016. They found that only 68/130 (52%) organizations reported this funding on their websites or in annual reports posted on the website—and few organizations reported how much funding was provided or how much of the organization's income came from industry. Four earlier studies, carried out between 2008 and 2012, looked at how often industry-funded patient groups in Australia, Italy, the US, and the UK reported industry funding on their websites, finding that only 27% reported this funding (Fabbri et al., 2020). In general, this research shows that there is a need for more openness and transparency about industry funding of patient organizations.

In Australia, pharmaceutical companies provided AU$34.51 million to patient organizations from 2013 to 2016 (Fabbri et al., 2019). Many of the most highly funded organizations represented conditions for which the company had a recently approved drug and was seeking public reimbursement. This included Macular Disease Foundation Australia, which received AU$2.36 million from Bayer, manufacturer of aflibercept, a drug for macular oedema. Over the study period, Bayer submitted five applications for public subsidy relating to new uses of the drug, two of which were rejected and three accepted. Aflibercept was the fifth highest cost drug in 2016–2017 in terms of public reimbursement (Fabbri et al., 2019). Similarly, other patient organizations receiving top tier industry funding represented conditions for which sponsors had drugs under consideration for reimbursement. This study did not directly examine whether the patient organizations had written letters of support or in other ways advocated funding of their sponsors' drugs, as these submissions about funding decisions are considered confidential in Australia. However, this funding pattern strongly suggests such a link.

Similar to Australia, the UK Association of the British Pharmaceutical Industry (ABPI) has required member companies to report their funding to patient organizations since 2012. Mulinari et al. (2020) examined companies' funding between 2012 and 2016. They found that the value of this funding increased over this period, from £8.18 million to £20.96 million. They also noted the number of drug companies making payments to patient organizations increased from 30 to 45, and the number of organizations receiving payment jumped from 229 to 277. This suggests that links between pharmaceutical companies and patient organizations strengthened over this 5-year period. Funding was concentrated on a select few patient organizations, with the top-funded organization for each of 30 conditions receiving around two-thirds of funding.

Both in Australia and the UK, industry associations have taken an important step in making funding relationships between drug companies and patient organizations more transparent. This is especially important given the finding from other studies that only one quarter to one half of patient organizations with industry funding report this on their websites (Lau et al., 2018; Fabbri et al., 2020). However, these transparency reports have some limitations. In both countries, each company posts reports of its funding separately, rather than making them available in a single searchable database. In the US, companies' reports on funding of patient organizations are also only provided on their own websites, rather than being centralized (Rothman et al., 2011). These scattered reports make it much harder to find out whether a specific organization is industry-funded, how much it receives, or which companies fund it. In addition, some drug companies are not members of their national industry association and are therefore not bound by their local guidelines. For example, MundiPharma, the Australian arm of Purdue, the US manufacturer of

Oxycontin (fined alongside its parent company for misleading marketing practices) is not a member of Medicines Australia (Medicines Australia, 2021).

Public disclosure of a conflict of interest does not mean it has less influence than a secret conflict, but at least the person accessing an organization's website, attending an event, or reading an organization's materials or research reports can know that such a relationship exists. In contrast to these scattered and incomplete reports on funding of patient organizations, all drug company reports of payments to doctors in the US are legally required to be publicly available in a centralized searchable database, allowing anyone to easily find out how much money each doctor received, which companies were involved, and which drugs were being promoted (Agrawal et al., 2013). This level of transparency is very different from that available for patient organizations. There is a strong argument for the need for similar levels of transparency of patient organization funding, especially given patient organizations' roles in research and advocacy (Kanter, 2018).

12.4 Why Is Industry Funding of Patient Organizations a Concern?

Patient organizations speak openly about the benefits of industry funding. Many say that they would not be able to do the good work they do without it (Jones, 2008). Others talk about the usefulness of having access to current information on products and clinical trials (Parker et al., 2019a). However, there is also evidence that some patient organizations feel pressure from their commercial funders. For example, O'Donovan's in-depth study of Irish patient organizations described how the CEO of *Aware*, an organization focused on depression, was becoming increasingly wary about pharmaceutical funders after experiences of an industry sponsor that wanted 'bang for its buck' (O'Donovan, 2007, 724). Our own study with leadership staff from 23 Australian patient organizations similarly reported pressure from company sponsors over their organization's activities, including diversion of activities towards funder priorities and seeking to influence an organization's newsletter content (Parker et al., 2021).

There is also evidence that commercial funding correlates with patient organization advocacy in favour of industry interests (Public Citizen, 2016; Jorgensen & Gotzsche, 2004). For example, Lin et al. (2017) studied submissions commenting on draft US opioid guidelines. The proposed changes recommended more restricted opioid use in chronic noncancer pain, aimed at reducing potentially harmful use to decrease addiction and overdose deaths. More restricted prescribing of opioids in this cohort could reduce profits of opioid manufacturers. Of the 31 patient organizations making comments on these draft guidelines, over half of those with funding from opioid manufacturers opposed the changes, whereas the large majority of those without industry funding supported them.

In another example, Perehudoff and Alves (2011) found an association between pharmaceutical industry funding and patient organizations' positions on advertising regulations. Direct-to-consumer advertising of prescription medicine is only allowed in the US and New Zealand. When this type of advertising took off in the 1990s and early 2000s, especially in the US, other countries were under pressure to change their laws to allow it. The European Commission introduced an initiative to allow advertising for diabetes and AIDS drugs in 2002, but it was voted down by the European Parliament. After this failure, a follow-up 'information for patient' initiative, which would have allowed companies more leeway to advertise prescription medicines to the public, was being considered. Perehudoff and Alves (2011) surveyed patient groups that were members of an advisory committee to the European Medicines Agency, on their positions on the 'information for patient' initiative. They found that all six industry-funded groups supported a change in law to allow more of an industry role in patient information; neither of the two non-industry funded groups did. Although this was a small study, it raises concerns about groups' support for a policy that was helpful to the industry but had strong opposition from independent consumer and health professional groups. The policy initiative was eventually abandoned.

Two recent situations involve pressure from patient organizations on the US Food and Drug Administration (FDA) to approve drugs with uncertain effectiveness and safety profiles. These raise concerns about the effects of industry sponsorship in framing how patient priorities are understood and how government agencies respond to these priorities.

The FDA's approval of aducanumab (*Aduhelm*) for Alzheimer's disease in June 2021 was controversial, as the FDA's own expert advisory committee had overwhelmingly recommended against approval. Three advisory committee members resigned over the drug's approval, including long term committee member Aaron Kesselheim, MD, JD, MPH, from Harvard Medical School who said, "This might be the worst approval decision that the FDA has made that I can remember" (Belluck & Robbins, 2021). Although the drug had shown an effect on the number of amyloid plaques, a biological change associated with Alzheimer's disease, the advisory committee had not found convincing evidence of benefit for cognitive decline and were concerned about serious side effects. In contrast, the U.S. Alzheimer's Association issued a press release "enthusiastically welcome[ing]" the drug's approval, saying it "delays decline due to Alzheimer's disease" (Alzheimer's Association, 2021a June 7). There was no mention in the media release of any serious harmful effects of aducanumab, nor of any controversy over whether the drug benefits patients, nor that in 2020 the Alzheimer's Association received more than half a million dollars from Biogen and Esai, the two companies producing aducanumab (Alzheimer's Association, 2021a, b). Peter Stein, the FDA's Director of the Office of New Drugs confirmed that patient testimony had played a role in the agency's decision to approve aducanumab, saying that the FDA, "heard very clearly from patients that they're willing to accept some uncertainty to have access to a drug that could provide meaningful benefit in preventing the progression of this disease" (Gingery, 2021). There is, however, concern that this decision will expose vulnerable patients and their families to false hope and harm due to the lack of clear clinical benefit and risk of serious adverse effects (Liu & Howard, 2021). Other patient organizations and patients may share the advisory committee's concerns about lack of confirmed benefit and serious risks, but the Alzheimer's Association—with its substantial industry funding—is able to proclaim its views loudly, potentially drowning out other voices.

A second example of a controversial drug approval in which patient testimony proved influential is the FDA's approval of flibanserin (*Adyii*) for women experiencing low levels of sexual desire. Flibanserin was originally developed as an antidepressant, but after research found it ineffective for that use, the manufacturer, Sprout Pharmaceuticals, then tested it for low sexual desire in women. The FDA rejected applications for market approval in 2010 and 2013 because of limited evidence of effectiveness and concerns about potential harmful effects. In 2015, with no new evidence of effectiveness, the FDA approved flibanserin (Mintzes et al., 2021). What had happened between 2013 and 2015? An intensive public relations campaign called 'Even the Score' initiated by Sprout claimed that sexism was behind the FDA's rejection of the drug, and that while there were 26 sex drugs on the US market for men there were none for women. Although the claim was inaccurate, the campaign garnered a lot of support. Sprout's role in this advocacy was not transparent. Additionally, women testifying before the FDA had their expenses covered by a group funded by Sprout and met beforehand to prepare their talking points (Mintzes et al., 2021). The expert advisory committee comments acknowledged the drug's limited effectiveness but highlighted the influence of women's testimony about their distress (Joffe et al., 2016). It is likely that the women's testimony would not have had the same impact if Sprout had not provided funding to bring together a set of women, given them information, and helped them frame talking points. The women who spoke may well have been genuinely distressed about their sex lives but a drug with limited effectiveness and risk of harm seems unlikely to be the answer.

Another major concern about industry funding of patient organizations is whether this funding buys silence when patients' and sponsors' priorities clash. The *EpiPen* case brought this issue to public attention. Many people with life-threatening serious allergies carry an auto-injector of epinephrine with them at all times to prevent anaphylactic shock. The market leader is *EpiPen*. These injectors have a short, 18-month shelf life, so need regular replacement even when not used. In the US, the company Mylan, which produces *EpiPen*, raised the price from $100 to $600, leading to a public outcry among people with severe allergies. However, in an exposé published by the Hastings Center, patient organizations that had been holding campaigns to raise awareness of allergy and asthma stayed silent (Batt & Fugh-Berman, 2016). These included major US patient organizations: the Food Allergy Research & Education, the Asthma and Allergy Foundation of America, and the Allergy & Asthma Network. All these organizations received substantial funding from Mylan—a total of over US $10 million to fund educational campaigns from 2011 to 2016. Batt and Fugh-Berman (2016) suggest that "money buys silence."

These are only a few examples of patient organizations who have either loudly spoken out in support of the need for a funder's drug—even when it has not been shown to be very effective and can cause serious harm—or who stayed silent about price gouging. Such examples highlight that although patients' and companies' priorities often align, for example when a new highly effective drug is being developed for a condition that did not previously have good treatments, they can also differ. Patient organizations may feel pressured to advocate in particular ways that align with their funders, and patient organizations whose views are aligned with industry may be more likely to attract industry money, in which case those groups are more likely to survive and prosper. This problem is especially acute due to limited available public funding for patient organizations in many countries (Hemminki et al., 2010; Jones, 2008). Either way, industry money translates to louder patient organization advocacy for industry aligned interests.

12.5 How Does Industry Funding of Patient Organizations Influence Research?

We noted at the outset of this chapter that patient organizations have many roles in research including research funding, conduct of research, and communication of research results to members. Industry funding of patient organizations can influence research agendas, methods, and/or communication in ways that benefit the sponsor.

A sizable proportion of industry money provided to patient organizations goes towards funding research projects led by others or by the organization itself. Ozieranski and colleagues from the UK reported that almost a quarter (24.6%) of industry money for patient organizations was used for research purposes including, for example, industry funding of patient organization grants for clinical research that use the sponsor's drugs (Ozieranski et al., 2019). An Australian study of industry-funded patient groups found that 28% of organizations received their funding for research, including for patient-organization-led research projects (Fabbri et al., 2019). Industry funding of patient organization research may be lower in other countries (Mulinari et al., 2020).

Research that is funded by industry-sponsored patient organizations can be problematic if it skews research agendas towards industry-friendly projects (Fabbri et al., 2018b). Industry-sponsored patient organizations may be more inclined to initiate or fund research projects that favour industry interests (Every-Palmer & Howick, 2014). This may mean a focus on product-oriented biomedical research rather than a more holistic focus. O'Donovan describes how some organizations that accept pharmaceutical industry money frame illness as 'a quest for biomedical solutions', largely ignoring social determinants of health (O'Donovan, 2007, 722). The example above of patients who spoke in favour of approving a drug for low sexual desire (Mintzes et al., 2021) highlights exactly this type of narrow technological solution to problems that often have their basis in a woman's previous experiences, and in social and cultural expectations.

We have already noted that industry-funded patient organizations are less likely to speak out in ways that might damage their sponsors' interests (Lin et al., 2017; Perehudoff & Alves, 2011). It seems highly probable then that conflicted patient groups will also sometimes avoid engaging in or funding research studies that do not align with industry interests, such as research on safety concerns (Batt, 2017), non-pharmacological prevention or management of health conditions (O'Donovan, 2007), or overdiagnosis and overtreatment (Jorgensen & Gotzsche, 2004).

Patient organizations that accept industry funding might also communicate about research with their members in ways that can be influenced by industry funders through selective publication and/or favourable 'spin' of results to present the findings in a positive light (Lexchin et al., 2003; Lundh et al., 2017). For example, organizations sometimes pass on pre-publication information about ongoing industry trials or accept industry-funded speakers at their seminars (Hemminki et al., 2010). There is little direct research on these types of communications within patient organizations. However, industry-funded research is more likely to generate outcomes that favour the sponsor's product compared with non-industry-sponsored research (Lundh et al., 2017), and academic publications are more likely to communicate favourably about pharmaceutical products if the authors are funded by the sponsors (Wang et al., 2010; Chiu et al., 2017). Information provided by company sales representatives to doctors has also been found to under-report harmful effects of medicines (Mintzes et al., 2013). It is therefore likely that these types of industry-generated communications within patient organizations also overemphasise benefits and under-report harms of sponsors' products.

12.6 How Could the Risk of Undue Influence from Industry Funders Be Managed?

Many patient organizations acknowledge the risks and dilemmas associated with accepting industry funding, including being pressured to act in industry interests and receiving reputational damage (Parker et al., 2019a, 2021; Jones, 2008). Groups use a variety of strategies to try and counteract those risks. Some have decided to completely refuse industry funding (Grey & Bolland, 2015; Parker et al., 2019a). Others rely on a variety of formal or informal policies. This might include guidance co-authored by industry and patient organizations (Parker et al. 2021; O'Donovan, 2007), such as the Australian 'Working Together' document (Consumers Health Forum and Medicines Australia, 2015), written by Medicines Australia (medicinesaustralia.com.au), the national umbrella group for pharmaceutical companies, in conjunction with Consumers Health Forum of Australia, the national umbrella group for patient organizations. This document describes a set of principles to guide organizational relationships and offers examples of successful relationships. Some organizations might also have formal policies that cover topics such as sole-company funding, product brand naming, company influence over organization agenda and/

or content, collaborative advocacy, and public disclosure of funding sources (Parker et al., 2021; Jones, 2008; McCoy et al., 2017) while other organizations use 'the pub test'—an informal thought experiment about the views of ordinary people—to think through the acceptability of interactions with companies as they arise (Parker et al., 2021). Many organizations rely heavily on industry to set the boundaries, trusting industry self-regulation in the form of Codes of Conduct that are written by national industry bodies for all company members, and that include direction for companies about their relationships with patient groups (Medicines Australia, 2022; ABPI, 2019). Companies that are members of the national industry body must comply with this Code or they risk losing their membership status. However, as discussed above, not all companies are members of their local industry body.

These strategies to manage industry funding are inconsistent and often lacking in transparency. There is no sector-wide consensus about policies and practices organizations should adhere to in order to safeguard independence or on the limits of acceptable funder behaviour (Parker et al., 2021). This might mean that some groups interact with industry in ways that put their independence at risk. Despite this, patient groups typically believe that they are not influenced by industry funding (Taylor & Denegri, 2017). This attitude is worryingly similar to physicians' beliefs that they are not influenced by pharma gifts when evidence clearly shows this is not the case (O'Donovan, 2007; Mitchell et al., 2021).

12.6.1 What More Could Be Done?

As a start, we recommend improved public information about industry funding of patient organizations. This should include better reporting from organizations themselves, and mandatory disclosure of patient advocacy group funding by the pharmaceutical industry by including them in the US Open Payments program established by the Physician Payments Sunshine Act (Section 6002 of the Affordable Care Act of 2010) (Moynihan & Bero, 2017; McCoy, 2018) and other national transparency databases. When included in a national database, funding information on patient organizations should be made accessible in a user-friendly, searchable format (Fabbri et al., 2018a). As noted above, researchers are encouraged to include patients in their research processes, and this kind of transparency would assist those researchers in selecting appropriate patient organizations for partnerships. Accessible national databases of patient organizations, including groups without industry funding, would also be helpful to researchers.

Independent education and guidance for patient organizations on how to think about and/or manage interactions with industry could also make a difference. US ethicist Susannah Rose has published a number of suggestions, including limiting industry funding to a small portion of the organization's budget (e.g., less than 25%), and separating out the roles of fundraiser and policy maker within the organization to minimise the likelihood that friendly personal relationships interfere with organizational policy-making around commercial funders (Rose, 2013). We have previously delivered workshops with patient advocacy groups on financial conflicts of interest (Moynihan et al., 2020), discussing the evidence around industry sponsorship of research and key health stakeholders including patient organizations, and introducing the publicly accessible databases of industry funding to doctors (Kirschner et al., 2014) and patient organizations (Parker et al., 2019b). Workshop attendees were enthusiastic and expressed a need for more public awareness and debate around the topics raised.

In 2020 we co-convened a public workshop with attendees from 22 Australian patient organizations to discuss principles and suggestions for best practices for interacting with industry (Parker et al., 2020a, b). The attendees highlighted the importance of principles such as consumer centredness, transparency, fairness independence, values alignment, and accountability. Examples of best practices that might affect patient organization research activities included:

- regularly consulting members about their views, which could include their research priorities;
- public reporting of all industry funding including actual dollar amounts and how money was spent;
- having independently written, publicly available, and regularly reviewed policies aimed at preserving independence, which might include rules about funder involvement in the design, conduct, or reporting of research projects;
- advocating for a pooled fund of industry money that could support research that the pharmaceutical industry would not otherwise be likely to fund;
- banning current or recent company staff from holding governance positions or other official roles in the patient organization;
- avoiding financial relationships with commercial entities with a poor social responsibility profile.

Finally, an important solution is to work towards financial independence from pharmaceutical and medical device companies, thus avoiding all conflicts of interest (Moynihan & Bero, 2017) .There are other funding models that might assist patient organizations (Moynihan et al., 2019). For example, the Italian government taxes drug company promotional spending to create a fund for public interest research (Italian Medicines Agency (AIFA) Research Development Working Group, 2010). Patient organizations could use a similar model to harness their significant power to request donations from pharmaceutical and medical devices into a centralized pool that could be managed independently from donors and fairly distributed among organizations for the purpose of providing research grants. Given the role that patient organizations have in providing needed healthcare services, such as helping patients and their families to navigate complex care situations, especially for chronic conditions, another model would be to finance such a fund out of general tax revenues.

12.7 Conclusions

We applaud the growing trend towards inclusion of patient advocacy organizations in biomedical research. Patient organizations can act as an independent voice, promoting research that is in their members' interests, without regard to commercial imperatives or professional advancement. However, we are deeply concerned that widespread industry funding of these organizations may interfere with this mandate. Groups that rely on industry funding may endorse and communicate research that makes their sponsors happy and avoid studies that embarrass or upset industry. This could contribute to unwarranted emphasis on biotechnical solutions over non-drug options, facilitate overdiagnosis and overtreatment, and perpetuate silences about safety concerns. We encourage patient organizations to maintain their independent voice rather than merge with the multiple blended voices already contained within the industry 'megaphone' (Bero, 2018). To do so, patient organizations could seek out independent education and advice on how to maintain distance from commercial funders and ultimately work towards disentanglement from industry.

Acknowledgements We would like to thank Lisa Bero, Alice Fabbri, Quinn Grundy and Joel Lexchin from the Evidence, Policy and Influence Collaboration, Charles Perkins Centre, University of Sydney; Anthony Brown, Health Consumers NSW; and Leanne Wells, Consumers Health Forum of Australia.

Conflict of Interest Declarations LP has no conflicts to declare. BM is an expert witness for Health Canada on a legal case involving marketing of an unapproved drug product.

References

Abola, M. V., & Prasad, V. (2016). Characteristics and conflicts of public speakers at meetings of the oncologic drugs advisory committee to the US Food and Drug Administration. *JAMA Internal Medicine, 176*(3), 389–391. <Go to ISI>://MEDLINE:26831527.

Association of the British Pharmaceutical Industry. (2019). *ABPI code of practice for the pharmaceutical industry.* http://www.pmcpa.org.uk/thecode/Documents/ABPI%20Code%20of%20Practice%202019.pdf

Agrawal, S., Brennan, N., & Budetti, P. (2013). The Sunshine Act—Effects on physicians. *The New England Journal of Medicine, 368*(22), 2054–2057. https://doi.org/10.1056/NEJMp1303523. http://www.ncbi.nlm.nih.gov/pubmed/23718163

Alzheimer's Association. (2021a, June 7). *Alzheimer's Association welcomes FDA approval of Aducanumab*. Press Release. Altzheimer's Association. Accessed Nov 10. https://www.alz.org/news/2021/alzheimers-association-fda-approval-aducanumab.

Alzheimer's Association. (2021b). *Pharmaceutical industry contributions: FY20*. Accessed Nov 18. https://www.alz.org/media/Documents/Pharmaceutical-Industry-Contributions-FY20.pdf

Angell, M. (2004). *The truth about drug companies – How they deceive us and what to do about it*. Random House.

Applebaum, K. (2009). Getting to yes: Corporate power and the creation of a psychopharmaceutical blockbuster. *Culture, Medicine and Psychiatry, 33*(2), 185–215. https://doi.org/10.1007/s11013-009-9129-3. https://www.ncbi.nlm.nih.gov/pubmed/19247823

Batt, S. (2017). *Health Advocacy, Inc.: How pharmaceutical funding changed the breast cancer movement*. UBC Press.

Batt, S., & Fugh-Berman, A. (2016). EpiPen furor: Patient groups take money, stay mum. *Hastings Center*.

Belluck, P., & Robbins, R. (2021). Three FDA advisers resign over agency's approval of Alzheimer's Drug. *The New York Times*.

Bero, L. (2018). Influences on evidence: Putting the cart before the horse. *Journal and Proceedings of the Royal Society of New South Wales, 151*(467/468), 59–68.

Chiu, K., Grundy, Q., & Bero, L. (2017). 'Spin' in published biomedical literature: A methodological systematic review. *PLoS Biology, 15*(9), e2002173. <Go to ISI>://MEDLINE:28892482.

Consumers Health Forum, and Medicines Australia. (2015). *Working together guide* (3rd ed.). Consumers Health Forum. Last Modified 24 March 2020. Accessed Mar 24. https://medicinesaustralia.com.au/community/working-together-guide/

den Oudendammer, W. M., Noordhoek, J., Abma-Schouten, R. Y., van Houtum, L., Broerse, J. E. W., & Dedding, C. W. M. (2019). Patient participation in research funding: An overview of when, why and how amongst Dutch health funds. *Research Involvement and Engagement, 5*(1), 33. https://doi.org/10.1186/s40900-019-0163-1

Edwards, K. T. (2017). The role of patient participation in drug approvals: Lessons from the accelerated approval of Eteplirsen. *Food & Drug Law Journal, 72*(3), 406–450.

Epstein, S. (2008). 21 Patient groups and health movements. In *The handbook of science and technology studies* (pp. 499–541).

Every-Palmer, S., & Howick, J. (2014). How evidence-based medicine is failing due to biased trials and selective publication. *Journal of Evaluation in Clinical Practice, 20*(6), 908–914.

Fabbri, A., La Santos, A., Mezinska, S., Mulinari, S., & Mintzes, B. (2018a). Sunshine policies and murky shadows in Europe: Disclosure of pharmaceutical industry payments to health professionals in nine European countries. *International Journal of Health Policy Management, x*(x), 1–6. https://doi.org/10.15171/ijhpm.2018.20

Fabbri, A., Lai, A., Grundy, Q., & Bero, L. A. (2018b). The influence of industry sponsorship on the research agenda: A scoping review. *American Journal of Public Health, 108*(11), e9–e16. https://doi.org/10.2105/AJPH.2018.304677. https://www.ncbi.nlm.nih.gov/pubmed/30252531

Fabbri, S. S., Lau, E., Vitry, A., & Mintzes, B. (2019). Pharmaceutical industry funding of health consumer groups in Australia: A cross-sectional analysis. *International Journal of Health Services, 49*(2), 273–293. https://journals.sagepub.com/doi/abs/10.1177/0020731418823376

Fabbri, L. P., Colombo, C., Mosconi, P., Barbara, G., Frattaruolo, M. P., Lau, E., Kroeger, C. M., Lunny, C., Salzwedel, D. M., & Mintzes, B. (2020). Industry funding of patient and health consumer organisations: Systematic review with meta-analysis. *BMJ, 368*, l6925. https://www.bmj.com/content/bmj/368/bmj.l6925.full.pdf

Gingery, D. (2021). Patient support may have helped push Aduhelm toward approval. *Pink Sheet Informa Pharma Intelligence*.

Grey, A., & Bolland, M. (2015). Web of industry, advocacy, and academia in the management of osteoporosis. *BMJ, 351*, h3170. https://doi.org/10.1136/bmj.h3170. http://ovidsp.ovid.com/ovidweb.cgi?T=JS&CSC=Y&NEWS=N&PAGE=fulltext&D=med8&AN=26198274

Hemminki, E., Toiviainen, H. K., & Vuorenkoski, L. (2010). Co-operation between patient organisations and the drug industry in Finland. *Social Science & Medicine, 70*(8), 1171–1175.

Hoddinott, P., Pollock, A., O'Cathain, A., Boyer, I., Taylor, J., MacDonald, C., Oliver, S., & Donovan, J. L. (2018). How to incorporate patient and public perspectives into the design and conduct of research. *F1000Research* 7.

Institute of Medicine. (2009). *Conflict of interest in medical research, education and practice*. The National Academies Press.

Italian Medicines Agency (AIFA) Research Development Working Group. (2010). Feasibility and challenges of independent research on drugs: The Italian medicines agency (AIFA) experience. *European Journal of Clinical Investigation, 40*(1), 69–86.

Joffe, H. V., Chang, C., Sewell, C., Easley, O., Nguyen, C., Dunn, S., Lehrfeld, K., Lee, L. M., Kim, M.-J., & Slagle, A. F. (2016). FDA approval of flibanserin—Treating hypoactive sexual desire disorder. *New England Journal of Medicine, 374*(2), 101–104.

Jones, K. (2008). In whose interest? Relationships between health consumer groups and the pharmaceutical industry in the UK. *Sociology of Health & Illness, 30*(6), 929–943.

Jorgensen, K. J., & Gotzsche, P. C. (2004). Presentation on websites of possible benefits and harms from screening for breast cancer: Cross sectional study. *BMJ, 328*(7432), 148. http://ovidsp.ovid.com/ovidweb.cgi?T=JS&CSC=Y&NEWS=N&PAGE=fulltext&D=med5&AN=14726344

Kanter, G. P. (2018). Extending the sunshine act from physicians to patient advocacy organizations. *American Journal of Public Health, 108*(8), 978.

Kirschner, N. M., Sulmasy, L. S., & Kesselheim, A. S. (2014). Health policy basics: The physician payment sunshine act and the open payments program. *Annals of Internal Medicine, 161*(7), 519–521.

Lau, E., Fabbri, A., & Mintzes, B. (2018). How do health consumer organisations in Australia manage pharmaceutical industry sponsorship? A cross-sectional study. *Australian Health Review, 43*(4), 474–480. https://www.ncbi.nlm.nih.gov/pubmed/30021601

Lexchin, J., Bero, L. A., Djulbegovic, B., & Clark, O. (2003). Pharmaceutical industry sponsorship and research outcome and quality: Systematic review. *BMJ, 326*(7400), 1167–1170. https://doi.org/10.1136/bmj.326.7400.1167. http://www.ncbi.nlm.nih.gov/pubmed/12775614

Lin, D. H., Lucas, E., Murimi, I. B., Kolodny, A., & Alexander, G. C. (2017). Financial conflicts of interest and the centers for disease control and prevention's 2016 guideline for prescribing opioids for chronic pain. *JAMA Internal Medicine, 177*(3), 427–428. https://doi.org/10.1001/jamainternmed.2016.8471

Liu, K. Y., & Howard, R. (2021). Can we learn lessons from the FDA's approval of aducanumab? *Nature Reviews Neurology*, 1–8.

Lofgren, H. (2004). Pharmaceuticals and the consumer movement: The ambivalences of 'patient power'. *Australian Health Review, 28*(2), 228–237. http://ovidsp.ovid.com/ovidweb.cgi?T=JS&CSC=Y&NEWS=N&PAGE=fulltext&D=med5&AN=15527403, http://www.publish.csiro.au/ah/pdf/ah040228

Lundh, A., Lexchin, J., Mintzes, B., Schroll, J. B., & Bero, L. (2017). Industry sponsorship and research outcome. *The Cochrane Database of Systematic Reviews, 2*, MR000033.

McCoy, M. S. (2018). Industry support of patient advocacy organizations: The case for an extension of the sunshine act provisions of the affordable care act. *American Journal of Public Health, 108*(8), 1026–1030.

McCoy, M. S., Carniol, M., Chockley, K., Urwin, J. W., Emanuel, E. J., & Schmidt, H. (2017). Conflicts of interest for patient-advocacy organizations. *New England Journal of Medicine, 376*(9), 880–885.

Medicines Australia. (2021). *Our members*. Medicines Australia. Accessed Oct 20. https://www.medicinesaustralia.com.au/about-us/our-members/

Medicines Australia. (2022). *Code of conduct, 19th ed.* Available at www.medicinesaustralia.com.au

Mintzes, B., Lexchin, J., Sutherland, J. M., Beaulieu, M.-D., Wilkes, M. S., Durrieu, G., & Reynolds, E. (2013). Pharmaceutical sales representatives and patient safety: A comparative prospective study of information quality in Canada, France and the United States. *Journal of General Internal Medicine, 28*(10), 1368–1375.

Mintzes, B., Tiefer, L., & Cosgrove, L. (2021). Bremelanotide and flibanserin for low sexual desire in women: The fallacy of regulatory precedent. *Drug and Therapeutics Bulletin*.

Mitchell, A. P., Trivedi, N. U., Gennarelli, R. L., Chimonas, S., Tabatabai, S. M., Goldberg, J., Diaz Jr, L. A., & Korenstein, D. (2021). Are financial payments from the pharmaceutical industry associated with physician prescribing? A systematic review. *Annals of Internal Medicine, 174*(3), 353–361.

Moynihan, R., & Bero, L. (2017). Toward a healthier patient voice: More independence, less industry funding. *JAMA Internal Medicine, 177*(3), 350–351.

Moynihan, R. & Henry, D. (2006). The fight against disease mongering: Generating knowledge for action. *PLoS Medicine, 3*(4), e191.

Moynihan, R., Bero, L., Hill, S., Johansson, M., Lexchin, J., Macdonald, H., Mintzes, B., Pearson, C., Rodwin, M. A., & Stavdal, A. (2019). Pathways to independence: Towards producing and using trustworthy evidence. *BMJ, 367*, l6576.

Moynihan, R., Fabbri, A., Parker, L., & Bero, L. (2020). Mixed methods evaluation of workshops for citizen health advocates about financial conflicts of interests in healthcare. *BMJ Open, 10*(5), e034195. https://doi.org/10.1136/bmjopen-2019-034195. https://bmjopen.bmj.com/content/bmjopen/10/5/e034195.full.pdf

Mulinari, S. (2016). Unhealthy marketing of pharmaceutical products: An international public health concern. *Journal of Public Health Policy, 37*(2), 149–159.

Mulinari, S., Vilhelmsson, A., Rickard, E., & Ozieranski, P. (2020). Five years of pharmaceutical industry funding of patient organisations in Sweden: Cross-sectional study of companies, patient organisations and drugs. *PLoS One, 15*(6), e0235021. https://doi.org/10.1371/journal.pone.0235021

National Health and Medical Research Council, and Consumers Health Forum of Australia. (2016). *Statement on consumer and community involvement in health and medical research*. National Health and Medical Research Council. Accessed Jan 4. https://www.nhmrc.gov.au/about-us/publications/statement-consumer-and-community-involvement-health-and-medical-research

National Institute for Health Research. (2020). *NIHR launches new centre for engagement and dissemination*. Department of Health & Social Care. Accessed Jan 4. https://www.nihr.ac.uk/news/nihr-launches-new-centre-for-engagement-and-dissemination/24576

O'Donovan, O. (2007). Corporate colonization of health activism? Irish health advocacy organizations' modes of engagement with pharmaceutical corporations. *International Journal of Health Services, 37*(4), 711–733.

Ozieranski, P., Rickard, E., & Mulinari, S. (2019). Exposing drug industry funding of UK patient organisations. *BMJ, 365*, l1806. https://doi.org/10.1136/bmj.l1806. https://www.ncbi.nlm.nih.gov/pubmed/31122928

Parker, L., Fabbri, A., Grundy, Q., Mintzes, B., & Bero, L. (2019a). "Asset exchange"—Interactions between patient groups and pharmaceutical industry: Australian qualitative study. *BMJ, 367*, l6694. https://doi.org/10.1136/bmj.l6694

Parker, L., Karanges, E. A., & Bero, L. (2019b). Changes in the type and amount of spending disclosed by Australian pharmaceutical companies: An observational study. *BMJ Open, 9*(2). https://doi.org/10.1136/bmjopen-2018-024928

Parker, L., Brown, A., & Wells, L. (2020a). Building trust and transparency – Health consumer organisation-pharmaceutical industry relationships. *Aus Health Review, 45(3)*, 393–394.

Parker, L., Brown, A., Wells, L., Joyner, S., Mintzes, B., Fabbri, A., Chiu, K., Wang, Z., & Bero, L (2020b). *Meeting report – Building trust and transprency*. Health Consumers NSW. Last Modified 23 September 2020. Accessed Sept 23. https://www.hcnsw.org.au/trust-and-transparency/

Parker, L., Grundy, Q., Fabbri, A., Mintzes, B., & Bero, L. (2021). 'Lines in the sand': An Australian qualitative study of patient group practices to promote independence from pharmaceutical industry funders. *BMJ Open, 11*(2), e045140. https://doi.org/10.1136/bmjopen-2020-045140

Patient-Centered Outcomes Research Institute (PCORI). (2022). *PCORI*. Accessed Jan 4. https://www.pcori.org/

Perehudoff, S. K., & Alves, T. L. (2011). *The patient & consumer voice and pharmaceutical industry sponsorship*. Health Action International. Accessed Jan 4. https://research.rug.nl/en/publications/the-patient-amp-consumer-voice-and-pharmaceutical-industry-sponso

Perry, S. (2016). New patient-advocacy group 'outed' by Minnesota-based website as 'Astroturf' campaign. *Minnpost*, Feb 16. https://www.minnpost.com/second-opinion/2016/02/new-patient-advocacy-group-outed-minnesota-based-website-astroturf-campaign/

Pinto, D., Martin, D., & Chenhall, R. (2016). The involvement of patient organisations in rare disease research: A mixed methods study in Australia. *Orphanet Journal of Rare Diseases, 11*(1), 1–15.

Public Citizen. (2016). *Patients' groups and big pharma.* Accessed 4 Aug 2020. Available at https://www.citizen.org/

Rose, S. L. (2013). Patient advocacy organizations: Institutional conflicts of interest, trust, and trustworthiness. *Journal of Law, Medicine & Ethics, 41*(3), 680–687.

Rose, S. L., Highland, J., Karafa, M. T., & Joffe, S. (2017). Patient advocacy organizations, industry funding, and conflicts of interest. *JAMA Internal Medicine, 177*(3), 344–350.

Rothman, S. M., Raveis, V. H., Friedman, A., & Rothman, D. J. (2011). Health advocacy organizations and the pharmaceutical industry: An analysis of disclosure practices. *American Journal of Public Health, 101*(4), 602–609.

Taylor, J., & Denegri, S. (2017). Industry links with patient organisations. *BMJ, 356*, j1251. https://doi.org/10.1136/bmj.j1251

Terry, S. F., Terry, P. F., Rauen, K. A., Uitto, J., & Bercovitch, L. G. (2007). Advocacy groups as research organizations: The PXE international example. *Nature Reviews Genetics, 8*(2), 157–164.

Wang, A. T., McCoy, C. P., Murad, M. H., & Montori, V. M. (2010). Association between industry affiliation and position on cardiovascular risk with rosiglitazone: Cross sectional systematic review. *BMJ, 340*, c1344.

Lisa Parker is a researcher, bioethicist, and practicing physician. Her research focus is on critical evaluation of health research, practice and policy, including research fraud, conflicts of interest, industry influence in health, and overdiagnosis. Lisa has expertise in qualitative research methodology.

Barbara Mintzes is an epidemiologist with a main research focus on pharmaceutical policy, including commercial influences on prescribing and medicine use. She has carried out systematic reviews of drug treatments and observational research on direct-to-consumer advertising, one-to-one sales visits in primary care and regulatory safety warnings on medicines.

Chapter 13
Representing and Protecting: Gatekeepers in Community-Engaged Research

Ryan Spellecy

13.1 Introduction

There are many reasons—ethical, scientific, and practical—for researchers to engage community and patient stakeholders, and many different roles in which they may serve. One particularly important role of community and patient organizations and representatives is to serve as gatekeepers, monitoring, and in some cases even determining, what research does and does not get conducted with their communities. Such gatekeeping can prevent "helicopter" research and community research fatigue. Gatekeeping can also aid in identifying and mitigating harms that might occur not only to individual participants but to third parties (who do not provide consent for participation) and or the community as a whole (or group harms; see Chap. 15, in this volume). Although individual informed consent and independent review both aim to protect against research risks, in research with identifiable communities these protections may be insufficient to protect from other types of harms.

Gatekeeping does not and cannot replace informed consent, which is given to permit researchers to collect data from and potentially experiment on (through the delivery of unproven interventions, randomization, etc.) an individual participant. Consent cannot be given on behalf of communities; however, gatekeepers can control researcher interactions with a community in a variety of ways, through formal and informal means. Additionally, gatekeeping can supplement (but not replace) independent review, as consideration of long-term risks to communities are not within institutional review boards' (IRBs') mandate (Ross et al., 2010).

R. Spellecy (✉)
Center for Bioethics and Medical Humanities, Medical College of Wisconsin, Milwaukee, WI, USA
e-mail: rspellecy@mcw.edu

E. E. Anderson (ed.), *Ethical Issues in Community and Patient Stakeholder–Engaged Health Research*, Philosophy and Medicine 146,
https://doi.org/10.1007/978-3-031-40379-8_13

Given the gaps in protection, the gatekeeping role of community research partners is an important supplement to informed consent and independent IRB review. To be sure, gatekeeping raises its own set of ethical challenges. For example, it is not clear how best to determine who can and should be the gatekeepers. Additionally, there is a real risk that a gatekeeper "endorsement" may pose a threat to individual informed consent. Here, we discuss the limitations of informed consent and independent review in research with identifiable communities, the benefits of gatekeeping for protecting third parties and groups, types of gatekeepers, and issues in the selection of gatekeepers.

13.2 The Limits of Informed Consent and Independent Review in Protecting Third Parties and Groups

Reliance on individual informed consent alone has been criticized as inadequate to protect third parties and entire communities. As Friesen et al. argue,

> Harm to these groups cannot be mitigated simply by securing informed consent from individuals according to *Belmont's* principle of respect for persons. This principle fails to take into account the unique harms that can be done to communities *qua* communities, such as violating widespread trust or taking ownership of a community's stories (Friesen et al., 2017).

In research that engages individuals from identifiable communities, whether these share geography, culture, personal characteristics, or illness (see Chap. 7, in this volume), there are risks to third parties, or members of the community in which the research is conducted who are not participants in the research (see Chap. 15, in this volume). Risks to third parties can include stigmatization and social harm. For example, research that reports risky sexual behavior among members of a community may reflect poorly and directly (e.g., result in discrimination in job hiring) on individuals beyond those who actually participated.

Community- or group-level harms can also result from research on identifiable communities. The now infamous Havasupai study (Mello & Wolf, 2010) has been strongly condemned due to its use of blood samples from a study on diabetes for other research purposes. Although tribal elders reviewed the study and gave permission for the research to continue, and individual participants provided informed consent, samples were later used without individual or tribal permission for schizophrenia research as well as research on the origins of the tribe that contradicted the tribes' oral traditions. According to a member of the Havasupai tribe,

> Though some Havasupai knew already that their ancestors most likely came from Asia, "when people tell us, 'No, this is not where you are from,' and your own blood says so—it is confusing to us," Rex Tilousi said. "It hurts the elders who have been telling these stories to our grandchildren."(Harmon, 2010)

Emotional harms and harms to tribal cohesion and identity occurred when DNA research refuted the tribe's origin story. To publish such findings essentially accused tribal elders—people's grandparents—of being liars. Some tribe members also feared dissemination of research findings related to ancestry could have the potential to jeopardize native land rights, as they were in part based on the tradition that the tribe originated from the Havasupai Falls area in Arizona.

Whether or not the Havasupai people originated from the waters of Havasupai Falls is the not the controversy here. What is at issue is that reliance solely on individual informed consent cannot protect third parties or groups; they have no voice in the process. Individuals considering research participation make a decision based on whether or not the research study is right for them, whether the risks are acceptable or too high, whether they would support the conduct and goals of the research, and other factors—but this process does not necessarily involve considering risks to others or communities/groups to which one belongs unless those happen to be priorities of the individual. In the case of the Havasupai, the tribal elders speak for the third parties, that is, they speak for all members of the tribe. It is the role of gatekeepers to safeguard against these unique harms that can befall third parties and entire communities when research results may be extrapolated to everyone. (It is, however, important to note that while the gatekeepers performed their role in this instance, the researcher broke their promises and did not follow the approved protocol. This demonstrates that there are limits to gatekeeping.)

How IRBs address social risks, including risks to third parties and groups, remains unclear and not well-studied (Resnik & Sharp, 2006; Klitzman, 2013). There has also been some debate regarding whether consideration of group harms is within IRB purview (Ross et al., 2010; Wikler, 2020). Institutional IRB members are likely not as familiar with the risks to third parties nor the appropriate protections to mitigate these risks, although this literature has recently somewhat proliferated (Shah et al., 2020; Kimmelman, 2020).

Community gatekeepers may serve the important goals of identifying and mitigating these types of harms as well as holding researchers accountable. Since risks to third parties and groups can be quite common in community-engaged research, as it involves conducting research on identifiable communities, gatekeepers are needed to ensure that the community in which the research in conducted is both protected and that the concerns and the collective interests of the community are considered.

To be clear, the solution to this problem of third-party harms in community research cannot be completely solved by gatekeeper permission. Community gatekeepers cannot consent for individuals, nor can they usually completely deny researchers access to a community; they can only raise concerns and questions about harms, provide access to community members for consultation and study recruitment, and provide accountability to ensure that accurate information about risks and benefits is presented to individuals. Gatekeepers can also seek to ensure that potential harms to third parties are mitigated, for example, by sharing decisions about what data from a given study are published (Israel et al., 2003).

13.3 Types of Gatekeepers

There are various entry points to any community, including community leaders as well as what you might call "everyday" community members. No matter who serves in this role, gatekeepers to research should represent the interests of the community. Gatekeepers can be divided into four groups: formal leadership organizations, community-created research gatekeeping organizations, informal community leaders, and researcher-created gatekeepers. Below, I will review each type and provide examples.

13.3.1 Formal Leadership Organizations

Formal leadership organizations include formal IRBs with Federal Wide Assurances from the Office of Human Research Protections. Some native tribes, including the Navajo Nation, Cherokee Nation, Choctaw Nation, and Chickasaw Nation, have such IRBs (Navajo Nation Human Research Review Board, 2022). The Navajo Nation Human Research Review Board (HRB) was the first IRB created by a native tribe (Brugge & Missaghian, 2006). Any research involving Navajo people on their land requires approval by their HRB. Like any other IRB, the Navajo Nation HRB reviews, approves, and disapproves research; unlike traditional IRBs, it prospectively reviews manuscripts prior to publication, and this is a requirement for all research.

The Navajo Nation created and adopted the Navajo Nation Health Research Code, which begins by stating that, "The purpose of this Code shall be to set forth conditions under which investigators, physicians, researchers, and others may perform research activities on living human subjects within the territorial jurisdiction of the Navajo Nation" (Navajo Nation Human Research Review Board, 2022). The Code includes traditional ethical principles for research, such as beneficence (Navajo Nation Human Research Review Board, 2022). It also states that research shall be "beneficial, community-based, and consistent with Navajo Nation priorities and concerns," in which it goes beyond the ethical requirements for research outlined in the *Belmont Report*. Importantly, any data generated remains the intellectual property of the Navajo Nation. This allows for tribal leaders to represent and protect the interests of the entire community, including those third parties who do not consent to research participation.

Importantly, the Navajo Nation Health Research Code clearly communicates how the Navajo Nation HRB aims to protect all members of their community from the potential harms of research, whether they are participants or not. The code states that the purpose of the HRB is to assure that both research and publication "are consistent with the health and education goals and objectives of the Navajo Nation" and "do not endanger the well-being of individuals or communities" (Navajo Nation Human Research Review Board, 2022). Thus, the code specifically charges the HRB with ensuring that the collection, dissemination, and publication of research results do not violate the health and education goals of the Navajo Nation as a whole. By setting their own conditions under which research may proceed on their land, the Navajo Nation HRB serves as a formal gatekeeper representing Navajo interests. This is an additional responsibility that IRBs that follow only the Common Rule and *Belmont Report* do not assume.

13.3.2 Community-Created Research Gatekeeping Organizations

Of course, most communities in which research takes place do not have formal structures like a tribal government that is recognized by treaties and has legal authority. In communities without formal structures, research gatekeeping organizations may be created by the community to fill this role (see Chap. 19, in this volume). For example, the Bronx Community Research Review Board (BxCRRB) seeks to:

> develop an independent research review board of volunteer community residents and representatives that will test a model of community consultation, dialogue, and "community-informed consent" by reviewing community-based research proposals, and to increase understanding of and participation in clinical research among residents of the Bronx. (Martin del Campo et al., 2013)

The BxCRRB is a gatekeeping organization that is comprised of community members who receive additional training in research ethics and study design to fulfill their role on the board. Unlike the Navajo Nation Human Research Review Board, the BxCRRB is not an IRB. The BxCRRB conducts its own review in addition to review by an institutionally-based IRB (e.g., the IRB at an academic institution with which the principal investigator of the study is affiliated).

Through community consultation, the BxCRRB seeks to prevent abuses and protect research participants, as well to protect and advance the interests of the community as a whole (Martin del Campo et al., 2013). According to their mission and vision, they are "focused on ensuring the proper representation of all Bronx residents during any community research projects, regardless of social status or economic standing" (Mission & Vision, 2022). By protecting and advancing the interests of the community and ensuring proper representation of all Bronx residents in community research, the BxCRRB addresses the shortcomings of individual consent in protecting third parties not enrolled in the research study.

In their reviews of proposed research, the BxCRRB aims to represent all Bronx residents in a variety of ways. For example, they make suggestions for how to shorten surveys, ensure that there are mechanisms in place for community involvement, and share results of research with the Bronx community. In one specific study, the BxCRRB noted that the researchers did not consider the feelings of potential research participants around risky sexual behaviors and issues of low views of self-worth and therefore suggested modifying the researcher's model to account for this as well as sexual violence (Martin del Campo et al., 2013). Such suggestions can serve to protect individual research participants, third parties, and the entire Bronx community. They also have the potential improve the quality of the research and its acceptability to the community.

13.3.3 Informal Community Leaders

Community leaders sometimes serve as informal gatekeepers to research when they control access to the community by virtue of their position. Community leaders hold profound influence in their community, to the extent that in some cases a research study may not succeed without their assistance and endorsement. This facilitates recruitment and continued participation in research by members of the community, providing access and improving implementation. Of course, if a community agency provides endorsement, researchers must proceed respectfully, as the actions of the study team will reflect on the leaders that "vouched" for them. This gatekeeping is formalized, for example, when researchers are required to obtain a letter of support or engagement from a community agency for a grant or an IRB protocol.

Community leader support can be integral to success, as these leaders, like other types of gatekeepers, will likely have a broader view and understanding of the community than most researchers, especially if the researchers have not previously worked in that community. While any individual member of a community might bring their perspective regarding the risks and benefits of a potential study, leaders may bring a broader perspective of the risks and benefits for the *entire* community informed by knowledge of the history of the community and past research studies in the community. Consider a scenario familiar to many researchers: A community partner and school district leader remarks that their school district is littered with the remains of research from investigators who came in, got their data, and left without ever telling the school district what they found. Such lack of respect can lead to a research institution developing a reputation among community members and community agencies as an untrustworthy research partner. Community leaders may have learned invaluable lessons from the mistakes of past researchers that provide insight into potential risks to third parties and the community as a whole as well as potential protections.

13.3.4 Researcher-Created Gatekeepers

Researchers often create community advisory boards (CABs) to obtain input and advice on specific features of a research study as well as how to engage the broader community in research. CABs advise on study design, recruitment, and retention of participants, interpretation of results, and other aspects of research. CABs are often convened by researchers; they are not generally convened by members of the community, although they can be (in which case they would be community-created gatekeeping organizations). Researchers create CABs sometimes in an ad hoc manner for a specific study or as a standing advisory committee for an institution (Newman et al., 2011; Stewart et al., 2019). When established and utilized properly, CABs can provide a structure for research partnerships that ensure the voices of the community are heard (Newman et al., 2011). In fact, CAB members have described their role in terms such as serving as the "voice of the community" (Ortega et al., 2018; Matthews et al., 2018). When CABs advise researchers regarding methods to ensure that they are "respectful and acceptable to the community" (Newman et al., 2011), they protect third parties and the community as a whole.

A CAB can advise researchers on the specific concerns of the community they represent, and even serve as a liaison between the researchers and the community, ensuring that potential participants understand their rights, including the right not to enroll or stop participation at any time (Strauss et al., 2001). When consulted early in the research project, CABs can help ensure that recruitment materials, consent forms, and the informed consent process adequately inform community members of study risks and benefits to ensure their voluntary informed consent and that these materials. Data suggest that many research participants, even after the informed consent process, do not understand the study to which they consented nor that they can stop participation at any time (Nishimura et al., 2013). The limitations of traditional informed consent to protect community members enrolled in community-based research have also been raised in the literature (Strauss et al., 2001).

13.4 Who Represents the Community?

The perspectives of everyday members of the community regarding what might be beneficial can differ from the perspectives of community leaders, so it is important to consider including both. Ultimately, researchers should engage with both community leaders *and* everyday community members—and do so early and often. A discussion of the advantages and disadvantages of engaging with these groups will describe a wholistic picture of community engagement and what researchers might reasonably seek and expect from such engagement.

When researchers engage with everyday members of the community, they will obtain important information regarding optimizing recruitment, understanding risks and benefits in the context of those who live in the community, and other insights they can use to improve their studies and the likelihood that such studies will be acceptable to members of the community. Engaging everyday community members helps lay the foundation for access to the community, as members of the study team will become known and recognized in the community through this process. Understanding the risks and benefits of a study from the perspective of community members in turn leads to more relevant and useful research for the community, as the benefits are optimized in the context of what is useful to and needed by the community, and risks can be foreseen and minimized. Authentic engagement that really listens and responds to community input—that takes the time to understand the needs and history of the community—demonstrates respect for the community and thus can repair mistrust based on historical abuses and recent negative interactions.

As noted above in the discussion of community leaders as gatekeepers, there are drawbacks to *exclusively* engaging everyday members of the community. Everyday members of the community might lack a historical perspective of research in the community (though surely not always) that leaders and organizations more readily grasp. Importantly, the study might need approval from community leaders to move forward; in native tribes with formal gatekeeping structures like tribal IRBs, approval is a pre-requisite for research to commence. Even in the absence of formal gatekeeping structures, community leaders might limit access to a key recruitment site such as a community center or school where their research will be conducted unless they are engaged and their input is sought.

Community leaders are in a position of prestige, and often have the power to prevent the research from moving forward, but they also possess knowledge regarding what their communities need as well as the values, perspectives, and priorities of different community members. The former is a necessity for the very possibility of conducting research, whereas the latter is truly what researchers should seek to improve their research.

13.5 Gatekeeping Threats to Voluntariness

In research that engages members of an identifiable community, the challenges to presenting information and ensuring comprehension are similar as in other types of studies. However, there are also unique challenges to voluntariness that arise when a study may have the apparent approval of a trusted community organization or leader. Such approval can obviously never replace individual determination about study participation. However, despite the earnest efforts of researchers, potential participants may not realize that they can truly decline participation in the research.

Consider for example research taking place at a substance abuse treatment center run by a community agency. In the U.S. there is a shortage of such treatment facilities leaving individuals desperate for treatment. Additionally, those seeking treatment are required to sign a number of documents in order to be treated. Imagine being in this situation and then being presented with an optional consent form for a research study by the same intake worker. The individual seeking treatment might not understand that they can decline participation in the study when each preceding form has been presented as a requirement.

This example illustrates the threats to voluntariness posed by some community-engaged research. Community members may be accustomed to signing multiple documents to access services at the community site, and a consent to participate in research, which they are free to decline without consequence to the services they receive, is an "outlier" in their usual experience. Endorsement by community leaders can also be a threat to voluntariness, as this endorsement carries immense weight. Of course, these threats can be addressed through a robust informed consent process and procedural steps (such as limited access to information about who participates in a study), but they must first be recognized.

13.6 Conclusion

There are numerous ways in which gatekeepers in communities protect not only research participants but third parties who are not enrolled as participants and the community as a whole. Formal and informal gatekeepers, identified by the community or by researchers, can represent community interests and address the shortcomings in protection from risks that reliance on individual consent alone presents in research on identifiable communities. While from an ethical, legal, and regulatory standpoint, gatekeepers are by no means a substitute for individual consent, when engaged correctly, they can improve the quality and acceptability of the research for the community, engender trust, and identify and mitigate potential harms.

References

Brugge, D., & Missaghian, M. (2006). Protecting the Navajo people through tribal regulation of research. *Science and Engineering Ethics, 12*(3), 491–507.

Friesen, P., Kearns, L., Redman, B., & Caplan, A. L. (2017). Rethinking the Belmont report? *The American Journal of Bioethics, 17*(7), 15–21.

Harmon, A. (2010). Indian tribe wins fight to limit research of Its DNA. *The New York Times* [Internet]. Apr 21 [Cited 2019 Jun 12]. Available from: https://www.nytimes.com/2010/04/22/us/22dna.html

Israel, B. A., Schulz, A. J., Parker, E. A., Becker, A. B., Allen, A., & Guzman, J. R. (2003). Critical issues in developing and following community-based participatory research principles. In *Critical issues in developing and following community-based participatory research for health* (pp. 56–73). Jossey-Bass.

Kimmelman, J. (2020). Why IRBs should protect bystanders in human research. *Bioethics, 34*(9), 933–936.

Klitzman, R. L. (2013). How IRBs view and make decisions about social risks. *Journal of Empirical Research on Human Research Ethics, 8*(3), 58–65. https://doi.org/10.1525/jer.2013.8.3.58

Martin del Campo, F., Casado, J., Spencer, P., & Strelnick, H. (2013). The development of the Bronx community research review board. *Progress in Community Health Partnerships, 7*(3), 341–352.

Matthews, A. K., Anderson, E. E., Willis, M., Castillo, A., & Choure, W. (2018). A community engagement advisory board as a strategy to improve research engagement and build institutional capacity for community-engaged research. *Journal of Clinical and Translational Science, 2*(2), 66–72.

Mello, M. M., & Wolf, L. E. (2010). The Havasupai Indian tribe case—Lessons for research involving stored biologic samples. *New England Journal of Medicine, 363*(3), 204–207.

Mission & Vision. (2022). [Internet] *Bronx Community Research Review Board.* [Cited 2022 Feb 11]. Available from: http://bxcrrb.org/who-we-are/mission-vision/

Navajo Nation Human Research Review Board. (2022). [Internet]. [Cited 2022 Jan 25]. Available from: https://www.nnhrrb.navajo-nsn.gov/resources.html

Newman, S. D., Andrews, J. O., Magwood, G. S., Jenkins, C., Cox, M. J., & Williamson, D. C. (2011). Community advisory boards in community-based participatory research: A synthesis of best processes. *Preventing Chronic Disease*, *8*(3).

Nishimura, A., Carey, J., Erwin, P. J., et al. (2013). Improving understanding in the research informed consent process: A systematic review of 54 interventions tested in randomized control trials. *BMC Medical Ethics, 14*(28). https://doi.org/10.1186/1472-6939-14-28

Ortega, S., McAlvain, M. S., Briant, K. J., Hohl, S., & Thompson, B. (2018). Perspectives of community advisory board members in a community-academic partnership. *Journal of Health Care Poor Underserved, 29*(4), 1529–1543.

Resnik, D. B., & Sharp, R. R. (2006). Protecting third parties in human subjects research. *IRB, 28*(4), 1–7.

Ross, L. F., Loup, A., Nelson, R. M., et al. (2010). Human subjects protections in community-engaged research: A research ethics framework. *Journal of Empirical Research on Human Research Ethics, 5*(1), 5–17. https://doi.org/10.1525/jer.2010.5.1.5

Shah, S. K., Miller, F., & Fernandez, L. H. (2020). The role of community engagement in addressing bystander risks in research: The case of a Zika virus controlled human infection study. *Bioethics, 34*(9), 883–892.

Stewart, M., Boateng, B., Joosten, Y., Burshell, D., Broughton, H., Calhoun, K., et al. (2019). Community advisory boards: Experiences and common practices of clinical and translational science award programs. *Journal of Clinical and Translational Science, 3*(5), 218–226. https://doi.org/10.1017/cts.2019.389

Strauss, R. P., Sengupta, S., Quinn, S. C., Goeppinger, J., Spaulding, C., Kegeles, S. M., et al. (2001). The role of community advisory boards: Involving communities in the informed consent process. *American Journal of Public Health, 91*(12), 1938–1943.

Wikler, D. (2020). Bystanders and ethical review of research: Proceed with caution. *Bioethics, 34*(9), 937–940.

Ryan Spellecy is the Ursula von der Ruhr Professor of Bioethics and also the Assistant Provost for Research and Director of the Human Research Protection Program at the Medical College of Wisconsin. His work focuses on research ethics, ethical issues in psychiatry, character in medical education, and community involvement in research.

Chapter 14
Paying Research Participants and Community and Patient Research Partners: An Engaging Ethical Issue

Lisa Ballance and Elizabeth Ripley

14.1 Introduction

Much health-related research requires human participants, making their recruitment and cooperation imperative to answering many important scientific questions. There is growing recognition that globally, human research focused on health outcomes is critical and therefore must include participants from diverse backgrounds, including the engagement of community partners. Beyond scientific issues of study design, data measurement, and analysis, the ongoing engagement of community and patient stakeholders has been clearly established as elemental to the quality, sustainability, and impact of health-related human research (Silberberg & Martinez-Bianchi, 2019, 589). Engaging in research—whether as a participant or as a research partner—takes time, and time is valuable. Beyond time, there may be actual costs or resources required for participation. Appropriate reimbursement for expenses incurred, compensation for time, and recognition of *research participants* (those persons who consent to participate in human research, which carries a degree of risk that must be balanced by potential future benefit to themselves or others) and *research partners* (organizations or individuals who represent the interests of individual research participants who engage with research teams to design, conduct, analyze, and/or disseminate research) is ethically imperative ("Payment and Reimbursement to Research Subjects | FDA", 2018).

L. Ballance (✉)
Office of the Vice President for Research and Innovation, Virginia Commonwealth University, Richmond, VA, USA
e-mail: lballance@vcu.edu

E. Ripley
School of Medicine, Virginia Commonwealth University, Richmond, VA, USA
e-mail: elizabeth.ripley@vcuhealth.org

E. E. Anderson (ed.), *Ethical Issues in Community and Patient Stakeholder–Engaged Health Research*, Philosophy and Medicine 146,
https://doi.org/10.1007/978-3-031-40379-8_14

While federal guidance states that compensation for research participation must never be "coercive" or "unduly influential," (45CFR46.116 (a)(2), what exactly constitutes "fair remuneration" is debated (Largent & Fernandez Lynch, 2017; Ripley et al., 2010a). For far too long, university and industry researchers have undervalued or ignored contributions of community partners, and only recently have guidelines for paying research partners emerged ("Financial Compensation of Patients, Caregivers, and Patient/Caregiver Organizations Engaged in PCORI-Funded Research as Engaged Research Partners", 2015). When money is involved, the concept of fairness is often subjective. A clear rubric to guide decision-making empowers research teams, institutions, Institutional Review Boards (IRBs), and regulatory bodies to fairly and equitably consider remuneration in a construct beyond simply "avoiding that which is coercive" (Bierer et al., 2021). Towards that goal, this chapter discusses ethical and regulatory considerations for appropriate compensation for both groups—research participants and research partners, explores the factors impacting remuneration, and identifies emerging best practices.

14.2 Applying Ethical Principles to Payments for Research Participants and Research Partners

In 1979, the United States National Commission for the Protection of Human Subjects in Biomedical and Behavioral Research published *The Belmont Report: Ethical Principles and Guidelines for the Protection of Human Research Subjects.* The *Belmont Report* is widely known for setting forth three basic ethical principles for human research: respect for persons, beneficence, and justice (National Commission, 1979). Building upon the ethical principles in the *Belmont Report*, the United States Code of Federal Regulations establishes that IRBs must review and issue an assurance that *risks are minimized, participation is equitable, and that consent is obtained* when required.

Each of the *Belmont* principles has some relevance for payment of research participants. Respect for persons requires that the IRB-approved informed consent form clearly outlines risks, benefits, and procedures as well as details of payment and any costs of participation. As discussed above, consent must be obtained in ways that *minimize the possibility of coercion or undue influence*. Beneficence requires that benefits outweigh the risks overall; in this calculus, payments are not to be considered benefits. Compensation for research participation can minimize the financial burden which may disproportionately impact some potential participants and limit access to the benefits of research. The principle of justice also suggests that payments to participants should be equitable—across studies and for similar procedures.

14.3 Federal Regulations and Guidance, State Laws, and Institutional Policies

United States federal regulations, state and local laws, and institutional policies guide payment for research participants and for research partners. Generally, the more restrictive requirement supersedes the less restrictive requirement. For example, if federal regulations permit a given approach but the state law does not, the more conservative approach should be followed—in this case, the state law.

In 2018, the U.S. Food and Drug Administration (FDA) published an information sheet, "Payment and Reimbursement to Research Subjects Guidance for Institutional and Review Boards and Clinical Investigators" ("Payment and Reimbursement to Research Subjects", 2018). This guidance noted that paying research participants in exchange for participation is a common and an acceptable practice. It is clear in the guidance that payments to research participants should *not* be considered a benefit but rather a recruitment incentive. It does not reference payment of research partners who are not considered human subjects in the research activity. Department of Health and Human Services (DHHS) guidance states that in addition to compensation, any anticipated costs to a participant should be discussed with the individual as well as clearly outlined in the informed consent document. FDA guidance requires that the IRB review not only the amount but the proposed method and timing of disbursement to assure that neither are coercive nor present undue influence (echoing the language of the Common Rule).

In response to this information sheet, the DHHS Secretary's Advisory Committee on Human Research Protections (SACHRP) issued their recommendations entitled, "Addressing Ethical Concerns Regarding Offers of Payment to Research Participants"("Attachment A – Addressing Ethical Concerns, Payment to Research", 2019). It recommended that the FDA and the Office of Human Research Protections (OHRP) issue clarifying guidance on reimbursement payments, compensation, and token appreciation payments. SACHRP further recommended that the FDA and OHRP issue guidance that outlines ways to minimize undue influence of incentive payments without necessarily eliminating payments or lowering the amounts. Both the FDA and SACHRP guidance documents are based on the understanding that the study would minimize risk, address enrollment of vulnerable populations, and provide adequate informed consent regardless of payment.

State laws as well as federal regulations govern areas including taxes for compensation, leading to additional requirements that pertain to the payment of human research participants. Because payments beyond reimbursement for research participation are considered compensation, institutions are required to collect U.S. Social Security Numbers (or U.S. Tax Identification numbers) for compensation or payment estimates expected to exceed $600/year. This amount is reported to the U.S. Internal Revenue Service on Form 1099-NEC. For individuals participating in more than one study in a year at an institution, this would be total compensation for all studies. As it is considered compensation, this may have other unanticipated impacts including becoming compensation that others can place liens on (e.g., child support or unpaid taxes) and as reportable income; it can also be considered in calculations for Supplemental Security Income (SSI) benefits and potentially impact the ability to qualify for financial benefit programs. The scope and authority of tax law for a given state should be considered when determining payments. For research teams at university or academic medical centers, typically state, as well as federal requirements, are incorporated or referenced in institutional policies. For compensation, the tax burden not only applies to cash payments, but also applies to gift cards, debit cards, and coupons, considered cash equivalents.

State regulations may also prohibit raffles, lotteries, or drawings where participation is rewarded or compensated by entry into an offering for a chance to win a larger item or payment to the participant. For example, Florida Statute Sections 849.0935(4)(b), (d) and (i) assert that it is unlawful to require consideration or contribution as a condition of entering a drawing or being selected to win. Thus, research studies in Florida cannot use lotteries to compensate research participants. California also has laws regarding lotteries. Thus, according to Human Subjects Protection Program guidance for the University of California, in order for a study to utilize a lottery, drawing, or raffle, the study must provide an arrangement for all individuals asked to be in the study to have an equal chance to win whether they decline to participate in the study, complete part of the study, or complete the entire study (Research Subjects Payments, Human Subjects Protection Program, University of California).

Universities and other research institutions have policies that dictate not only payment amounts but forms and timing of payments to research participants. IRB guidance may require where payment should be included in the consent form, what information about payment must be outlined in the protocol, when payments should be prorated, and whether completion bonuses are acceptable. IRBs may also have policies related to the manner in which compensation is addressed as part of recruitment, such as a prohibition on referencing specific dollar amount within advertisements.

The policies of institutional financial and/or grants and contracts offices may cover things such as the use of petty cash, what to do if participants do not want to provide their Social Security number (in keeping with federal and state department of taxation requirements), how to deliver funds to individuals or groups, and how to track those funds. While no federal regulations or state laws address payment of research partners, institutional policies will influence these payments. We recommend that all researchers familiarize themselves with their institution's finance and compliance rules for payment and when appropriate, request a consultation regarding the current procedures for compensating research participants and research partners.

Beyond rules for appropriate payment amounts and methods, tracking payments can be time-consuming and include additional, somewhat hidden requirements. Examples include requirements to collect social security numbers or tax IDs, tracking of names and distribution of coupons and gift cards, and limits on amounts provided in gift cards or cash. Different institutions manage these requirements differently. Resources have emerged in the form of software, payment cards, and third-party services to support this process, but rules and requirements may change and therefore should be monitored closely by research teams. If your financial office and/or IRB approves an approach that you think would be of benefit to establish as a best practice model, request that the IRB document the approach as a guideline or model to which research teams and IRB members can refer, thereby streamlining the review of compensation and recompense strategies in future studies.

14.4 Research Funders' Payment Guidelines

Agencies that fund research, such as the National Institutes of Health (NIH), have specific guidelines for budget expenditures and allowable expenses. For instance, the NIH Grants Policy Statement provides details on allowable expenses that justify the payment of individual participants as well as research partners. For individual research participants, the Grants Policy Statement allows for the coverage of incentive costs, patient care costs, childcare costs for research participants, and payment for medical care ("7.9 Allowability of Costs/Activities", 2021). Exhibit 5 categorizes 'Advertising and Public Relations' as allowable costs related to "program outreach and other specific purposes necessary to meet the requirements of the Federal award." The policy statement further identifies the meaning of "public relations" to include community relations, meaning remuneration for activities dedicated to maintaining "relations with the community or public at large or any segment of the public." In addition, "professional service costs" can support the payment of representatives of community groups where the service is needed to achieve the goals of the federal award.

There is emerging realization from funding organizations that research partners should be considered in determining the study budget. The Patient Centered Outcomes Research Institute (PCORI), a non-profit funding agency focused on clinical comparative effectiveness research, sets forth the expectation "that any research proposal submitted to PCORI will include a plan and related budget for fairly compensating patients, caregivers, and patient/caregiver organizations engaged as partners in the project" ("A Framework for Financial Compensation for Patient Partners in Research", 2015). PCORI recognizes the importance of financial compensation of research partners as a separate consideration beyond compensation for research participants. They also advise that the nature, amount, and details of compensation should reflect the skill level, experience, commitment and input of the engaged research partners. They expect community partners to be compensated ("Financial Compensation of Patients, Caregivers, and Patient/Caregiver Organizations Engaged in PCORI-Funded Research as Engaged Research Partners", 2015).

14.5 Guidance from Professional Organizations

Many professional organizations, including licensing bodies, have published norms and standards for the payment of research participants as part of broader ethical guidance for research. For instance, the American Psychological Association's Ethical Principles for Psychologists and Code of Conduct standards ("Ethical Principles of Psychologists and Code of Conduct", 2017) require that student pools provide options to earn the same course credit by completing equitable alternatives that do not require research participation and that students be protected if they decline or withdraw from participation.

14.6 Additional Considerations for Paying Research Partners

The Council for International Organizations of Medical Sciences, in their 2016, discuss the benefits of research for community research partners as well as for individual participants (Council for International Organizations of Medical Sciences and World Health Organization, 2016). According to Guideline 2, sponsors and researchers are obligated to assure fair distribution of benefits and burdens. On a community level, this includes benefits like investments in the local health infrastructure, training of laboratory personnel, education of the public, and financial gain from developing a successful product. Guideline 8 discusses capacity building, which includes building research infrastructure and research capacity, educating personnel, sharing in publications, authorship and data sharing, and preparing for future economic gains from the research. A research study should determine not only the financial costs and benefits but also non-financial benefits which should be shared with their community research partners. Bedeker et al. have expanded on the concept of ethical benefit sharing to include infrastructure, equipment, learned skills to do tasks and work, knowledge growth, ability to provide services to their community, career development and attribution and recognition of the contributions to the research (Bedeker et al., 2022).

PCORI calls for research partners to be appropriately and equitably compensated for their time, "at rates reflecting their level of engagement consistent with other members of the research team," that is, consistent with academic researchers ("Financial Compensation of Patients, Caregivers, and Patient/Caregiver Organizations Engaged in PCORI-Funded Research as Engaged Research Partners", 2015). This is a crucial point that has, in part, served as a primary catalyst for change in not only how research participants and groups are viewed but also has led to a greater recognition of the importance of consulting with the community about ways to approach compensation for individuals as well as community partners.

For example, community partners have real costs for engaging in research such as use of facilities, resources like printing, labor for cleaning, and security. Consider a group of academic researchers partnering with a local community organization that plans to utilize the organization's conference room for an event. The organization normally charges for these events to cover utilities, cleaning, and maintenance. Academic partners should recognize these costs and work with the community partners to plan for and reimburse these costs. If the community partner is a sub-awardee on a grant, the indirect costs for the organization should cover these expenses. If, however, the organization is not receiving a sub-award or a portion of the budget for participation, academic partners should discuss these costs with the organization and at a minimum acknowledge their cost as in-kind support and recognize their contribution to the success of the activity. If a community group is asked to visit your institution, reimbursement for those travel costs should be considered.

In research that engages community organizations, academic researchers must determine not only what budget will be necessary for community partners but also how those funds will be distributed and managed. Subcontracts may pose barriers for community organizations with limited resources for financial management. The time delay for reimbursement of actual expenses may also create financial stress for research partner organizations and individuals (Huff-Davis et al., 2018). Additionally, academic research institutions usually have predetermined indirect cost rates which may not have been established for community partner organizations. Including certain expenses on the academic institution's budget may limit the financial benefit to the partner organization due to the need for an increase to cover indirect costs.

Helping community partners get ready to participate with academic partners can strengthen collaborations (Darling et al., 2015). Resources exist to inform community organizations about research-related financial issues, such as the University of North Carolina's fiscal readiness guide: *The Community Partner's Guide for pre- and post-award grants management when conducting community engaged research* (Carter-Edwards et al., 2018) .

14.7 Proposed Models for Ethical Payment of Research Participants

Payments for research participation are ethical, fair, and appropriate if the amount is thoughtfully considered and well justified. Underpaying or simply not paying at all in an effort to avoid the perception of undue influence is unacceptable (Bierer et al., 2021). Ultimately, payment for participating in research could be a combined model considering reimbursement of any expenses, compensation for time (influenced by certain market considerations), and incentives (including opportunity cost to the individual or group) (Gelinas et al., 2018).

Individuals consider opportunity costs when determining whether to participate in research. In the case of human research, opportunity costs may include lost wages for missed work for study visits or the inability to pursue other sources of income or personal activities due to time dedicated to the research activities, which have become increasingly complex including daily diaries, nutrition logs, and digital check-ins between study visits. Yet, the focus remains on standard approaches as in equitable compensation using either a wage model (assignment of an hourly wage-like value) or a market-value model (a more complex view of the availability of research participants and the importance of their engagement) (Dickert & Grady, 1999).

While the goal of equitable compensation for time has merit, this singular approach has not resulted in equitable engagement of research participants by gender, race, ethnicity, and socio-economic factors. Ultimately, participants in a study may have very different opportunity costs depending on a multitude of factors, including their jobs, skills, and training. Attempts to cover actual opportunity costs would require a sliding scale compensation depending on actual or potential labor wages, providing participants with higher compensation for the same research procedures, raising ethical concerns. In practice, a fair approach is to provide the same compensation to participants who undergo the same study visits and procedures. This amount may vary by geographic area and should be considered for multisite studies. This does not include providing different payments for urban and suburban research sites in the same town but rather a recognition of the cost-of-living differences across states and geographic areas.

Incentive payments are designed to encourage an individual to participate or continue to participate through to the completion of the study. These payments can increase participation or assist with retaining participation in activities that may become particularly burdensome over time, such as annual follow-up visits or completion of nutritional or activity logs.

No individual or group should be further economically disadvantaged by participating in a clinical study. However, some groups may face specific financial barriers to research participation that others do not experience, and it is widely understood that failing to consider socioeconomic factors has led to a lack of diversity in clinical research (Bierer et al., 2021; Largent & Lynch, 2020). A simple reimbursement model has the potential to be inequitable. Requiring research participants to ask for reimbursement (e.g., by submitting receipts for transportation costs) may also be inequitable because some people may be less comfortable asking for reimbursement. Payment strategies that require federal reporting may impact social benefits if remuneration causes reported income to exceed the federal threshold (Bierer et al., 2021).

Inclusivity may require a variable remuneration model that considers different expenses for different individuals associated with research participation, such as childcare expenses, opportunity lost by not working when paid vacation is not available, or additional costs related to travel, such as added travel time due to bus transfers (Persad et al., 2019).

As an ethical imperative to human research resulting in public impact, representatives of and/or advocates for potential participants should be meaningfully engaged to provide input not only on the design of the study, consent process risks, and recruitment and data collection approaches but also recruitment and payment strategies. Consideration should be given to context, such as community factors that may be outside the lived experience of the original protocol design team. The engagement of community partners in determining participant payments can help provide both the context as well as help establish transparency and trust.

14.8 Comprehensive Frameworks for Determining Payments for Research Participants and Research Partners

Payment amounts for individual research participants and for research partners are part of an overall study budget and must be determined early in the planning process. Given the lack of comprehensive guidelines on acceptable payment amounts for specific research activities (Ripley et al., 2010a, b), here we provide comprehensive frameworks with guiding questions for determining payments for research participants and research partners. For studies that engage community research partners, obtaining their input on questions related to payment can not only establish equitable payment schemes it can also build trust and transparency.

For research participants, IRBs must first determine that the risk to the participants has been minimized and that the consent form and process is adequate. This creates the ethical foundation for appropriate consideration of participant payments. Ideally, investigators will determine the reasons and logistics for payment in collaboration with their community partners (Fig. 14.1).

For community partners, there is no ongoing oversight of the payments by the IRB. Funding agencies and institutions may have guidelines for how payments can be determined and distributed. Involving community partners in determining necessary payments and development of the budget can help increase transparency and trust (Fig. 14.2).

14.9 Case Study: When Research Partners Are Also Research Participants

For some studies that take place in communities, certain individuals may be both research participants and research partners. For purposes of IRB submission and payment, this requires clarification regarding which activities fall into each category. Study teams must be prepared to address issues that arise when these roles and activities merge. The case study below, which involves a community-based participatory research study that was separate from but related to a clinical trial, shows

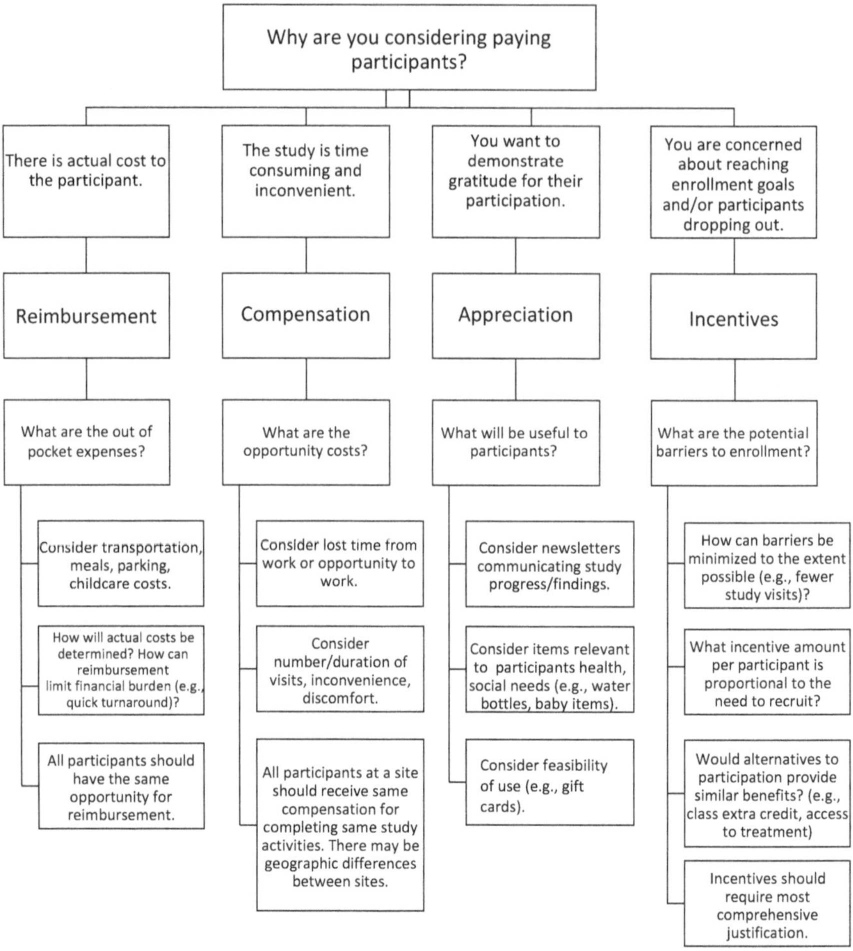

Fig. 14.1 Determining research participant payment
Reimbursements for expenses incurred are not considered compensation under the IRS Tax code sect. 62 – as such not taxable

the complexities of paying individuals as both research participants and partners. The case also highlights issues that can arise related to payments for research participants and community partners.

EFIC (pronounced "E-fik") clinical trials are those that seek to request an "exception from informed consent." Often conducted in emergency medical settings, these trials involve participants who, due to the nature of their health condition, are unable to give consent but who may require immediate enrollment—likely before legally authorized representatives can be reached. Specific federal regulations apply to such studies ("CFR—Code of Federal Regulations Title 21", 1996) that outline unique requirements. Because informed consent cannot be obtained prior to enrollment,

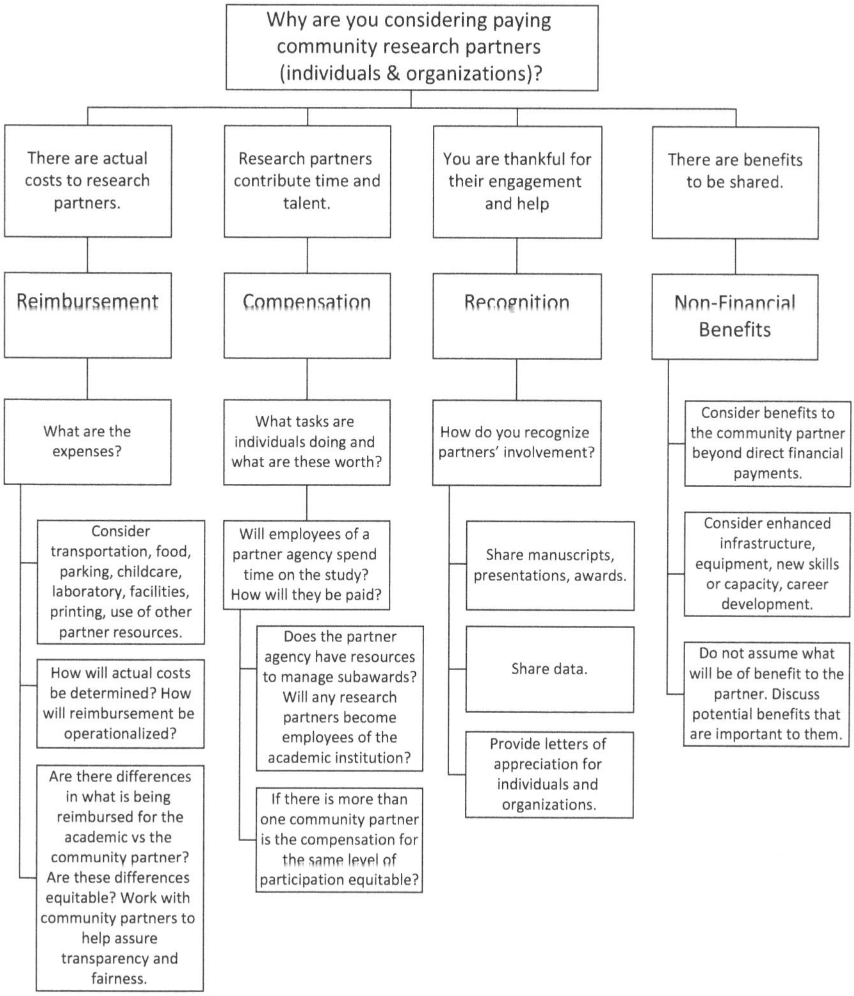

Fig. 14.2 Determining community partner payment
Reimbursements for expenses incurred are not considered compensation under the IRS Tax code section 62—as such not taxable.

researchers must consult the local community to determine concerns about the research and general willingness to participate. Additionally, community members must be notified regarding procedures to opt out of the trial. Community consideration, involvement, and voice are critical in these studies.

An academic medical center received a federal grant to evaluate developing community advocates for research as a method of improving community consultation for a trial that would request an exception from informed consent (EFIC). The clinical trial aimed to test the muscle injection of a medication for active seizures to be given by Emergency Medical System (EMS) providers (Shtull-Leber et al., 2017). Researchers engaged community partners, called Community Advocates for

Research (CARs), who represented key stakeholder communities, included a leader of a church, an EMS provider, a parent of an adult child with seizures, a parent of a child with seizures, a nurse manager who worked with seizure patients, a member of a community organization, a community advocate, and employees of two organizations serving the homeless population (Ramsey et al., 2011). The CARs partnered with the university investigators to learn about human subjects research and the planned study, to develop communication strategies, to gather opinions about research and the study among their communities, and to eventually provide consultation to another EFIC study that was being planned. In a supplemental study, researchers also studied the CARs and their activities to inform how best to engage community research partners in the planning and implementation of EFIC studies. Individuals with multiple roles were involved in varied activities. To delineate between a study of the CARs and the clinical trial itself, there were several consultations with the university IRB before and during the study.

The CARs served both as study personnel for the EFIC clinical trial and the supplemental study on the impact of CARs on community consultation and notification and as participants in the supplemental study. CARs provided informed consent for their participation in the supplemental study; for those that represented community organizations, this also required discussions and agreement from organizational leaders. The CARs received a stipend as compensation and reimbursement for some expenses. They also served as coauthors on several of the papers and presented study results at national meetings. Following the study, they received letters of appreciation and as requested their supervisors were copied.

The CARs study included two anonymous community surveys. The CARs as study personnel recruited participants and gathered the survey responses. During the first community survey, each respondent was to receive a \$1 coupon for a fast-food restaurant for responding to the survey. The academic investigators had determined this token without adequate discussion with the CARs. Several issues arose. First, the \$1 coupons were considered cash equivalents by the university and required careful documentation of the distribution of the coupons. With the approval of the university, each CAR received 100 coupons that were assigned to them with individual identifiable numbers. They then verified the use of the coupons for individuals completing the survey without gathering specific information about each survey respondent. This created a significant amount of logistical work which was difficult to explain to community members who were unaware of the policies. One of the individuals working with a community population also thought that those participants could best use bus passes and without discussion with the university investigators conducted drawings for bus passes for those that completed the survey. While it was not considered to create a risk to the respondents, this was a protocol violation which required reporting to the IRB. While the importance of following an IRB protocol had been discussed with the CARs, further education was required on paying research participants, ethical concerns, and protocol deviations. For the second survey, the CARS assisted in determining the best token for their populations. As a group, they decided small flashlights with the study logo to be the most useful. Cost-wise when bought in bulk, the flashlights were a little cheaper than the coupons and easier to manage.

One of the CARs was particularly interested in gaining research skills. He joined one of our IRB panels and became an affiliate faculty member which provided access to our library resources. He also helped author a manuscript about getting started in research in EMS settings. As part of the study, a qualitative study of EMS personnel was conducted to determine their opinions regarding participating in an EFIC trial. As a show of appreciation for the ambulance authority's participation in the EFIC trial and our CAR study, for EMS week the CARs and academic researchers provided a pancake breakfast for those finishing the night shift and starting the day shift. It was offered to all members of the community organization as a way of showing appreciation, building connections, and communication rather than direct payment for individual or the organization's participation.

CARs were invited to host our monthly meetings at their facilities or in their communities. This was not a requirement although the majority did host a meeting. This allowed others to see their organizations and learn more about their communities. Meeting costs were discussed with the host CAR and reimbursed by the study when possible.

The program received a community engagement research award from the academic institution. The academic investigators assured that the community partners were recognized in the award and invited to the award assembly and included in pictures.

There are many lessons to be learned from this case study for discussion of payment with community partners and the research team. Key items to discuss include:

1. Consider whether your community partners are participants and/or research personnel and what payment is reasonable for each of the roles.
2. Work with your community partners to determine the best options for appreciation, if offered for the participation of community members.
3. Remember to explain to community partners that compensation is considered taxable income.
4. Recognition of the contribution of community partners is important, and when appropriate, invite community partners to work with you as authors on manuscripts and presentations.
5. When meetings occur over mealtime, consider providing meals or reimbursing for the cost of the meal.
6. Invite community partners to host research study meetings at their facilities or in their communities and acknowledge any costs to the individual or their organization.
7. If community partners are involved with recruitment and the conduct of study procedures, assure that they understand key human subjects principles and IRB policies. This includes the voluntary nature of participation, the consent process, and following the approved study design. If the community partner will be obtaining consent and interacting with other research participants, consider what training your institution or IRB requires for them.

14.10 Conclusion

So much health research relies on the humans to participate. Additionally, when research studies engage and partner with community organizations or community members, this provides opportunities to translate research findings into transformative practices. Recognizing and appreciating these contributions—and their value—is critical.

Specific federal, state, and institutional guidelines and regulations regarding payment to research participants must be understood in the context of ethical principles. We supplement this limited guidance with frameworks (Figs. 1 and 2) that consider the why, the what, and the how of payment for both research participants and community partners.

References

"7.9 Allowability of Costs/Activities". (2021). Accessed 19 June 2022. https://grants.nih.gov/grants/policy/nihgps/HTML5/section_7/7.9_allowability_of_costs_activities.htm

"A Framework for Financial Compensation for Patient Partners in Research". (2015). *PCORI*. Accessed 19 June 2022. https://www.pcori.org/blog/framework-financial-compensation-patient-partners-research

"Attachment A – Addressing Ethical Concerns, Payment to Research". (2019). *HHS.gov*. Accessed 19 June 2022. https://www.hhs.gov/ohrp/sachrp-committee/recommendations/attachment-a-september-30-2019/index.html

Bedeker, A., Nichols, M., Allie, T., Tamuhla, T., van Heusden, P., Olorunsogbon, O., & Tiffin, N. (2022). A framework for the promotion of ethical benefit sharing in health research. *BMJ Global Health, 7*(2), e008096. https://doi.org/10.1136/bmjgh-2021-008096

Bierer, B. E., Bierer, B. E., White, S. A., Gelinas, L., & Strauss, D. H. (2021). Implementation, policy and community engagement special communication fair payment and just benefits to enhance diversity in clinical research. *Journal of Clinical and Translational Science, 5*, 159–160. https://doi.org/10.1017/cts.2021.816

Carter-Edwards, L., Enga, Z., Millar, E., Hyman, K., Washington, C., Quarles, E., Mitchell, M., et al. (2018). *Fiscal readiness initiative community partner's guide fiscal readiness guide for community partners fiscal readiness guide for community partners*.

"CFR – Code of Federal Regulations Title 21". (1996). Accessed 19 June 2022. https://www.accessdata.fda.gov/scripts/cdrh/cfdocs/cfcfr/cfrsearch.cfm?fr=50.24

Council for International Organizations of Medical Sciences and World Health Organization. (2016). *International ethical guidelines for health-related research involving humans*.

Darling, M., Gonzalez, F., Graves, K., Sheppard, V. B., de Mendoza, A. H., Leventhal, K. G., & Caicedo, L. (2015). *Practical tips for establishing partnerships with academic researchers: A resource guide for community-based organizations*. https://doi.org/10.1353/cpr.2015.0042.

Dickert, N., & Grady, C. (1999). What's the price of a research subject? Approaches to payment for research participation. *The New England Journal of Medicine, 341*(3), 198–203. https://doi.org/10.1056/NEJM199907153410312

Ethical Principles of Psychologists and Code of Conduct. (2017). Accessed 20 June 2022. https://www.apa.org/ethics/code

"Financial Compensation of Patients, Caregivers, and Patient/Caregiver Organizations Engaged in PCORI-Funded Research as Engaged Research Partners". (2015). *PCORI*. https://www.pcori.org/document/compensation-framework

Gelinas, L., Largent, E. A., Glenn Cohen, I., Kornetsky, S., Bierer, B. E., & Lynch, H. F. (2018). A framework for ethical payment to research participants. *New England Journal of Medicine, 378*(8), 766–771. https://doi.org/10.1056/NEJMsb1710591

Huff-Davis, A., Cornell, C. E., McElfish, P., Kim, K. H., & Yeary. (2018). Strategies to facilitate equitable resource sharing in community-engaged research. *Progress in Community Health Partnerships: Research, Education, and Action, 12*(2), 173–177. https://doi.org/10.1353/cpr.2018.0037

Largent, E. A., & Lynch, H. F. (2017). Paying research participants: Regulatory uncertainty, conceptual confusion, and a path forward. *Yale Journal of Health Policy, Law, and Ethics, 17*(1), 61–141.

Largent, E. A., & Lynch, H. F. (2020). Paying participants in COVID-19 trials. *The Journal of Infectious Diseases, 222*(3), 356–361. https://doi.org/10.1093/infdis/jiaa281

National Commission for the Protection of Human Subjects of Biomedical and Behavioral Research. (1979). *The Belmont Report: Ethical principles and guidelines for the protection of human subjects of research.* Accessed 19 June 2022. https://www.hhs.gov/ohrp/regulations-and-policy/belmont-report/index.html

"Payment and Reimbursement to Research Subjects". (2018). *FDA.* Accessed 19 June 2022. https://www.fda.gov/regulatory-information/search-fda-guidance-documents/payment-and-reimbursement-research-subjects

Persad, G., Lynch, H. F., & Largent, E. (2019). Differential payment to research participants in the same study: An ethical analysis. *Journal of Medical Ethics, 45*(5), 318–322. https://doi.org/10.1136/medethics-2018-105140

Ramsey, C. A., Quearry, B., & Ripley, E. (2011). Community consultation and public disclosure: Preliminary results from a new model. *Academic Emergency Medicine, 18*(7), 733–740. https://doi.org/10.1111/j.1553-2712.2011.01102.x

"Reporting Payments to Independent Contractors". (2022). IRS.gov. Accessed 19 June 2022. https://www.irs.gov/businesses/small-businesses-self-employed/reporting-payments-to-independent-contractors

"Research Subject Payments | Human Research Protection Program (HRPP)". (2022). Accessed 19 June 2022. https://irb.ucsf.edu/research-subject-payments#Special-rules-that-apply-to-drawingslotteriesraffles

Ripley, E., Macrina, F., Markowitz, M., & Gennings, C. (2010a). Who's doing the math? Are we really compensating research participants? *Journal of Empirical Research on Human Research Ethics, 5*(3), 57–65. https://doi.org/10.1525/jer.2010.5.3.57

Ripley, E., Macrina, F., Markowitz, M., & Gennings, C. (2010b). Why do we pay? A national survey of investigators and IRB chairpersons. *Journal of Empirical Research on Human Research Ethics, 5*(3), 43–56. https://doi.org/10.1525/jer.2010.5.3.43

Shtull-Leber, E., Silbergleit, R., & Meurer, W. J. (2017). Pre-hospital midazolam for benzodiazepine-treated seizures before and after the rapid anticonvulsant medication prior to arrival trial: A national observational cohort study. *PLoS One, 12*(3), e0173539. https://doi.org/10.1371/journal.pone.0173539

Silberberg, M., & Martinez-Bianchi, V. (2019). Community and stakeholder engagement. *Primary care, 46*(4), 587–594. https://doi.org/10.1016/j.pop.2019.07.014

Lisa Ballance is associate vice president for strategy and regulatory affairs and has over 25 years of experience in nearly every aspect of university research management and operations. She oversees critical aspects of the VCU research enterprise, including guiding the One VCU Research Strategic Priorities Plan and the regulatory affairs programs, including the human research protection program, the animal care and use program, and clinical research regulatory affairs. She has a master's degree from Old Dominion University.

Elizabeth Ripley is professor, vice dean, and senior associate dean for faculty affairs.

Chapter 15
Rethinking Risks and Benefits in Stakeholder-Engaged Research: Lessons from HIV, Substance Use, and Sexual Health Research with Marginalized Communities

Adrian Guta, Peter A. Newman, and Adam Bourne

15.1 Introduction

The SARS-CoV-2 (COVID-19) pandemic has dramatically impacted individual countries and global geopolitics. Throughout history, viruses, plagues, and pandemics have come and gone, influencing culture along the way. For example, the bubonic plague impacted most of Europe in waves that had wide cultural influences, such as the writings of William Shakespeare produced in sixteenth-century lockdown and in Renaissance architecture as can still be seen in Italy's 'wine windows.' The bubonic plague also changed the material conditions of millions, as evidenced by the increased wage bargaining power of those who survived. Other viruses were bounded within places or communities, like the so-called "Middle East respiratory syndrome-related coronavirus" (MERS). That COVID-19 spread as fast and far as it did reflects not only its transmissibility (with newer variants spreading even faster than the original) but a crisis of leadership in many countries following the rise of populist and authoritarian leaders and declining investments in public health. While many citizens diligently followed public health orders and isolated themselves in their homes, others ignored the risks, considering the pandemic 'fake news.' Numerous research studies have captured the range of opinions, attitudes, beliefs,

A. Guta (✉)
School of Social Work, University of Windsor, Windsor, Canada
e-mail: aguta@uwindsor.ca

P. A. Newman
Factor-Inwentash Faculty of Social Work, University of Toronto, Toronto, ON, Canada

A. Bourne
Australian Research Centre for Sex, Health and Society, La Trobe University, Melbourne, VIC, Australia

E. E. Anderson (ed.), *Ethical Issues in Community and Patient Stakeholder–Engaged Health Research*, Philosophy and Medicine 146,
https://doi.org/10.1007/978-3-031-40379-8_15

and preferences related to COVID-19 risk and prevention (Albarracin & Jung, 2021; Kleitman et al., 2021; Lee et al., 2021; Troiano & Nardi, 2021). As with many infectious diseases, COVID-19 disproportionately impacted communities that experience historical barriers to the social determinants of health and healthcare, especially racialized communities (Upshaw et al., 2021). Certain communities, such as people who use drugs (PWUD), the homeless, sex workers, and migrant workers, became viewed with increasing concern and suspicion over the perceived risk they posed to others (Guta & Newman, 2021; Newman & Guta, 2020).

The COVID-19 pandemic has highlighted the role of culture and politics in health, such as how information is shared and consumed across traditional and social media by diverse groups and communities. The COVID-19 pandemic has also highlighted the important role of political leaders, such as those who tell their communities to resist mask and vaccines mandates (Guta & Newman, 2021; Newman et al., 2022). Where governments failed to mobilize to protect the most vulnerable, or where the administrative requirements to access government aid programs effectively barred many from access (Chakrapani et al., 2021), community groups formed and mobilized to collect food and supplies to distribute to those in need. Some produced community-relevant public health messaging to better communicate the risks, as they were known at the time, with various marginalized groups. Such lessons are important, but certainly not new to those who work with community stakeholders to promote health, and who collaborate on research, program, and policy development.

We, the authors of this chapter, have been conducting stakeholder-engaged, community-based research (CBR) and collaborating with community, clinical, and policy stakeholders for decades. Stakeholder-engaged research is a broad umbrella term that covers a range of activities used to engage stakeholders throughout the research process that aim to increase the impact of research (Boaz et al., 2018). Guta has training in social work, public health, and bioethics, and has been conducting HIV, LGBTQ+, sexual health, and harm reduction research for nearly two decades in Canada. Newman has training in social psychology and social work and has been conducting HIV, LGBTQ+, sexual health and human rights research in Canada, India, South Africa, Thailand and across Southeast Asia. Bourne, with training in health psychology, has been conducting research on HIV, LGBTQ+, and sexual health and substance use research in the U.K., Australia, sub-Saharan Africa and Southeast Asia. We conduct stakeholder-engaged research because of the tremendous and multifaceted benefits of collaboration (which we have discussed in our respective writings), but also to address the complex ethical issues that arise when academic, clinical, and community stakeholders collaborate on research involving sensitive issues. Our shared interest in HIV and the communities most impacted provides us with a shared lens and history rooted in the activism of people living with and dying of AIDS at the beginning of the epidemic, and how in collaboration with clinicians, scientists, pharmaceutical companies, and policy and government leaders they changed the way research is done and who is expected to be around the proverbial 'table.'

In this chapter, we discuss the ways in which the weighing of risks and benefits in stakeholder-engaged research is similar *and* different from other forms of research involving human 'subjects.' Drawing on HIV CBR, we consider established risks, such as physical and emotional harm that may impact individual research participants, as well as social harms that may impact individuals, organizations and coalitions, communities, and entire populations. We consider how the active involvement of diverse stakeholders, with varying degrees of influence and power, can complicate traditional understandings of risks and benefits, and raise questions about academic ethics and social justice. We have training in research ethics and follow our respective national research ethics guidance and university research ethics policies and procedures, but also bring an understanding of bioethics, clinical ethics, and public health ethics. As we discuss further, stakeholder-engaged health research often necessitates more than one lens to make sense of the increasing complexity of projects; these may involve interdisciplinary research teams, clinical and community-based partners, community advisory boards, individuals with lived experience of the issue being researched—in community outreach and/or data collection roles, as well as trainees and staff. Stakeholder-engaged research also traverses various designs, included mixed methods (i.e., qualitative and quantitative) and multi-methods (i.e., more than one qualitative method), and expectations that the research results will be broadly disseminated and translated into improved programming at partner sites.

In the context of HIV, we are seeing a greater intensification of formalized partnerships between universities, research funders, public health agencies (at the local and national level), and global health organizations like UNAIDS, UNICEF, and the World Health Organization. Such alignments can be beneficial as in the case of initiatives to scale up HIV prevention and treatment, but they can also necessitate collaborations which may bring research goals into conflict with community needs (Guta et al., 2016a, b) and with government restrictions (Newman et al., 2021). Expectations in social science research for objectivity may clash with community expectations that research is a tool for advocacy, for example, when researchers are reluctant to make claims that are not directly supported by the results. Additionally, researchers and communities with shared goals may find themselves in conflict with government regulations. This has occurred when stakeholder-engaged HIV and sexual health research has occurred in religiously conservative sociopolitical contexts.

Much has already been written about tensions over the suitability of traditional research ethics review mechanisms (institutional review boards, research ethics boards, ethics review committees, etc.) (See Chaps. 18 and 19, this volume). These ethics review bodies typically privilege biomedical research models—expecting all research to have the specificity of a randomized controlled trial; however, the challenges faced by research teams conducting community-based, participatory, and action-oriented forms of research with marginalized communities may require greater flexibility and critical assessment of stereotypes that presume inability to safely engage in research (Guta et al., 2010, 2013; Tufford et al., 2012; see Chap. 18, in this volume). The purpose of this chapter is to move beyond these important but well debated and in some cases settled procedural issues (e.g., where ethics guidance and review boards have explicitly recognized such research in their guidelines and forms) to expand discussion about risks and benefits in stakeholder-engaged research.

We move beyond procedural understanding of ethics review and draw on conceptions of ethics rooted in critical traditions attuned to history, power, and discourse (Guta et al., 2016a, b; Murray & Holmes, 2009), feminist and communitarian approaches attuned to the embodied, relational, and collective (Ellis, 2016; Fry et al., 2005), and empirical research on human research ethics which seeks to understand, measure, and describe community preferences (Newman et al., 2015; Rubincam et al., 2016). Our engagement with different ethical lenses and published research combined with our collective experiences across dozens of research teams reflects our commitment to accountability and pluralism in research.

In the following section we consider risks and benefits in terms of the entire research cycle, from the partnership to the research and engagement methods, through to knowledge translation and dissemination activities. While we provide several categories as signposts, many of the issues we discuss intersect and should not be understood as discreet and compartmentalized. Rather, stakeholder-engaged research has evolving complexity, which shapes risks and benefits over the life of a project with implications for researchers, participants, partner organizations, and communities.

15.2 Stakeholder-Engaged Research: Lessons from HIV CBR

There are many histories of stakeholder-engaged research, depending on one's disciplinary training. We understand stakeholder-engaged research to have evolved from the writings of Kurt Lewin (Lewin, 1946), which advanced action research, then feminist and participatory research (Maguire, 1987) and community-based participatory research in public health (Minkler, 2010). What were once marginal approaches in health research have become mainstream (Horowitz et al., 2009) and may even be used to complement clinical trials (McFarlane et al., 2021). Our focus will be the HIV CBR movement, which is defined by a commitment to power sharing between academic and community partners, a recognition of diverse forms of scientific and experiential knowledge, and a commitment to capacity building and reciprocity (Guta et al., 2014; Harris, 2006). Not only was COVID-19 vaccine research built on the 40-year infrastructure of HIV vaccine research, the enduring importance of lessons from the HIV sector, including those from the early days marked by denial and scapegoating, have been evident throughout the COVID-19 pandemic. For example, numerous commentaries warned of unequal access to COVID-19 vaccines and healthcare, and the stigma that could come as specific risk groups were identified (Guta & Newman, 2021; Vasan & Pitisuttithum, 2021).

HIV CBR evolved from calls for the "greater involvement of people with AIDS" (GIPA) (Travers et al., 2008) into an entire research infrastructure which, in many countries, often requires multi-stakeholder collaborations to secure funding. In the Canadian province of Ontario, where Guta and Newman work, we can access funds from a provincial HIV funder, a federal funder with HIV-specific funding portfolios (which has expanded in recent years to include other bloodborne and sexually transmitted infections), and a federal funder focused on global health research. Available funding opportunities range from small developmental grants to international partnerships but typically have high expectations for collaboration across the entire research cycle—from the development of the research questions to data collection and analysis, dissemination, and implementation of results. In Bourne's work in the Australian state of Victoria, government funding routinely requires a consortium of university-based researchers and community organisations. This level of collaboration can make the difference between research projects that do not get funded or fail to garner attention from the target participant group (social media recruitment efforts that go unnoticed) and projects that mobilize the leadership of key organizations, their clinicians and staff, and clients. The latter includes supposedly 'hard to reach' communities, sometimes characterized as difficult to recruit because of stigma or access issues: for example, people engaged in sex work who may be unwilling to identify themselves, and people living in poverty who may not have telephones (for a critique of this concept in HIV see Moen et al., 2012). In our experience, stakeholder-engaged research is very effective at finding creative solutions to reach the supposedly 'hard to reach' on their own terms (Bungay et al., 2015). When stakeholders are willing to lend their time and respective professional and lived expertise to generate data about an emerging issue, the impact of an intervention, or the efficacy of new drug treatments or candidate vaccines, research can provide important data and promote community development and social justice. However, in coming together, and the sometimes-necessary blurring of boundaries (which we will discuss), numerous questions arise over research ethics and the weighing of risks and benefits.

15.3 Setting the Stage: Complicated Research/Researcher/Researched Entanglements

Classical approaches to research imagine a detached and neutral scientist who follows the scientific method and listens only to specific forms of evidence. However, this ignores the reality that science does not occur in a vacuum and that evidence does not speak—it is interpreted by researchers, governments, and publics who approach it through their own lens. The handling of the COVID-19 pandemic in the U.S. provides a troubling case study into how even bench science can become highly politicised. The SARS-COV-2 vaccine was among the most tested vaccines in history, with more than 70,000 participants across over 150 sites in initial trials of

Oxford-AstraZeneca and Pfizer-BioNTech vaccines alone; yet through bipartisan politics a narrative was constructed that these vaccines were untested and dangerous, which contributed to mass underutilization.

Dr. Anthony Fauci, famed physician and director of the U.S. National Institute of Allergy and Infectious Diseases, experienced public backlash in the 1980s when he was the face of the federal government's inaction on AIDS and was perceived to be holding up access to lifesaving therapeutics. Fauci reached out to his detractors, including radical AIDS activists, in ways that changed the relationship between science, activism, and governments and created communication and partnership pathways (McNeil Jr., 2020). While democratizing science and promoting public input is generally recognized as beneficial, there may be risks for stakeholders. Concerns have been raised about multi-sector partnerships eroding research standards and leading to the sublimation and bureaucratization of community advocacy (e.g., where previously radical grassroots organizations become hierarchical or 'professionalised' to access funding). In the HIV sector, this led to critiques about the privileging of community stakeholders whose perspectives align with governmental agendas at the expense of others who may be calling for structural change and radical interventions (the latter are less likely to be invited to participate in planning). Concerns have also been raised that partnerships lead to dependency from both researchers and community stakeholders who become reliant on funding streams, which limits their ability to be critical of the state and pharmaceutical companies (McClelland et al., 2018; Newman et al., 2015).

In terms of stakeholder-engaged research, questions about project sponsors, conflicts of interest and dual roles fail to capture the complexity of the global health infrastructure that sets priorities, which trickle down to the national and local level (Biesma et al., 2009; Pfeiffer & Nichter, 2008; Guta et al., 2016a, b; see Chap. 12, in this volume). The involvement of multiple stakeholders in creating the conditions of funding can improve the relevance of individual funding calls (e.g., when persons with lived experience help identify funding priorities), but it can also contribute to unrealistic expectations for researchers and community partners down the line, for example, expectations that research findings will impact practice within the life of the grant or that the research can accomplish more than is feasible given resource constraints. University-based researchers, especially those seeking tenure, are under ever growing pressure to secure funding and publish. Their continued success may require community partners to obtain grants. Those same community partners are often struggling to maintain program funding and staffing levels and must show evidence of success to do so. When these university-based researchers and community organizations come together, collaborative research can be mutually beneficial, with both partners obtaining the data they need for publication and program evaluation purposes. Or, two stakeholders might be forced together with competing expectations and interests - leading to conflict. Community partners may feel saddled with the burden of logistical issues which are typically left out of grants – and research budgets. This includes all the things that must happen before someone walks in and fills out a survey or participates in a focus group, such as building trust, demonstrating respect for local cultures, and ensuring voluntariness and comprehension of informed consent (Slack et al., 2016). Community agencies may also be responsible for identifying who the recognized community stakeholders are (Newman et al., 2015) or ensuring open communication after research is completed (Koen et al., 2013). This can be challenging to navigate and lead to misunderstandings on the part of community, particularly if there is lack of communication from researchers—for example when clinical trials are stopped early (Koen et al., 2013; Newman et al., 2011).

For their part, academic partners may feel pressured to produce flattering research about an organization with which they are partnering. In the Canadian context, many university-based researchers collaborate with AIDS service organizations and community-health centres which offer HIV programing. This can be a 'win-win' for the researchers who require access to potential participants and the organizations that must show evidence of their impact to program funders. However, conflict can arise over what kinds of questions to ask, who to ask, and how to interpret results when the organization's reputation and future funding might be at stake (for a discussion of issues related to a specific funding mechanism see Guta et al., 2014). As well, many administrative and regulatory processes which govern funding and research are ill-designed to include community partners in decision-making and to respond to changing community input (e.g., clinical trials which failed because community input was not integrated into the design) (Newman, 2006; UNAIDS, 2021). One of our chief concerns is when the momentum behind these partnerships and the need for data supersedes the needs of community members and risks overburdening them (Bungay et al., 2022). There are so called 'over researched' communities who continue to be researched despite not always seeing the benefit of previous research (Clark, 2008; Damon et al., 2017; Goodman et al., 2018; Koen et al., 2017). The issue is so pervasive that some communities have developed alternative ethical guidelines or processes (Neufeld et al., 2019; see Chaps. 19 and 20). In Victoria, Australia, Thorne Harbour Health, the leading HIV and LGBTQ+ health organisation, has for more than a decade convened a Community Research Endorsement Panel. This panel is tasked with reviewing all requests from researchers for the organisation to engage with research (such as by facilitating recruitment) and to ensure the research aligns with the sensitivities and needs of HIV-affected and LGBTQ+ communities. It was established after repeated research projects were seen to conflict with the right to self-determination of these communities and were insufficiently affirming of the identities and values of LGBTQ+ people or those living with HIV. Similar approaches of community research review or ethical approval are evident in other parts of Australia and in Canada. These systems can complicate and elongate project approvals and timelines, as well as foster disagreement between researchers and community organisations, but they can also be a valuable check and balance that research is meeting community need.

Researchers drawn to approaches that engage community members and other stakeholders may be members of the 'target' community (e.g., themselves identifying as LGBTQ+, living with HIV, have lived/living experience of drug use), may have been a practitioner (physician, nurse, social worker), have strong ties to the partner organization (perhaps even founded it and/or served on the Board), and may be known to the broader community through their research and activism. The 'multi-hat' wearing researcher is not uncommon in our experience, and the three of us have multiple positionalities which we bring to our research. This may bode well for the quality of the proposed research and strength of the partnership, but it also may place researchers in a tenuous situation. Whereas traditional non-stakeholder engaged approaches to research promote distance and boundaries between researchers and participants, and between research and care (e.g., a clinician should not recruit their own patients for a research study they are leading), this ignores the reality that research participants from very marginalized communities may want overlapping relationships. For example, we have encountered situations in which community members want assurances that the partnering organization (perhaps the only one serving them) is partnering with researchers with strong ties to the organization and community (those researchers who wear multiple hats), and may even prefer to integrate research activities into care to support their ability to participate (e.g., having nurses facilitate research participation because the community advisory board identified them as trusted sources and requested their assistance) (Strike et al., 2016).

Additionally, stakeholder-engaged research about complex health issues often requires interdisciplinary (medicine, public health, social work, nursing) expertise and community partnerships. While having a diversity of perspectives at the table can help challenge power hierarchies (Fauci at the same table with people living with HIV) there remains the risk that longstanding power hierarchies may be reproduced (i.e., that physicians dominate the discussions and set the research agenda with community members serving as merely symbols of stakeholder engagement) (Pantelic et al., 2022). A longstanding tradition within stakeholder-engaged research, especially within feminist participatory approaches (Williams et al., 2003), is the need to reflect on power and positionality and ask difficult questions about the partnership such as whose needs are being met and who is in control of the process (Muhammad et al., 2014; Travers et al., 2013). We have raised these issues to offer a backdrop for the subsequent analysis of risks and benefits in stakeholder-engaged research, which presents both opportunities and challenges in terms of procedural and relational ethics.

15.4 Scientific Review and Adaptation

Most funded research undergoes some form of scientific review to assess the quality of the research design and proposed activities. While typically considered to be outside of the purview of research ethics review, the quality of scientific review is an important ethical issue in stakeholder-engaged research. Scientific review is typically focused on the rationale, objectives, and research questions/hypotheses, and methods in a grant, but does not assess the quality or appropriateness of stakeholder engagement beyond ensuring that basic grant requirements are met (e.g., clear description of what the individual stakeholders bring to the project where this is required). Reviewers may be working on different issues in different contexts, and they may not understand the intricacies of a project set in a particular community. That is, scientific reviewers may be in a position to assess the quality of science generally but not the appropriateness of the scientific methods for the community/context, nor the quality of the engagement processes that led to the research questions/instruments. One important consideration at the funding stage is whether grants were developed in consultation with advisory boards who reviewed research questions and instruments, and who have a sense of the real world risks and benefits and feasibility (Quinn, 2004).

Following scientific review and funding approval, all research must undergo a certain level of post-funding adaptation in order to transform from a great idea into something that can be executed, particularly where the amount of funding requested does not align with the funds awarded. Stakeholder-engaged research may require additional post funding work to ensure that decisions made during the proposal phase are still relevant by the time funding is secured. In our experience, community research partners who gladly offered up their staff time and space for a worthwhile research project at the time of proposal submission may now, six or more months later, be facing new pressures, may have changed leadership, or may have reprioritized other initiatives. Our own work funded during the pandemic required considerable discussion among the project stakeholders and 'pivoting' to ensure participant safety and minimize disruptions at our partner sites, which were managing public health protocols that were changing on a weekly basis. Some projects, for the sake of the community and partners, were paused for one to two years to ensure the research would not disrupt care and services.

15.5 Power in Partnerships

What differentiates stakeholder-engaged research is the role of the team and partners, especially where community advisories and peer researchers are involved, the combination of methods, and the impact on participants. The need to examine power is not limited to project stakeholders and should be considered in all aspects of the research, including the design, combination of methods, and in data collection. For example, an extension of bringing together interdisciplinary researchers is that a growing number of projects combine biomedical and traditional social science techniques with more novel approaches like arts-based methods. Each of these have their own ethical dimensions, but when different research approaches are combined, this can create new risks for individual research participants who also access care and services from a partner organization. The use of venues that are considered safe spaces for research activities may understandably confuse or create challenges for participants; in fact, such spaces may be neither stable nor consistently safe, and hold different meanings for participants across intersectional sexual, class, and racial lines. Such issues emerged in our HIV research partnership including men who have sex with men (MSM) as participants and community-based organizations that serve MSM in South Africa amid pervasive anti-gay stigma and discrimination (Hassan et al., 2018). For example, while the provision of temporary (e.g., once monthly) safe spaces for Black African and 'colored' MSM in low-income areas facilitates engagement in HIV prevention research and advocacy amid otherwise heteronormative community environments, it also introduces individual risks. Unintentional disclosure of MSM's sexual behavior or identities in local communities can result in threats and physical violence, social disapprobation, and financial consequences (Hassan et al., 2018).

Stakeholder-engaged research often mobilizes the experiential knowledge and connections of persons with lived experience who may serve in community advisory roles or as peer researchers who may recruit participants and collect data (Philbin et al., 2021). (Also see Chap. 8, this volume.) This is a very popular approach in HIV, harm reduction, and in other research areas because of the ability of peers to gain access to networks that have previously been considered 'hard to reach' and communicate in ways that resonate with other community members. Peer-driven outreach and research with marginalized communities may entail both risks to participants and unique opportunities (Hassan et al., 2018). For example, the presence of peers may influence participants to share information they might not have otherwise (Guta et al., 2013). In a Canada-South Africa partnership focused on HIV prevention, the need emerged for peer training directed to developing safe and positive peer-MSM relationships, including attention to confidentiality and potential risks to participants outside the project's safe space. However, the emancipatory potential of safe spaces and peer training, even temporarily nurtured by time-limited research programs, emerged as a potentially strategic tool for promoting queer visibility and empowering MSM and community-based organizations that serve them (Hassan et al., 2018). As well, organizations often need research to show that their programs are working, and research budgets may become entangled with program budgets; for example, a single staff member may be funded through a combination of both program and research funding. Participants may understand the implications of hearing that a program is being "evaluated" and that the success of a peer initiative will determine the likelihood of it being sustained. This is not to say that a particular method is *a priori* "unethical," but that the risks must be considered for the individual method, the combination of stakeholders and methods, and how they might be experienced by participants within various contexts of care and multiple programs of research.

15.6 Compensation and Research Economies

The growth of stakeholder-engaged research with marginalized communities has gone so far from the margins to the mainstream that concerns have been raised about the impact of over-research and survival research economies, where marginalized participants support themselves on research work as advisory members, peers, and participants. We do not take issue with participants supporting themselves through research, and their knowing that their data, lived experience or expertise is currency to researchers, and advocating for better compensation (Collins et al., 2017; see Chap. 14, in this volume). Rather, we can become concerned when there are multiple projects being conducted at the same time leading to situations in which individual participants might be required to disclose traumatic experiences multiple times in a single day as they move from project to project (e.g., filling out surveys, sitting through focus groups, and drawing body maps; see Chaps. 19 and 20, in this volume).

Although stakeholder-engaged research is highly touted for asking better questions, tapping into better recruitment networks, and collecting better data, involvement in multiple projects can undermine trust within those networks. For example, when a staff person or peer working at an organization recruits clients to participate based on their understanding of a project (which may vary from the actual project goals), participants may be left having to deal with the emotional consequences (e.g., using drugs to cope with their feelings after filling out an invasive survey about their sexual assault history because the invitation came from a trusted source) (Bungay et al., 2022). Clinicians and staff have reported discomfort with the use of incentives and the blurring of research and clinical care and the use of incentives in stakeholder-engaged research (Gagnon et al., 2020). Where possible, we try to ensure staff and clinicians are at least aware that research is being conducted, in case a participant requires support after the data collection (e.g., a focus group becomes heated, which will impact programs for the rest of the day), but this may not be possible depending on staffing capacity.

15.7 The Risk of Unrecognized Risk

Under-estimating risks and overstating benefits may contribute to tensions in stakeholder-engaged research. We are committed to stakeholder-engaged research and recognize its benefits, but we are concerned about the risks that come with this work. Guta and Newman have served on research ethics boards and observed the pendulum swing from 'these people are inherently vulnerable and should not participate in research' because of their status as people living with HIV, MSM, people who use drugs, or sex workers, to what seems like *carte blanche* in the zealous pursuit of better data. That communities have emerging health issues which need to be understood is important, as is the potential for stakeholder-involved research to ensure the research is conducted ethically; but such determinations require a holistic weighing of risks and benefits which are typically eclipsed by practical considerations such as the needs for funding and evidence.

Stakeholder-engaged research typically involves research topics which by their nature require participants to explore emotionally complex issues such as illness and disease, poverty and hunger, and intimate partner violence. Our HIV research requires us to confront the intersections of poverty, colonization, racism, homophobia, gender-based violence, and stigmatized and criminalized activities, with further complexities added across different cultures and global settings. These issues certainly are part of many individuals' everyday lived experience; HIV stigma may follow people everywhere from their own homes to workplaces to healthcare settings. However, discussing these issues in the context of a project that involves numerous and diverse stakeholders can change the dynamic. The success of recruitment strategies using community-embedded stakeholders such as healthcare providers, faith leaders, and other people living with HIV from one's own ethnic community may entice individuals who might not otherwise feel ready to share their experiences or who might regret it afterwards (e.g., Hassan et al., 2018). Of course, this may be true of all research, but we argue there may be a difference between participating in research that takes place in psychology labs or hospitals and projects that take place at the sole organization that serves one's health and social needs. Should someone become upset, or if conflict escalates, that formerly 'safe space' may become compromised. Ideally, the collective expertise of the stakeholders should be mobilized to understand, to the extent possible, all contingencies, but even well-planned projects may lose sight of the complexities of bringing research into healthcare, service delivery, and social spaces where multiple issues may converge in unexpected ways. Furthermore, capacity-building of community-based organizations and peer researchers should inherently address these potential risks and enhance their skills in managing challenges, some of which may arise after researchers' involvement is completed.

Well-intentioned studies that seek to mobilize 'the community' may find divisions, fractures, or even multiple communities, which can be exacerbated by the presence of researchers. This may require changing project goals to better reflect the diversity of needs and changing methods (Switzer et al., 2015). It is one thing to be approached to do research on the street or on social media by a stranger with an affiliation to a university or research centre; it is another to be approached by someone from your own community or organization to contribute to a shared goal. Our point is not that any of these approaches are inherently 'unethical.' Indeed, they may be considered necessary and culturally appropriate. Rather, the combination of stakeholders, of research and practice considerations, of the target individuals, groups, communities, and contexts moderates the levels of risk. In countries as large and diverse as Canada, Australia, and South Africa, projects that try to reproduce a research activity across multiple sites may encounter completely different politics and dynamics wherever they go. This is fundamentally different than the prototypical lab-based research typically conducted in universities. Of course, such differences are also ever-present in international research partnerships, particularly in research such as HIV prevention that is considered sensitive with marginalized and stigmatized communities.

Certain aspects of HIV such as diverse forms of sexual expression and substance use are not just stigmatized but also criminalized. Collecting data, either from individuals or groups, can shine a spotlight on the participants, partnering organizations, and the entire community. Individual participants may be at risk of social and legal harms, and research has been used as a tool to misrepresent and shame communities, for example, when media and politicians manipulate research findings (Wenzel et al., 2017). When working with marginalized and stigmatized communities it is important to consider what kinds of data are collected and how they are used. For example, Guta was part of a team that worked with a specialty HIV hospital to explore the needs of their clients who use drugs. The results pointed to open substance use in clinical spaces, safety issues for non-substance using clients, and the challenging image of a patient in a medical gown buying drugs in sub-zero weather in front of the facility (Strike et al., 2014). In this case, the risk of collecting "unflattering data" was discussed in advance. What constitutes "unflattering data" is subjective, but the term has been used to describe data which may portray already stigmatized communities and the organizations that serve them in a negative light and lead to "victim blaming" if the media picks up on research findings (Brugge & Kole, 2003). In HIV and substance use, there is a history of reporting on risk behaviours (e.g., not using condoms and sterile injection equipment) without important contextual information (e.g., they are not accessible or are criminalized). In the case of the hospital study, the findings were discussed in relation to regulatory constraints which restrict opioid prescribing and harm reduction options and contribute to the reliance on illicit drugs that need to be used in precarious ways. To our knowledge, the results from this study did not lead to further stigmatization of patients or greater awareness and surveillance from the surrounding community and police involvement. However, arrests have happened in other projects that used stakeholders to bring sex workers and people who use drugs out into the open (Kazatchkine, 2014).

In Newman's community-based research with sexual and gender minority youth, young sex workers, and young people who use drugs in southeast Asia, the social and particularly the legal risks of participation were vastly different for young people in Indonesia than those in Thailand or the Philippines. Conducting research with adolescents and youth on HIV prevention and sexual health and rights required active awareness in project implementation that far exceeded what might be anticipated or addressed in a protocol prepared for an IRB/REB (Newman et al., 2021). In addition to careful procedures to protect the anonymity of youth key informants—some of whom might not have considered their own risk as high as that deemed by the research team—it was essential to also take special care to protect the anonymity of adult staff of various high-profile community and international organizations. Maintaining anonymity enhanced the veracity of the information shared (some of which could not be articulated in audio recordings but was revealed off-script and after recording was terminated) and provided important insights into the complex positionality of key staff in government ministries with clear dedication to serving young people amid repressive political and religious systems.

15.8 Managing Sensitive Data and Data Sensitivities

Across many of our projects, we have been acutely aware of the ways in which bonds built with community research partners have given us access to sensitive data, such as places where people hide and use drugs when they are hospitalized, which we have not shared with certain project stakeholders (e.g., clinical partners) or reported on in publications to protect community interests. Stakeholder-engaged research may have requirements for data sharing between partners to ensure the data are used in ways which benefit and do not harm the community. This may necessitate conversations within research teams about which partners have access to what data. In the Canadian context, research with Indigenous communities requires that they retain control of their data to ensure it is not used in ways which undermine Indigenous sovereignty and reproduce stigmatizing research which fails to account for the ongoing legacy of colonisation (Schnarch, 2004). Data protection is also salient in Canada because of unfortunate examples of authorities trying to obtain research data as evidence in court cases (Lowman & Palys, 2000; Palys & MacAlister, 2016). Such incidents have certainly caused distress to researchers, individual participants, and possibly resulted in a research chill across communities. Not all stakeholders will be able to fight subpoenas and protect data in the same way.

Stakeholder-engaged research can also create economic risks for participants, communities, and organizations. For example, research about sex work and drug use can shine a spotlight on certain practices such as drug selling and using venues or the intricacies of how or where sex is covertly sold on social media. When multiple stakeholders are involved, different conceptions of ethics may influence how such issues are viewed and handled. For example, if research partners include law enforcement, there may be a tension between a commitment to producing research evidence vs. protecting a community's safety. Again, some of these same issues may be present in research that does not engage stakeholders, but where it becomes especially complicated is when research funding is closely linked to service provision, and the economic risks of research extend to the sustainability of entire programs and organizations. If research does not gather deep and rich data or does not show improvements in key health outcomes, then funding may dry up. This will impact community members who rely on the research to supplement their incomes and organizations that may use research funds to pay staff salaries. As well, should these issues garner the attention of the news, politicians, and the public, there could be backlash that leads to entire programs of research and human service programming being shut down if deemed too controversial or a poor use of funding.

Neoliberalism has created conditions where small community-based organizations compete for state funding to provide services and must demonstrate evidence of their effectiveness (Grundy & Smith, 2005). They rely on research partners to evaluate their programs, but negative findings are often seen as evidence of a 'poor return on investment' rather than need of greater state investment. This can create situations where researchers may feel pressured to provide flattering accounts of partner organizations (Guta et al., 2014). Of course, positive research does not automatically result in long-term funding and systemic change. That community programs are unable to obtain core funding and must rely on research should not be accepted and normalized. This issue is especially pressing when advisory members and peers are involved and have become reliant on the salaries they receive from these projects. Hiring marginalized individuals to inform the research process and even collect data may be understood as short term and transactional by project leads, but those involved may experience considerable distress and be economically impacted when they are 'fired' from projects or promised work does not come through because of funding gaps or when projects end (Guta et al., 2013; MacKinnon et al., 2021; Newman et al., 2015).

Finally, concerns have also been raised in the literature about the validity of stakeholder-engaged research that involves community partners because of claims from some who have been involved in these initiatives that rigour has taken a back-seat to community preferences and agendas (Guta et al., 2014). Here research ethics starts to blend with scientific ethics, and when academic (e.g., publish or perish) and organizational (e.g., keeping programs funded) agendas compete, there may be unexpected risks for the communities whose realities and needs the research is meant to identify and articulate. When partnerships fall apart, or projects are stopped early, those who rely on the programs being offered may be hurt most—for example, HIV research in which participants receive food and money for attending appointments that combine care and research goals (Gagnon et al., 2020); peer researchers who relied on the income from collecting surveys (Guta et al., 2013); and biomedical HIV prevention trials with participants reliant on project-supported healthcare (Chakrapani et al., 2012).

15.9 Dissemination and Knowledge Translation

Finally, social, legal, and economic considerations extend into knowledge translation and dissemination. Dissemination has not always been framed as a core ethical consideration, except perhaps ensuring that participants will hear about results; but expectations for publication and dissemination of health research are now considered necessary for researcher accountability (Council for International Organizations of Medical Sciences 2017). Stakeholder-engaged research in health often follows publishing standards from medicine and public health, and it is not unusual to see academic authors, clinical and service providers, and even community members listed on grants and publications. This co-authorship is meant to recognize different kinds of expertise and what it takes to make these complex projects succeed. However, various stakeholders may share different ideas of what constitutes authorship and there may be conflicts over who is included, particularly in stakeholder contexts where 'authorship' is reflected as the organisation, rather than as individuals. The extent to which such inclusion and participation of stakeholders is meaningful is contested and hard to discern given publishing conventions that do not typically require such reporting (Pantelic et al., 2022).

As well, tensions may flare over what is included in publications related to the social, economic, and legal issues discussed previously. As illustrated by the example of "unflattering data" related to substance use in hospitals, the potential for these issues to emerge should be discussed in advance of data collection and agreements should be made about how the data will be collected and written about (see Chap. 16, in this volume). Early stakeholder engagement may be necessary to anticipate certain challenges of which researchers, particularly those new to a topical area or local community, themselves may be unaware. Here, too, we remind readers to consider inflated expectations of what a single project can achieve in terms of the impact of publishing a single article or community report. Despite our best intentions to marshal research into policy change, this may not happen and can lead to further disappointment.

15.10 Conclusion

In this chapter we have reflected on stakeholder-engaged research, with a focus on the HIV community-based research for which we share an interest and decades of experience. Our analysis of risks and benefits has been rooted in our own experience doing this work. We remain ardent advocates for the benefits of stakeholder-engaged research, especially when it involves interdisciplinary, inter-professional, and inter-sectoral collaborations which centre the needs of those most affected by a health issue. We have seen our work lead to policy change in individual organizations and contribute to shifts in clinical care. Sometimes these victories are small: a study on adolescent sexual health leads to a 'know your rights' document for youth, which ends up being presented prominently in health clinics; invitations to present findings to national and international organizations responsible for funding, researching, and introducing new forms of biomedical HIV prevention; and opportunities to discuss our research in national and international media outlets. However, this work requires thoughtful reflection on standard research risks—those found in all social science and biomedical health research—and attention to relational and process ethics, power between stakeholders, and the role of culture, space and place.

We are not the first to reflect on ethical tensions in stakeholder-engaged research and invite readers to explore and contribute to this literature. There is a growing evidence base which covers the spectrum of stakeholder-engaged research beyond what we have been able to address in our accounting of these issues based on our own experience. However, we leave readers with the advice to embrace ethical and methodological reflexivity, transdisciplinarity, and a commitment to inquiry and dialogue about the entire research cycle and imagined future projects. We wish to end where we started, by discussing the importance of stakeholder-engaged research for responding to global health issues like HIV and COVID-19. Currently other infectious diseases, such as monkeypox and polio, are spreading, with growing attention from global health and public health leadership and media, and questions about the responsibilities of those within the communities most affected. Much of this is top down without input from those most affected (e.g., MSM in the case of monkeypox) and those who care for them and fails to account for well-established stigma, barriers to healthcare, and even criminalization and violence in some contexts. The stigmatizing of HIV and COVID-19 do not need to be repeated, and stakeholder-engaged research conducted ethically may go a long way to promoting open lines of communication, dialogue, and trust.

References

Albarracin, D., & Jung, H. (2021). A research agenda for the post-COVID-19 world: Theory and research in social psychology. *Asian Journal of Social Psychology, 24*(1), 10–17. https://doi.org/10.1111/ajsp.12469

Biesma, R. G., Brugha, R., Harmer, A., Walsh, A., Spicer, N., & Walt, G. (2009). The effects of global health initiatives on country health systems: A review of the evidence from HIV/AIDS control. *Health Policy and Planning, 24*(4), 239–252. https://doi.org/10.1093/heapol/czp025

Boaz, A., Hanney, S., Borst, R., O'Shea, A., & Kok, M. (2018). How to engage stakeholders in research: Design principles to support improvement. *Health Research Policy and Systems, 16*(1), 60. https://doi.org/10.1186/s12961-018-0337-6

Brugge, D., & Kole, A. (2003). A case study of community-based participatory research ethics: The healthy public housing initiative. *Science and Engineering Ethics, 9*(4), 485–501.

Bungay, V., Oliffe, J., & Atchison, C. (2015). Addressing underrepresentation in sex work research: Reflections on designing a purposeful sampling strategy. *Qualitative Health Research, 26*(7), 966–978. https://doi.org/10.1177/1049732315613042

Bungay, V., Guta, A., Slemon, A., Varcoe, C., & Comber, S. (2022). The ethics of financial Incentivization for Health Research participation among sex Workers in a Canadian Context. *Qualitative Health Research, 0*(0), 10497323221089877. https://doi.org/10.1177/10497323221089877

Chakrapani, V., Newman, P. A., Singhal, N., Jerajani, J., & Shunmugam, M. (2012). Willingness to participate in HIV vaccine trials among men who have sex with men in Chennai and Mumbai, India: A social ecological approach. *PLoS One, 7*(12), e51080. https://doi.org/10.1371/journal.pone.0051080

Chakrapani, V., Newman, P. A., Sebastian, A., Rawat, S., Shunmugam, M., & Sellamuthu, P. (2021). The impact of COVID-19 on economic Well-being and health outcomes among transgender women in India. *Transgender Health*. https://doi.org/10.1089/trgh.2020.0131

Clark, T. (2008). `We're over-researched here!': Exploring accounts of research fatigue within qualitative research engagements. *Sociology, 42*(5), 953–970. https://doi.org/10.1177/0038038508094573

Collins, A. B., Strike, C., Guta, A., Turje, R. B., McDougall, P., Parashar, S., & McNeil, R. (2017). "We're giving you something so we get something in return": Perspectives on research participation and compensation among people living with HIV who use drugs. *International Journal of Drug Policy, 39*, 92–98. https://doi.org/10.1016/j.drugpo.2016.09.004

Council for International Organizations of Medical Sciences. (2017). International ethical guidelines for health-related research involving humans. *World Health Organization*.

Damon, W., Callon, C., Wiebe, L., Small, W., Kerr, T., & McNeil, R. (2017). Community-based participatory research in a heavily researched inner city neighbourhood: Perspectives of people who use drugs on their experiences as peer researchers. *Social Science & Medicine, 176*, 85–92.

Ellis, C. (2016). Compassionate research: Interviewing and storytelling from a relational ethics of care. In *The Routledge international handbook on narrative and life history* (pp. 441–455). Routledge.

Fry, C. L., Treloar, C., & Maher, L. (2005). Ethical challenges and responses in harm reduction research: Promoting applied communitarian ethics. *Drug and Alcohol Review, 24*(5), 449–459.

Gagnon, M., Guta, A., Upshur, R., Murray, S. J., & Bungay, V. (2020). "it gets people through the door": A qualitative case study of the use of incentives in the care of people at risk or living with HIV in British Columbia, Canada. *BMC Medical Ethics, 21*(1), 105. https://doi.org/10.1186/s12910-020-00548-5

Goodman, A., Morgan, R., Kuehlke, R., Kastor, S., Fleming, K., & Boyd, J. (2018). "We've been researched to death": Exploring the research experiences of urban indigenous peoples in Vancouver, Canada. *International Indigenous Policy Journal, 9*(2).

Grundy, J., & Smith, M. (2005). The politics of multiscalar citizenship: The case of lesbian and gay organizing in Canada. *Citizenship Studies, 9*(4), 389–404. https://doi.org/10.1080/13621020500211388

Guta, A., Wilson, M. G., Flicker, S., Travers, R., Mason, C., Wenyeve, G., & O'Campo, P. (2010). Are we asking the right questions? A review of Canadian REB practices in relation to community-based participatory research. *Journal of Empirical Research on Human Research Ethics, 5*(2), 35–46. https://doi.org/10.1525/jer.2010.5.2.35

Guta, A., Nixon, S. A., & Wilson, M. G. (2013). Resisting the seduction of "ethics creep": Using Foucault to surface complexity and contradiction in research ethics review. *Social Science & Medicine, 98*, 301–310. https://doi.org/10.1016/j.socscimed.2012.09.019

Guta, A., & Newman, P. A. (2021). Virality, desire and health assemblages: Mapping (dis)continuities in the response to and management of HIV and COVID-19. *Culture, Health & Sexuality, 23*(11), 1516–1531. https://doi.org/10.1080/13691058.2021.1981453

Guta, A., Flicker, S., & Roche, B. (2013). Governing through community allegiance: A qualitative examination of peer research in community-based participatory research. *Critical Public Health, 23*(4), 432–451. https://doi.org/10.1080/09581596.2012.761675

Guta, A., Strike, C., Flicker, S., Murray, S. J., Upshur, R., & Myers, T. (2014). Governing through community-based research: Lessons from the Canadian HIV research sector. *Social Science & Medicine, 123*, 250–261. https://doi.org/10.1016/j.socscimed.2014.07.028. https://www.sciencedirect.com/science/article/pii/S0277953614004572

Guta, A., Murray, S. J., & Gagnon, M. (2016a). HIV, viral suppression and new Technologies of Surveillance and Control. *Body & Society, 22*(2), 82–107. https://doi.org/10.1177/1357034x15624510

Guta, A., Murray, S. J., Strike, C., Flicker, S., Upshur, R., & Myers, T. (2016b). Governing well in community-based research: Lessons from Canada's HIV research sector on ethics, publics and the Care of the Self. *Public Health Ethics, 10*(3), 315–328. https://doi.org/10.1093/phe/phw024

Harris, G. E. (2006). Practicing HIV/AIDS community-based research. *AIDS Care, 18*(7), 731–738.

Hassan, N. R., Swartz, L., Kagee, A., De Wet, A., Lesch, A., Kafaar, Z., & Newman, P. A. (2018). "There is not a safe space where they can find themselves to be free": (un)safe spaces and the promotion of queer visibilities among township males who have sex with males (MSM) in Cape Town, South Africa. *Health & Place, 49*, 93–100. https://doi.org/10.1016/j.healthplace.2017.11.010

Horowitz, C. R., Robinson, M., & Seifer, S. (2009). Community-based participatory research from the margin to the mainstream: Are researchers prepared? *Circulation, 119*(19), 2633–2642.

Kazatchkine, M. (2014). TO PROTECT AND SERVE: How police, sex workers, and people who use drugs are joining forces to improve health and human rights.

Kleitman, S., Fullerton, D. J., Zhang, L. M., Blanchard, M. D., Lee, J., Stankov, L., & Thompson, V. (2021). To comply or not comply? A latent profile analysis of behaviours and attitudes during the COVID-19 pandemic. *PLoS One, 16*(7), e0255268. https://doi.org/10.1371/journal.pone.0255268

Koen, J., Essack, Z., Slack, C., Lindegger, G., & Newman, P. A. (2013). 'It looks like you just want them when things get rough': Civil society perspectives on negative trial results and stakeholder engagement in HIV prevention trials. *Developing World Bioethics, 13*(3), 138–148. https://doi.org/10.1111/j.1471-8847.2012.00338.x

Koen, J., Wassenaar, D., & Mamotte, N. (2017). The 'over-researched community': An ethics analysis of stakeholder views at two south African HIV prevention research sites. *Social Science & Medicine, 194*, 1–9. https://doi.org/10.1016/j.socscimed.2017.10.005

Lee, J.-K., Bullen, C., Amor, Y. B., Bush, S. R., Colombo, F., Gaviria, A., Abdool, S. S., Karim, B. K., Lavis, J. N., Lazarus, J. V., Lo, Y.-C., Michie, S. F., Norheim, O. F., Juhwan, O., Reddy, K. S., Rostila, M., Sáenz, R., Smith, L. D. G., Thwaites, J. W., Were, M. K., & Xue, L. (2021). Institutional and behaviour-change interventions to support COVID-19 public health measures:

A review by the lancet commission task force on public health measures to suppress the pandemic. *International Health, 13*(5), 399–409. https://doi.org/10.1093/inthealth/ihab022

Lewin, K. (1946). Action research and minority problems. *Journal of Social Issues, 2*(4), 34–46.

Lowman, J., & Palys, T. (2000). Ethics and institutional conflict of interest: The research confidentiality controversy at Simon Fraser University. *Sociological Practice, 2*(4), 245–264.

MacKinnon, K. R., Guta, A., Voronka, J., Pilling, M., Williams, C. C., Strike, C., & Ross, L. E. (2021). The political economy of peer research: Mapping the possibilities and Precarities of paying people for lived experience. *The British Journal of Social Work*. https://doi.org/10.1093/bjsw/bcaa241

Maguire, P. (1987). *Doing participatory research: A feminist approach*. University of Massachusetts Amherst.

McClelland, A., Guta, A., & Greenspan, N. (2018). Governing participation: A critical analysis of international and Canadian texts promoting the greater involvement of people living with HIV & AIDS. *Seeing Red: HIV/AIDS and Public Policy in Canada*, 195–214.

McFarlane, J., Soroya, A. O., Peng, W., Awonuga, O., & Morgan, S. E. (2021). Community-based participatory research (CBPR) to enhance participation of racial/ethnic minorities in clinical trials: A 10-year systematic review. *Health Communication, 1-18*. https://doi.org/10.1080/10410236.2021.1943978

McNeil, D. G. Jr. (2020). 'We loved each other': Fauci recalls Larry Kramer, friend and nemesis. *The New York times*, 2020. https://www.nytimes.com/2020/05/27/health/larry-kramer-anthony-fauci.html

Minkler, M. (2010). Linking science and policy through community-based participatory research to study and address health disparities. *American Journal of Public Health, 100*(S1), S81–S87.

Moen, K., Aggleton, P., Leshabari, M. T., & Middelthon, A.-L. (2012). Not at all so hard-to-reach: Same-sex attracted men in Dar Es Salaam. *Culture, Health & Sexuality, 14*(2), 195–208. https://doi.org/10.1080/13691058.2011.632825

Muhammad, M., Wallerstein, N., Sussman, A. L., Avila, M., Belone, L., & Duran, B. (2014). Reflections on researcher identity and power: The impact of positionality on community based participatory research (CBPR) processes and outcomes. *Critical Sociology, 41*(7–8), 1045–1063. https://doi.org/10.1177/0896920513516025

Murray, S. J., & Holmes, D. (2009). Critical interventions in the ethics of healthcare: Challenging the principle of autonomy in bioethics.

Neufeld, S. D., Chapman, J., Crier, N., Marsh, S., McLeod, J., & Deane, L. A. (2019). Research 101: A process for developing local guidelines for ethical research in heavily researched communities. *Harm Reduction Journal, 16*(1), 41. https://doi.org/10.1186/s12954-019-0315-5

Newman, P. A. (2006). Towards a science of community engagement. *Lancet, 367*(9507), 302. https://doi.org/10.1016/s0140-6736(06)68067-7

Newman, P. A., & Guta, A. (2020). How to have sex in an epidemic Redux: Reinforcing HIV prevention in the COVID-19 pandemic. *AIDS and Behavior, 24*(8), 2260–2264. https://doi.org/10.1007/s10461-020-02940-z. https://www.ncbi.nlm.nih.gov/pubmed/32500463

Newman, P. A., Logie, C., James, L. L., Charles, T., Maxwell, J., Salam, K., & Woodford, M. (2011). "Speaking the dialect": Understanding public discourse in the aftermath of an HIV vaccine trial shutdown. *American Journal of Public Health, 101*(9), 1749–1758. https://doi.org/10.2105/AJPH.2011.300208

Newman, P. A., Rubincam, C., Slack, C., Essack, Z., Chakrapani, V., Chuang, D. M., Tepjan, S., Shunmugam, M., Roungprakhon, S., Logie, C., Koen, J., & Lindegger, G. (2015). Towards a science of community stakeholder engagement in biomedical HIV prevention trials: An embedded four-country case study. *PLoS One, 10*(8), e0135937. https://doi.org/10.1371/journal.pone.0135937

Newman, P. A., Prabhu, S. M., Akkakanjanasupar, P., & Tepjan, S. (2021). HIV and mental health among young people in low-resource contexts in Southeast Asia: A qualitative investigation. *Global Public Health, 1-15*. https://doi.org/10.1080/17441692.2021.1924822

Newman, P. A., Reid, L., Tepjan, S., Fantus, S., Allan, K., Nyoni, T., Guta, A., & Williams, C. C. (2022). COVID-19 vaccine hesitancy among marginalized populations in the US and Canada: Protocol for a scoping review. *PLoS One, 17*(3), e0266120.

Palys, T., & MacAlister, D. (2016). Protecting research confidentiality via the Wigmore criteria: Some implications of parent and Bruckert v the Queen and Luka Rocco Magnotta. *Canadian Journal of Law and Society/La Revue Canadienne Droit et Société, 31*(3), 473–493.

Pantelic, M., Steinert, J. I., Ayala, G., Sprague, L., Chang, J., Thomas, R. M., Nininahazwe, C., Caswell, G., Bach-Mortensen, A. M., & Bourne, A. (2022). Addressing epistemic injustice in HIV research: A call for reporting guidelines on meaningful community engagement. *Journal of the International AIDS Society, 25*(1), e25880. https://doi.org/10.1002/jia2.25880

Pfeiffer, J., & Nichter, M. (2008). What can critical medical anthropology contribute to Global Health? A health systems perspective. *Medical Anthropology Quarterly, 22*(4), 410–415. http://www.jstor.org/stable/25487843

Philbin, M. M., Guta, A., Wurtz, H., Kinnard, E. N., Bradley-Perrin, I., & Goldsamt, L. (2021). How black and Latino young men who have sex with men in the United States experience and engage with eligibility criteria and recruitment practices: Implications for the sustainability of community-based research. *Critical Public Health, 1-12*. https://doi.org/10.1080/09581596.2021.1918329

Quinn, S. C. (2004). Ethics in public Health Research. *American Journal of Public Health, 94*(6), 918–922. https://doi.org/10.2105/AJPH.94.6.918

Rubincam, C., Lacombe-Duncan, A., & Newman, P. A. (2016). Taking culture seriously in biomedical HIV prevention trials: A meta-synthesis of qualitative studies. *Expert Review of Vaccines, 15*(3), 331–347. https://doi.org/10.1586/14760584.2016.1118349

Schnarch, B. (2004). Ownership, control, access, and possession (OCAP) or self-determination applied to research: A critical analysis of contemporary first nations research and some options for first nations communities. *International Journal of Indigenous Health, 1*(1), 80–95.

Slack, C., Thabethe, S., Lindegger, G., Matandika, L., Newman, P. A., Kerr, P., Wassenaar, D., Roux, S., & Bekker, L. G. (2016). I've gone through this my own self, so i practice what i preach. *Journal of Empirical Research on Human Research Ethics, 11*(4), 322–333. https://doi.org/10.1177/1556264616675202

Strike, C., Guta, A., de Prinse, K., Switzer, S., & Carusone, S. C. (2014). Living with addiction: The perspectives of drug using and non-using individuals about sharing space in a hospital setting. *International Journal of Drug Policy, 25*(3), 640–649. https://doi.org/10.1016/j.drugpo.2014.02.012

Strike, C., Guta, A., De Prinse, K., Switzer, S., & Carusone, S. C. (2016). Opportunities, challenges and ethical issues associated with conducting community-based participatory research in a hospital setting. *Research Ethics, 12*(3), 149–157.

Switzer, S, Adrian Guta, de K Prinse, S Chan Carusone, C Strike. 2015. "Visualizing harm reduction: Methodological and ethical considerations." Social Science & Medicine 133: 77–84.

Travers, R., Wilson, M. G., Flicker, S., Guta, A., Bereket, T., McKay, C., van der Meulen, A., Cleverly, S., Dickie, M., & Globerman, J. (2008). The greater involvement of people living with AIDS principle: Theory versus practice in Ontario's HIV/AIDS community-based research sector. *AIDS Care, 20*(6), 615–624.

Travers, R., Pyne, J., Bauer, G., Munro, L., Giambrone, B., Hammond, R., & Scanlon, K. (2013). 'Community control' in CBPR: Challenges experienced and questions raised from the trans PULSE project. *Action Research, 11*(4), 403–422. https://doi.org/10.1177/1476750313507093

Troiano, G., & Nardi, A. (2021). Vaccine hesitancy in the era of COVID-19. *Public Health, 194*, 245–251. https://doi.org/10.1016/j.puhe.2021.02.025

Tufford, L., Newman, P. A., Brennan, D. J., Craig, S. L., & Woodford, M. R. (2012). Conducting research with lesbian, gay, and bisexual populations: Navigating research ethics board reviews. *Journal of Gay & Lesbian Social Services, 24*(3), 221–240. https://doi.org/10.1080/10538720.2012.697039

UNAIDS. 2021. Ethical considerations in HIV prevention trials.

Upshaw, T. L., Brown, C., Smith, R., Perri, M., Ziegler, C., & Pinto, A. D. (2021). Social determinants of COVID-19 incidence and outcomes: A rapid review. *PLoS One, 16*(3), e0248336. https://doi.org/10.1371/journal.pone.0248336
Vasan, S., & Pitisuttithum, P. (2021). Vaccine development lessons between HIV and COVID-19. *The Lancet Infectious Diseases, 21*(6), 759–761. https://doi.org/10.1016/S1473-3099(21)00274-7
Wenzel, A., Gerson, D., Moreno, E., Son, M., & Hawkins, B. M. (2017). Engaging stigmatized communities through solutions journalism: Residents of South Los Angeles respond. *Journalism, 19*(5), 649–667. https://doi.org/10.1177/1464884917703125
Williams, J., Brinton, M., & Lykes. (2003). Bridging theory and practice: Using reflexive cycles in feminist participatory action research. *Feminism & Psychology, 13*(3), 287–294.

Adrian Guta has training in social work, public health, and bioethics, and has been conducting HIV, LGBTQ+, sexual health, and harm reduction research for nearly two decades in Canada.

Peter A. Newman has training in social psychology and social work and has been conducting HIV, LGBTQ+, sexual health and human rights research in Canada, India, South Africa and across Southeast Asia.

Adam Bourne has training in health psychology and has been conducting research on HIV, LGBTQ+ communities, sexual health, and substance use in the U.K., Australia, sub-Saharan Africa, and Southeast Asia.

Chapter 16
Data Decisions and Ethics: The Case of Stakeholder-Engaged Research

Melody S. Goodman, Kristyn A. Pierce, James M. DuBois, and Vetta Sanders Thompson

16.1 Introduction

The established standard frameworks of ethical review used by institutional review boards (IRBs), which are designed to maintain compliance with regulations and to protect individual research participants from harm, do not always adequately address the ethical challenges that arise within research relationships and projects. The shortcomings of the "one-size-fits-all" ethical frameworks used in traditional research are especially apparent regarding data-related decisions in stakeholder-engaged research (SER). Therefore, normative ethical guidelines are needed to ensure ethical conduct related to data ownership, use, publication, and sharing in SER (Wilson et al., 2017).

Kouper and colleagues conducted a study among individuals who work with data, the majority of whom were from social science disciplines, to understand how

M. S. Goodman (✉)
Department of Biostatistics, School of Global Public Health, New York University, New York, NY, USA
e-mail: melody.goodman@nyu.edu

K. A. Pierce
Department of Pediatrics, NYU Langone Health, New York, NY, USA
e-mail: kristyn.pierce@nyulangone.org

J. M. DuBois
Center for Clinical and Research Ethics, Division of General Medical Sciences, Washington University School of Medicine, Saint Louis, MO, USA
e-mail: duboisjm@wustl.edu

V. S. Thompson
Brown School, Washington University in St. Louis, Saint Louis, MO, USA
e-mail: vthompson22@wustl.edu

E. E. Anderson (ed.), *Ethical Issues in Community and Patient Stakeholder–Engaged Health Research*, Philosophy and Medicine 146,
https://doi.org/10.1007/978-3-031-40379-8_16

various stakeholders work together to make decisions regarding data sharing (Kouper et al., 2020). Almost a quarter of participants perceived funding agencies as being responsible for making key decisions regarding data. However, when asked who should take on this responsibility, 65% said individual researchers should be responsible for the governance of the data. The research team ultimately concluded that data governance should be shared by the "data ecosystem" (Kouper et al., 2020). The complexity of this ecosystem is defined by the following:

> 1) the varied and substantial number of organizations and institutions involved, 2) individual actors who act both on behalf of their employing organizations and the larger collective communities, 3) the presence of organizations with economic interests, 4) the belief that everyone is responsible for data governance, 5) and the absence of a shared vision and collective action organizations that balance the influences of the various actors. (Kouper et al., 2020, p. 133)

Overall, data governance in the United States, and globally, is a complex issue with serious implications for society. Here, we will focus on ethical challenges involving ownership, use, and publication of data collected during a stakeholder-engaged research study.

Several ethical challenges may arise during SER, but the potential benefits will outweigh the challenges if researchers plan accordingly. By establishing meaningful partnerships with community stakeholders, researchers can act in a sensitive, ethical manner when collecting, managing, sharing, and publishing data obtained in SER. Investigators should take the time to help the community understand funders' expectations for data ownership and availability. If there are requirements to deposit data, the community must know that the data may be available to be analyzed by parties with whom they have no agreement or relationship and when this might occur. Beyond issues of funding, important negotiation topics include budgets and barriers to community participation in research, data sharing, and dissemination. The discussion is not simply whether data are shared, but also the format and method of sharing. How data and findings are shared affects whether they are useful to the community and meet community needs and SER expectations. Without these discussions, unexpected dissemination of findings may undermine trust and violate informal assumptions and understandings based on SER principles (see Chap. 3, this volume).

16.1.1 Definition of Data

The National Institutes of Health (NIH) defines *data* as "recorded information, regardless of the form or media on which it may be recorded" (National Institutes of Health, 2021, par. 1). Based on this definition, data include "writings, films, sound recordings, pictorial reproductions, drawings, designs, or other graphic representations, procedural manuals, forms, diagrams, workflow charts, equipment descriptions, data files, data processing or computer programs (software), statistical records, and other research data" (National Institutes of Health, 2021, par. 1).

Policies and practices related to data ownership, publication, and sharing must consider all of these forms of data.

16.1.2 Ownership, Stewardship, Use, Publication, Sharing, Repository, and Open Access

Before addressing the myriad ethical challenges surrounding data in SER, we will broadly discuss the terms *ownership*, *steward*, *use*, *publication*, *sharing*, *repository*, and *Open Access*, and their applications to research data (Table 16.1).

First, the entity who has ownership, or the legal right to make decisions regarding the data, may be determined by institutional policies, contracts, case law, and how the project is funded (DuBois et al., 2018a; National Institutes of Health, 2021; Blum, 2015). The owner of research data is usually the institution where the research takes place (Blum, 2015). A data steward is the individual who is responsible for making data findable, accessible, interoperable, and reusable on a long-term basis (Jansen et al., 2019). The challenge with SER is that the data steward (e.g., Principal Investigator), not the data owner (e.g., institution), negotiates with nonacademic stakeholders on how the data will be used, stored, and shared (Glass & Kaufert, 2007; Flicker et al., 2007). Although the data steward controls data use, it is unclear who will make the ultimate decision about data storage and sharing: the data steward or the data owner (Blum, 2015).

Data use refers to the set of processes, conditions, and contexts in which the steward uses the data, such as in certain analyses or to answer various research questions (Coburn & Turner, 2011). In SER, it is important to make sure that all partners have access to the data in useful formats and have permission to use the data for their needs (e.g., program evaluation, advocacy, grant writing, publication). Every partnership should have clear guidelines on how the data will be used and should ensure that the guidelines are appropriate for and applied consistently across all members of the partnership (Minkler, 2004).

Table 16.1 Definitions of key terms related to data

Key term	Definition
Data ownership	Individual or entity that has the legal right to possession of data and is allowed to make decisions regarding data
Data Steward	Individual or entity responsible for activities regarding the long-term care of and access to data
Data use	Various ways in which the owner employs the data
Data publication	Making publicly available the results derived from data
Data sharing	Making data available for use by other individuals or entities
Data repository	A digital "warehouse" where data are deposited, stored, managed, and made available to other individuals or entities
Open access data	Data that are made available to be freely accessed and used without any restrictions

Publication occurs when the data steward has made the results derived from the research study publicly available via scientific journals or other public forums (National Institutes of Health, 2021). The NIH defines data sharing as the process of making data as "widely and freely available as possible while safeguarding the privacy of participants, and protecting confidential and proprietary data" (National Institutes of Health, 2003b, par. 3). A data repository, where data are often shared, is a central domain where datasets may be submitted and then stored, maintained, archived, and shared with other researchers (National Institutes of Health Office of Data Science Strategy, 2022). Finally, open access data are data that are available for free and are unrestricted in terms of how they may be used (United Nations Educational Scientific and Cultural Organization, 2022).

In SER, it is important to make a distinction between data sharing within the project team among the contributing stakeholders and making data publicly available. Sharing data between academic researchers and community partners is inherent in SER, as stakeholders contribute to the interpretation and validation of data (Minkler, 2005). However, broader data sharing—with those who have not been involved in the collection of data—should be discussed with community partners early in collaborations. It may cause some concerns, as community partners may lose control over secondary analyses, yet making the data available for such analyses may be mandated by funding agencies. Case 16.1, "Just Because You Can, Doesn't Mean You Should," illustrates how perspectives on secondary data use may differ between academic and community stakeholders.

Case 16.1: Just Because You Can, Doesn't Mean You Should

Dr. Joseph Gone, a community psychologist and a member of the Gros Ventre tribal community of the Fort Belknap Indian reservation in Montana (Gone, 2017), reflected on a time when during a presentation at a tribal college in Montana, hoping to critically discuss Indigenous research methodologies, he described a Crow Indian religious tradition and included a photo to supplement the description. Conference audience members who were American Indian did not receive his presentation well. Dr. Gone later learned from his audience that his presentation was viewed as unethical, due to Indigenous beliefs that sacred knowledge and sacred objects should not be publicized. In his reflection, he notes that all the historical data he shared, including images of various sacred items, were openly available from public sources, although one audience member suggested that seeing the photograph "felt like violence." In this situation, Dr. Gone grapples with his identity as a part of the American Indian community and his need to be sensitive to their sacred beliefs, while also maintaining his dedication to academic inquiry as a researcher. This account further underscores two key considerations for data sharing. First, the way data are interpreted and shared is meaningful to the community to which they belong. Second, researchers can never be certain of the effects of their research unless they consult with the individuals who created the knowledge in the first place.

16.2 Benefits of Sharing Data

The NIH posits that "data sharing is essential for expedited translation of research results into knowledge, products, and procedures to improve human health" (National Institutes of Health, 2003a, par. 2). The NIH's stance rests on several principles. First, by allowing public access to data, researchers demonstrate transparency as well as their accountability and dedication to sound scientific methods, encourage public oversight, and foster public trust (DuBois et al., 2018a; Langat et al., 2011). Second, when making data publicly available, researchers also pave the way for novel research to be conducted. A variety of researchers can diversify analyses and opinions on a particular set of data and, therefore, support the collaborative nature of contemporary science (DuBois et al., 2018a; Chauvette et al., 2019; Langat et al., 2011). Third, allowing previously collected data to be "repurposed" in secondary analyses is also economically responsible for institutions, trainees, and those who funded the original research (e.g., taxpayers, health organizations) and demonstrates good stewardship of the data (DuBois et al., 2018a; Chauvette et al., 2019; Langat et al., 2011). Finally, sharing of data supports data democratization and, therefore, has the potential to broaden our ability to produce knowledge and promote social justice for communities and society as a whole (Reynolds & Sariola, 2020; Langat et al., 2011).

16.3 Responsible Use of Data in Stakeholder-Engaged Research

The main goal of SER is to make meaningful improvements for the community or group that is the focus of the research. Therefore, researchers must be mindful of how data are used. To ensure data are used in a way that positively affects the community, researchers must ensure that community partners are actively involved in the dialogue regarding the analysis, interpretation, and dissemination of the study's findings (Minkler, 2004). As the popularity of SER methods grows, so does the demand to share these data with government and funding agencies and to publish findings in academic journals (Fienberg et al., 1985; Office of Science and Technology Policy, 2013; Shelby, 2000). Before making decisions about publication or data sharing, however, research teams must determine and consider who owns the data, possible benefits and burdens of sharing data, and how to share data safely. These considerations may be difficult to discern, as there is no explicit policy in the United States that entails guidelines on how to share data (Langat et al., 2011).

16.3.1 Data Ownership

Before any governing decisions can be made regarding data collected in SER, it is important to identify who has the legal right to make such decisions. Several factors influence who owns data. First, most research grants are given to an institution rather than to an individual or group of researchers. Therefore, when a project is funded by a grant, the data are typically owned by the grantee—that is, the institution that is the primary recipient of funds (DuBois et al., 2018a). According to the NIH Grants Policy Statement, the grant recipient institution owns the rights to the data resulting from the project (National Institutes of Health, 2021). However, when research is funded by an internal grant within an institution, rules regarding ownership are typically dictated by institutional policy (DuBois et al., 2018a) but may be negotiated when third parties (e.g., community partners) are involved (Blum, 2015). Ownership ordinarily confers significant rights and responsibilities, and in SER, community partners usually want some control over how data are used and shared. Negotiating this control can pose challenges.

When project teams discuss data ownership, these conversations are had in good faith. However, in grant-funded research, the players involved in the discussion (e.g., academic researchers, community stakeholders) do not own the data collected; the institution owns the data. For projects not funded by grants but conducted by researchers at academic institutions with institutional resources, data ownership may fall within the university's intellectual property and copyright policies (Carroll, 2015). It is important that researchers are transparent with their stakeholders about such policies and that they continue to act in good faith. It should be clear to stakeholders that their ownership rights to data are equivalent to the ownership rights of the researchers on the study team. It should also be clear to all stakeholders that academic researchers may not have the final decision about ownership rights, as demonstrated in Case 16.2, "Data Ownership of Biological Samples."

Case 16.2: Data Ownership of Biological Samples
A thought-provoking outlook on the complexity of data ownership is offered in the case of Washington University vs. Catalona (Wash. Univ. v. Catalona, 437 F.Supp.2d 985, 1002 [E.D.Mo.2006], 2006). The case was opened to determine the lawful owner of biological samples that individuals had contributed to the Washington University (WU) Genito-urinary (GU) Biorepository for cancer research. The founder of the GU Biorepository, Dr. William J. Catalona, eventually left WU for a different institution and, unable to gain permission to take the samples with him, urged former research participants and patients to consent to the re-location of their samples. Ultimately, the court found that based on the original consent forms signed at WU, WU was the sole owner of the samples. Under the facts of the case, the "donors" of the biospecimens did not retain any ownership that allowed them to authorize the transfer of their samples to a third-party individual. Although the

(continued)

Case 16.2 (continued)
biological samples were literally part of the participants at one point, the signed informed consent forms at WU ultimately were the basis for determining who owned the data.

Since this case, to avoid future lawsuits, most research institutions have instituted "template" language in their consent forms and contracts clarifying matters of data ownership and sharing. Researchers and community partners may wish to initiate early discussions with oversight offices when changes to template language are desired. When data are complex or qualitative, such as biologic specimens or interview recordings, participants may feel especially "connected" to these data and assume ownership over them. Therefore, in SER, it may be important to revise template language to clearly define who owns the research data and who has the right to grant permission for secondary data users. It may be useful to also attempt to outline the intended lifecycle of these data to ensure there is no confusion among researchers and stakeholders.

16.3.2 Data Decisions

Stakeholder engagement principles direct researchers toward equitable interaction with communities, but what constitutes an equitable interaction is not self-evident (Minkler, 2005; Wallerstein & Duran, 2006). Arguably, equitable interaction requires community participation in decision-making in addition to researcher commitment to share data and study findings with the community in ways that support social change (Ansley & Gaventa, 1997). Increasingly, funders require that grantees share data to the extent possible with the broader research community, so these expectations should then be conveyed to stakeholder partners and included in formal agreements. However, the conditions and requirements of data repositories may affect the ability of community organizations and other stakeholders to access data that they assisted in generating. Community organizations may not be able to demonstrate that they have adequate capacity to secure the data as required, the ability to obtain regulatory approvals, or the background and credentials to conduct analyses deemed of value. For example, it is possible that the community may not have the infrastructure to store and protect the data or an ethics board in place to ensure proper use of the data. Because of these constraints, it may be difficult for researchers to ensure community access to the data, given funders' repository access guidelines. However, if researchers provide support to community organizations to try to overcome these infrastructural and regulatory barriers, repositories may be helpful in promoting ongoing community access to the data. Repositories offer long-term data preservation and sharing, but even still, project teams lose control over who can access the data and what types of questions are explored with the data once the data are made available in a repository. As research environments change, such as the type of community (e.g., grouped by diagnosis or geographic location), type of data being collected, where the data are stored, or research question being explored, other issues and concerns may arise.

Minkler (2004) discusses that a community or community partner organization may desire to suppress findings—for instance, findings that are perceived as negative and/or damaging to the community. In addition to encountering community impressions of the implications of the findings for community well-being and image, researchers may encounter ethical dilemmas, such as community backlash or pressure from industry, if they have not considered the policy impact of their work (Minkler, 2004). On the other hand, suppression of results may be considered antithetical by researchers given the importance of "open science" and transparency in academic research. However, it is reasonable for communities to be concerned about the ways that research, interpretation of findings, and their dissemination may affect legislative and political activities. Yet researchers may be less aware of legislative and policy activities and, thus, less prepared to address community concerns about these issues.

In consideration of the SER call for researchers to commit to work for social change, community voice matters. However, Wang et al. (2016) note that in any partnership, there may be disagreement about the type or scale of the change sought from the project (also see Chap. 2, in this volume). Conflicts related to the nature of the sought change may exist within the community and can lead to differences among stakeholders in their beliefs about how the data should be used, analyzed, published, and shared. It is important for researchers to discern how differing perspectives may affect the work of the partnership and to have processes in place to resolve any conflicts that may arise. It is important that conflict resolution does not mute minority voices, especially related to ethical concerns. Case 16.3, "Balancing the Scales Between Advocate and Academic," outlines a situation when a researcher faced conflict regarding study outcomes as well as conflict regarding protection of study participants. The researcher sought small changes to improve quality of life for a community but was met with backlash when the results of the study catalyzed policy change that could have jeopardized the livelihoods of some community members.

Case 16.3: Balancing the Scales Between Advocate and Academic
A perspective offered by Dr. Steve Wing, an epidemiologist at the University of North Carolina (UNC), sheds some light on the many ethical dilemmas researchers may face in regard to policy and social change (Wing, 2002). In the late 1990s, Dr. Wing and his team partnered with the Concerned Citizens of Tillery (CCT), a local grassroots organization in rural North Carolina, to study the effect of industrialized hog production on environmental health and quality of life for those in the community. The expansion of confined animal feeding operations (CAFOs) at the time in Halifax County caused concerns for residents about economic development, environmental pollution, and contamination of drinking water. With funding from the National Institute of Environmental Health Sciences (NIEHS), the SER project found evidence that CAFOs were more concentrated in low-income, predominately Black areas as well as in areas where residents relied on well water for drinking.

(continued)

Case 16.3 (continued)
Furthermore, individuals in these areas reported increased negative health symptoms due to CAFO emissions.

With the support of his CCT partners, Dr. Wing presented these findings at a large academic meeting and shared them with the press. While the release of information was both exciting and empowering to his stakeholder partners, Dr. Wing faced severe backlash from pork industry leaders and state legislative bodies. The North Carolina Pork Council demanded copies of all of the study documents under the North Carolina Public Records Statute. Although Dr. Wing was determined to maintain the confidentiality of participants, lengthy legal action eventually led the UNC attorney to agree to release the de-identified study documents. Although the released documents did not contain any explicit identifying information, there remained a concern for loss of community trust and breach of confidentiality due to the sparse population in which the research was conducted.

Dr. Wing describes two complex ethical dilemmas he faced while working on this important environmental justice project. First, the results would differentially impact the community. The outcomes from the project were intended to improve the quality of life of individuals who were ill from the CAFO-produced environmental contaminants. However, the project also had the potential to jeopardize the livelihoods of community members who relied on the pork industry for income. Second, Dr. Wing grappled with the tensions between his obligation to protect the confidentiality and trust of participants and the essential scientific culture of data transparency and availability for re-analysis.

16.3.3 Data Publication Decisions

Project teams should establish dissemination guidelines that address who can publish project information, what information can be shared outside of the project team, when information can be shared, what contributions qualify for authorship on publications, the standard acknowledgements that are included for project publications, who makes decisions about what can be published, and how conflicts about publication will be resolved (Holkup et al., 2004; Minkler, 2005; Israel et al., 1998). It is recommended that partnerships discuss these intended outputs (e.g., publications or press releases) of the project in the early phase of the research project (Prehoda et al., 2019; Glass & Kaufert, 2007). These conversations should result in mutual agreement between researchers and community partners regarding how the data are analyzed, interpreted, and then disseminated. Moreover, community members must be included in the decisions regarding what is published after the project ends.

Both formal and informal ways exist to ensure that publication is mutually agreeable to both the researchers and stakeholder partners. For example, in their collaboration with a Native research team, Holkup and colleagues implemented a policy whereby all team members edit, review, and are listed as co-authors on every publication resulting from their research (Holkup et al., 2004). However, some journals

Table 16.2 Authorship criteria as outlined by ICMJE

Recommended guidelines for authorship (must meet all criteria):
Significant contribution to concept or design of the study; or collection, analysis, or discussion of the data for the manuscript
Critically drafting or editing the manuscript for key intellectual content
Approval of the final body of work to be submitted for publication
Acceptance of accountability for the published work and dedication to ensure any questions regarding the legitimacy or scholarship of the work are resolved appropriately

Table adapted from International Committee of Medical Journal Editors (2022)

require more than recruitment and data collection participation to qualify for authorship, which will exclude some partnership members depending on their specific contributions to the work (International Committee of Medical Journal Editors, 2022). This stipulation leaves the potential for inequity between collaborating parties; therefore, requirements for authorship (Table 16.2) should be conveyed to stakeholders as early as possible in research partnerships and all partners should be given the opportunity to participate in all activities necessary for authorship.

One option in cases where the contributions of individual partners may not warrant authorship per journal guidelines is to consider "corporate authorship" in which one or more byline authors write an article "on behalf of" a group, and group members are all listed within the article; alternately, many journals now publish the names of nonauthor contributors (International Committee of Medical Journal Editors, 2022). Contributors who do not qualify as authors are typically listed either individually, or in a group, under a single heading with their contributions specified (International Committee of Medical Journal Editors, 2022).

Nevertheless, policies must be in place for determining how to proceed when researchers and stakeholders cannot reach an understanding about publication of certain findings. It is necessary for project teams to develop conflict resolution procedures as part of the partnership development process (Minkler, 2004; Mikesell et al., 2013; Han et al., 2021; Wilkins, 2011). A dissemination plan should be created in order to ensure all partners are on the same page regarding the study outputs and so that information that may be harmful to the community is not published (Bodison et al., 2015; Glass & Kaufert, 2007). For example, communities who are already stigmatized, such as racial subgroups or individuals with certain medical diagnoses, would face even more stigma if study results depicted them in a bad light. Ethical SER should always maximize benefits and minimize risks to communities, so the implications of the results of the study should be heavily considered.

16.3.4 Data Agreements

Once the researchers and stakeholders negotiate the data use issues outlined previously, they should create a mandatory formal agreement, or memorandum of understanding (MOU), which outlines how the partnership will handle the data (Glass &

Kaufert, 2007; Flicker et al., 2007; Mikesell et al., 2013). It is recommended that memoranda of understanding detail information regarding data ownership, decision-making processes, roles of each involved party, interpretation and analysis of the data, control and use of the data, and publication and dissemination of the results (Flicker et al., 2007; Glass & Kaufert, 2007). To be consistent with the ever-evolving relationship between researchers and community stakeholders, these agreements should retain some flexibility and be regularly re-negotiated as necessary (McDavitt, 2019).

16.4 Barriers to Responsible Data Sharing

16.4.1 Lack of Infrastructure

Given the varying, sometimes conflicting, guidelines on data sharing, it is common that the individual who is responsible for a dataset, most commonly the Principal Investigator (PI), may end up being the sole steward of said data (Kouper et al., 2020). Data are typically shared via submission to a data repository, along with any contextual materials (e.g., codebooks, field notes, interview recordings, drawings by participants, data collection protocols) required for meaningful interpretation of data (McLeod & O'Connor, 2020; Meyer, 2018). Repositories in the United States and other regions have their own specific data-sharing guidelines, and processes and requirements may differ (DuBois et al., 2018a). Given limited funding for research in general, it may be difficult to allocate research funds—and also time—to properly and responsibly prepare the data for repository sharing (McCurdy & Ross, 2018). McLeod and O'Connor argue that much current guidance regarding data sharing does not acknowledge how unique and complex qualitative data and their accompanying ethical and methodological dilemmas can be; instead, more of the guidance applies to quantitative data (McLeod & O'Connor, 2020). Regulations from the Health Insurance Portability and Accountability Act (HIPAA) specifically list all of the identifiers to remove from the dataset, but these guidelines have varied local interpretations and, thus, leave data sharing, whether qualitative or quantitative, to be prone to risk (United States Department of Health and Human Services, 1996; Freymann et al., 2012). Due to the general lack of consistent guidance, much of the responsibility for data stewardship is placed into the hands of the researcher and, therefore, could leave room for variable, questionable, or even (unintentionally) harmful data-sharing practices (Kouper et al., 2020).

Regardless of funders' guidelines, researchers may be inclined to take individual ownership over the data and to be reluctant to share (Broom et al., 2009). Due to the "competitive reality of science" and the growing demands on researchers from their own institutions, they may also be reluctant to share what they consider to be their hard-earned data (Langat et al., 2011). The withholding of "intellectual property" may be particularly tempting regarding qualitative data collected during SER, due to the investments of time, resources, and effort required to establish meaningful partnerships and to cultivate the trust required for knowledge sharing (Langat et al., 2011).

Although data sharing is crucial to increasing the production of knowledge and improving public health, sharing data may not be appropriate in some situations. Given the lack of general guidance regarding sharing data with repositories and the concern for breach of confidentiality, researchers partnering with communities may be inclined to request a data-sharing exemption from the funder (Kouper et al., 2020; McLeod & O'Connor, 2020; United States Department of Health and Human Services, 1996; Freymann et al., 2012; Sturges et al., 2015). Investigators may request an exemption due to risk of identification of individuals in small communities or the potential for exploitive analyses and reporting by outside investigators (Holkup et al., 2004; Guishard, 2018). The NIH's Final Policy on Data Management and Sharing, which went into effect in 2023, states that researchers should consider control of access to certain data when re-identification of participants poses the risk of increased harm (National Institutes of Health, 2020). However, the policy lacks explicit guidance on how to properly apply the sharing exceptions or how to request full exemption from data sharing to safeguard sensitive data (U.S. Department of Health and Human Services, 2020). Given the lack of clear-cut guidance on responsible data sharing, it is recommended that investigators become familiar with laws and regulations regarding human subjects' data and that they exercise caution when drafting agreements for data sharing with their community partners. Relevant laws and regulations for research data are outlined in Table 16.3.

Table 16.3 Laws and policies governing the stewardship of human subjects' research data

Law/policy	Agency	Brief summary
Health Insurance Portability and Accountability Act (HIPAA)	U.S. Department of Health and Human Services	Federal law to protect patients' protected health information
Family Educational Rights and Privacy Act (FERPA)	U.S. Department of Education	Federal law to protect students' education records
Federal Policy for the Protection of Human Subjects ("Common Rule")	U.S. Department of Health and Human Services	Federal policy to protect individuals who volunteer to participate in research studies
NIH Data Sharing Policy (effective until January 25, 2023)	National Institutes of Health	Policy requiring all grantees to include a data-sharing plan in their grant proposal and share their final research data
NIH Policy for Data Management and Sharing (effective January 25, 2023)	National Institutes of Health	Update to policy (as above) requiring grantees to submit a Data Management and Sharing plan with their grant application
NSF Data Sharing Policy	National Science Foundation	Policy requiring all grantees to share their research data with other researchers

Sources: National Institutes of Health (2003a, 2020), U.S. Department of Health and Human Services (2016), U.S. Department of Education (2021), National Science Foundation (2022), and United States Department of Health and Human Services (1996)

16.4.2 Ethical Considerations

In addition to the structural challenges that arise regarding the sharing of data, various ethical hurdles must also be considered. Stewards of data collected during community-academic partnered projects have an obligation to ensure that participants' privacy is safeguarded when they make decisions regarding data sharing and dissemination. Concerns regarding re-identification of the data can vary from participant to participant, based on the contextual implications of being identified (Banks et al., 2013). Even if data are de-identified using the HIPAA requirements, recent studies have shown just how easy it can be to re-identify data by using obscure additional data such as genome sequence or credit card metadata (Gymrek et al., 2013; de Montjoye et al., 2015). Chauvette and colleagues posit that full anonymization can never actually be guaranteed (Chauvette et al., 2019).

On the other hand, some research participants may want to be identified with the information that they share with researchers and may even be displeased if their contributions are diminished or even invisible because of de-identification practices (DuBois et al., 2018b). However, a participant can self-identify with published data and even share this information in public domains, which may put other participants and collaborators who want their identities to remain confidential at risk for identification (McCurdy & Ross, 2018). For instance, an individual who discusses their participation in a study on their publicly available social media account may lead to other participants being easily identified. Breaches of confidential information, such as immigration or disease status, can put individuals at risk for legal problems, blackmail, stigmatization, and psychological harms, among others (DuBois et al., 2018a, b; McCurdy & Ross, 2018). For example, individuals participating in a study of criminal behavior could face risk of imprisonment or even the death penalty if they are connected with their data.

In the case of qualitative data collected via key informant interviews or focus groups in community-academic partnerships, the complexity and variability of these data pose additional challenges. First, qualitative data are dependent on the context in which they were collected and the relationships that existed between researchers and the community at the time of data collection (Chauvette et al., 2019). When research participants are also research partners, often many things are left out of the record (DuBois et al., 2018a; McCurdy & Ross, 2018). Although contextual evidence, such as field notes, are encouraged to be archived with qualitative datasets in data repositories, it may be hard for a researcher who was not involved with the project to understand the notes of another researcher. Further, the subjectivity of qualitative data leaves room for bias, which ultimately could lead to misinterpretation of the data and the possibility of negative outcomes for the community (DuBois et al., 2018a; McCurdy & Ross, 2018). Additionally, in secondary analysis, mechanisms are not in place to ensure quality and meaningfulness of the findings (Chauvette et al., 2019). For example, in a re-analysis of their own data after some time had passed, Mauthner et al. (1998) found that even though they were aware of the context in which the data were collected, deriving meaningful answers to the questions posed in secondary analysis was difficult. There are no "checks and balances" in secondary analysis of data to ensure results are contextualized appropriately.

The duty to disseminate results must be balanced with duties to protect and respect community partners (Minkler, 2004). The risk of data misuse is an important consideration when preparing any type of data to share, especially qualitative data. Current data use policies do not guard against researchers using secondary sources to examine inherently racist hypotheses or research questions, essentially using data resources as "a modern tool of exploitation and scientific racism" (Guishard, 2018, p. 404). In cautious anticipation of such issues when sharing data, researchers should discuss these risks with community stakeholders in the early stages of the project (Minkler, 2004). Furthermore, it is necessary for repositories to consider the potential misuse of data and implement safeguards against this into their processes for accessing data.

16.5 Community Engagement to Strengthen Ethical Data Practices

Engaging with community members is important to ensure data are ethically handled. Because data-related decisions occur at many stages of the research project, there are several opportunities to seek input from community stakeholders to strengthen these decisions. We will focus on the benefits of including community advisors in discussions of informed consent, data collection methodology, and participant confidentiality, as well as the various issues to be considered in these conversations about research data.

16.5.1 Informed Consent

Informed consent documents have implications for data use, ownership, and sharing (DuBois et al., 2018a). When considering open access for research data, it is impossible to predict the future "life cycle" of the data (Chauvette et al., 2019). Therefore, it may not be easy for researchers to adequately inform participants about the specifics of how their data may be used down the line (DuBois et al., 2018a). Further, participants may wish to contribute their insights only to the specific research question outlined in the informed consent process (Chauvette et al., 2019). Case 16.4, "Context of Consent Matters," outlines a situation in which researcher-stakeholder discussions about data ownership could have informed the consent process to prevent unforeseen conflict later in the data lifecycle.

Case 16.4: Context of Consent Matters

Banks et al. (2013) describe the story of a project manager at a museum working on a stakeholder-engaged project with individuals to create their digital stories to be accessioned and displayed by the museum. During the consent process, the museum staff informed potential participants that if they agreed to participate, the museum would have a copyright over the digital material and the stories would be 'fixed,' or unchanged from the original submission. After the project ended and their stories had already been displayed, two participants requested either complete deletion, or amendment to their stories, which challenged the original agreement to the museum's definitive ownership and 'fixity' of the digital stories. It also challenged the manager's dedication to the important tenets of co-production of knowledge in research, forcing them to balance the terms of the project's regulatory agreements while also respecting participants' wishes regarding their data. Ultimately, the situation raised the question about whether the digital data of these participants should be treated as "regular museum objects." This situation raises an interesting dialogue about the ownership of unconventional forms of data. If the museum sought stakeholder input regarding ownership of the stories from study inception, they may have been more equipped to mitigate ethical conflicts down the line. Finally, this case illustrates differences between legal and ethical solutions; if the museum legally owned the stories, they thus had the legal right and arguably the ethical responsibility to consider making exceptions to their initial agreement.

16.5.2 Data Collection Methodology

Community voice (i.e., input from individuals within the community) can affect the research methodology used and ultimately the data collected. Academic researchers may be constrained by their usual ways of collecting data, whereas community members may recognize the need to use alternative strategies to gain information (Black et al., 2018). They may be aware of community-based resources to facilitate data collection (e.g., community theater, religious gatherings, recreational sporting events) as well as alternative methods (e.g., photovoice, digital narratives). Alternatively, community participation in research may be influenced by the research method (Adhikari et al., 2019). In other words, community members may be reluctant to contribute their data based on the protocol and the time and effort required to participate. Engagement in qualitative methods is common, but that does not mean that quantitative strategies cannot sustain community engagement. The measure selection and data collection processes complicate engagement because of time requirements for participation in the decision-making, as well as skill and capacity considerations. Therefore, research teams must engage in conversations with the community during study inception to ensure the protocol includes data collection methods that are reasonable to the community and allot resources to facilitate this. For example, community members may be able to participate along with organizational members and research consultants as long as they are provided relevant training and adequate compensation for their participation (Israel et al., 1998; Komaie et al., 2017, 2018; Goodman et al., 2018; McGowan et al., 2015; Coats et al., 2015).

16.5.3 Protection of Participants

Meaningful engagement with community co-researchers can increase protection of participants' anonymity. Since regulations direct IRBs to consider protection of individuals, potential risks to the community may not be obvious and, thus, not considered. As experts, stakeholders can inform researchers on certain vulnerabilities of individuals in the community and, therefore, can help identify ways to ensure that these individuals are included with the appropriate protections in place (Adhikari et al., 2019). If a study offers incentives or "singles out" a marginalized community in a way that is perceived to be excessive by outsiders, stigma toward that community may be compounded (Adhikari et al., 2019). In addition, community members can inform researchers about risks that may not be obvious and can help to ensure that the appropriate measures are taken to mitigate these risks (King et al., 2014). For example, stakeholder partners may be able to identify certain data, such as general location or personal narratives, that are not obvious to researchers that could implicate participants, and they could advise that these data are to be omitted in the data de-identification process.

16.5.4 Removing "Non-traditional" Identifiers from the Dataset Before Sharing

It is important to note that meeting HIPAA regulations is a minimum requirement and that these regulations do not represent the gold standard for data de-identification before submission to a data repository, especially regarding SER and qualitative research (United States Department of Health and Human Services, 1996; Freymann et al., 2012). Researchers have described several situations in which they made certain data available that seemed harmless to them, such as metadata in biomedical images, descriptions of experiences, genomic data, and even general location, only to later realize that this jeopardized the anonymity of all study participants (Banks et al., 2013; Chauvette et al., 2019; Wing, 2002; McCurdy & Ross, 2018; Meyer, 2018; Zimmer, 2010; Gymrek et al., 2013). For instance, anonymous users were able to triangulate publicly available, de-identified genomic data with surname and additional metadata, like age and state, to identify the owner of the genomic sequence (Gymrek et al., 2013). It is recommended that investigators share all reports and outputs with community collaborators to check for identifying information (Holkup et al., 2004). Engaging with community partners during the data preparation phase, and when drafting the data management plan, can ensure that all nonobvious identifiers are omitted from the data.

16.6 The Road to Responsibly Shared Data: Roles and Responsibilities

16.6.1 Role and Responsibilities of the Principal Investigator

As the primary stewards of the data collected during community-academic partnered projects, PIs play a key role in preparing these data for sharing. To start, PIs should include a data-sharing plan in the initial grant proposal; oftentimes, the funder may require this. The NIH recommends that the data-sharing plan outline the "expected schedule for data sharing, the format of the final dataset, the documentation to be provided, whether or not any analytic tools also will be provided, whether or not a data-sharing agreement will be required…and the mode of data sharing" (National Institutes of Health, 2003b). A data-sharing agreement should be considered in all SER partnerships (National Institutes of Health, 2003b; Jarquín, 2012). The data-sharing agreement should be developed with clear communication among all members of the partnership and should contain information that distinctly outlines the intended data-sharing process with well-developed content (Jarquín, 2012). In candid conversations with stakeholders, the PI can gain a better understanding of any indirect identifiers in the data that may not be obvious to remove before sharing and also whether or not they need to request a data-sharing exemption in the case of sensitive content (National Institutes of Health, 2003b; Holkup et al., 2004). Finally, the PI should ensure that the de-identified data are shared in a timely manner. The PI should share the data with community partners as soon as the data are available and with those outside of the partnership when the main findings are accepted for publication (National Institutes of Health, 2003b).

Given the myriad barriers to data sharing, conversations among researchers and stakeholders about potential barriers can begin to diminish the reluctance to share. Researchers can discuss the benefits of data sharing in their respective sector and open a dialogue surrounding standards and best practices for sharing (National Institutes of Health, 2003b). It is important that each of the stakeholders in the partnership has access to the data in a format that is useful for them. Given the time and resources expended by both communities and researchers to facilitate successful SER projects, it is especially important to share SER data to maximize their potential benefits. As SER data are shared, the potential exists for an emergence of common data elements that may aid in data harmonization and may increase partnership synergy and research outputs for the engagement science field (Holt & Chambers, 2017).

Sharing data in a manner that is responsible and respectful can be time-consuming and expensive. Many funding agencies, including the NIH, allow investigators to budget for data-sharing costs. As new requirements go into effect, investigators will want to budget accordingly, both for data-sharing costs and for the time and effort required to obtain input from community partners about the data-sharing plan.

16.6.2 Role and Responsibilities of Funders

While some U.S. funding agencies (e.g., Centers for Disease Control and Prevention, Food and Drug Administration) require grant recipients to submit a data-sharing plan as part of the yearly renewal application, it is clear that this is not yet the norm (Tenopir et al., 2020). In their review of over 300 academic research papers, Terry and colleagues found that 65% of these papers did not include any information about how to locate or access the data (Terry et al., 2018). In other words, almost two-thirds of the papers reviewed did not provide access to the data on which they were written, conflicting with the emerging demand by funders to share data. Funding agencies must engage with researchers and other stakeholders to clearly define the benefit of data sharing, and journals must do their part in encouraging data sharing. It is recommended that funders take steps to support the development of good practice standards for data sharing and for a strong infrastructure to host data (Terry et al., 2018). Funders must also provide adequate funding for data preparation, sharing, and archiving (National Institutes of Health, 2003a, b). The funders who do require data-sharing plans should make them publicly accessible and should even standardize them in order to encourage and aid researchers in their preparation for data sharing (Terry et al., 2018).

Funders may want to consider whether "traditional" data-sharing policies must always apply to SER. Current data-sharing policies are vague and do not specify where or how data should be shared, only that the plan for sharing be included in the application for funding, which is typically before researcher-stakeholder partnerships have had some of these important discussions (Pearce & Smith, 2011; Langat et al., 2011). SER requires trust between researchers and nonacademic stakeholders about who will have access to the data and how the data will be used; ultimately, the timelines for building trust and developing the data-sharing plan are often in conflict. In submitting an official data-sharing plan before funding is granted, the researcher becomes the sole steward of the data, and the tenet of equality in SER may be violated before the partnership even begins (Pearce & Smith, 2011; Kouper et al., 2020). Therefore, funders should allow some flexibility in the timeline to submit the data-sharing plan for SER projects to allow project teams adequate time to discuss and decide on how the data will be shared. It is important that the funder's requirements for data sharing be aligned with stakeholder engagement principles. Funders should allow sufficient time for discussions surrounding data stewardship after the partnership is formed and should allow for flexibility to change and adapt the data-sharing plan as the project progresses (Israel et al., 1998). Researchers work hard to establish partnerships with nonacademic stakeholders, and these partnerships have been beneficial to both the scientific process and scientific discovery (Balls-Berry & Acosta-Pérez, 2017). Therefore, it is important that data-sharing policies not cause partnership conflicts that can derail progress and damage relationships.

16.6.3 Roles and Responsibilities of Nonacademic Stakeholders

Community voice is important to the process of data sharing, but it must always be balanced against the norms of open science. Community partners and researchers should work together to develop protocols to protect the community from the harmful effects of sharing information inappropriately (Holkup et al., 2004). Community partners act as liaisons between the researchers and the community when negotiating the MOU, the data-sharing plan, and the dissemination plan (Glass & Kaufert, 2007; Flicker et al., 2007; Mikesell et al., 2013; McDavitt, 2019; Bodison et al., 2015). The scientific knowledge held by investigators and the cultural knowledge of stakeholder partners are both necessary to prevent unnecessary repercussions to community members by identifying what could happen if data are released prematurely, if they are released in an insensitive manner, or if the data contain any indirect identifiers (Flicker et al., 2007; National Institutes of Health, 2003b; Holkup et al., 2004). In addition, nonacademic stakeholders are crucial to the dissemination of data in ways that are useful and actionable to the community, key constituencies, and other project stakeholders (Israel et al., 1998; Boyer et al., 2007). Beyond dissemination of results, community members can provide input on interventions or policies that would be beneficial to their community. The nonacademic stakeholders' contribution to data interpretation is inherent in SER, and it is important for stakeholders to contribute to the development of contextual documents for data sharing, including the identification of limitations for secondary analysis.

16.7 Conclusion and Recommendations

It is clear that there is still a lot of work to be done in order to address the ethical concerns and lack of consensus regarding the sharing of data collected in SER. In order to respect community stakeholders while also allowing open access to data to support transparency in science, several recommendations for the ethical use of data in SER have been discussed, at many different levels in the data ecosystem. On a macro scale, regulatory agencies should establish data governance guidelines that are tailored more appropriately to nonquantitative data (especially data in unconventional forms). Institutions should work to reduce barriers for data sharing—for instance, by increasing funding and resources allotted for data repository preparation (DuBois et al., 2018b). They should also create standard operating procedures to guide researchers in their data-related decisions (Chauvette et al., 2019). Journals and other platforms that disseminate scientific knowledge should provide researchers with adequate time to properly prepare the data for sharing. Additionally, these entities should implement policies to ensure proper credit is given to the original researchers when data are used in secondary analyses (Chauvette et al., 2019). Finally, researchers have an important obligation to engage in an open dialogue with diverse stakeholders in the community (Wilson et al., 2017). The dialogue between researchers and community stakeholders should ultimately result in a consensus regarding the lifecycle of the data collected from the project, which should be reflected in the MOU and other partnership agreements, as outlined below.

16.7.1 Ethically Guided Solutions: Memorandum of Understanding and Partnership Agreements

Formal (e.g., MOU, partnership agreement) and informal (e.g., partnership meeting and communication practices) methods exist for addressing the ethical considerations for research data that emerge in SER. For these methods to reduce ethical missteps, transparency and information sharing are important aspects of implementation. Implications for data use, sharing, and ownership must be considered during discussions regarding funding transparency for both the funder and institution, research implementation, and of course, data management and use. The requirements and details of the discussion will vary, depending on the individual project and setting (Adhikari et al., 2019). Table 16.4 summarizes topics for discussion regarding research data and provides examples of leading questions that should be considered when researchers and stakeholders begin cultivating their partnership and developing their formal agreements.

Although the principal investigator is usually the one to secure and manage funding, it is important to be transparent regarding allocation of funds and to share the responsibility and decision-making power with stakeholder partners (Israel et al., 1998). Budgetary discussions can help teams forecast the costs incurred at several stages of the project, such as compensation for team members and cost of data preparation for sharing (Adhikari et al., 2019; McCurdy & Ross, 2018). Once an understanding is established regarding budget usage, partners will then be able to consider aspects of the project that will affect implementation and conduct of the project such as community representation, social and human capital, and regulatory requirements (Glass & Kaufert, 2007; Holkup et al., 2004; Gilbert, 2006; Adhikari et al., 2019). Ultimately, researcher-stakeholder partnerships should discuss several data-related decisions such as intended outcomes, data ownership and usage, authorship opportunities, and dissemination to ensure that the community's interests are

Table 16.4 Memorandum of understanding and partnership agreements regarding data use, sharing, and publication: ethical considerations and questions to lead discussions between partners

	Topics of importance	Questions to consider
Funding transparency		
Funder	Funder's allowable and nonallowable expenses	How much time and effort will be required to prepare the data for submission to a repository? Is this time and effort accounted for in the budget?
	Funder's policies and implications for individual and organizational partners	Will the community partners have indefinite access to the data? What is the timeline for finalization and submission of the data-sharing plan?
Institution	Options to share indirect amounts	How will the indirect costs be used? Can some of these funds be used to support data preparation activities?
	Institutional policies and implications for individual and organizational partners	What are the institution's requirements for sharing data with outside groups?
Research implementation		
	Community partner participation	Who will represent the community? Who will serve as a liaison? Are community partners aware of the guidelines for data sharing?
	Community partner capacity	Do the community partners have the time and social capital to actively participate? Are the community partners appropriately compensated for their time and contributions to the work (e.g., data-sharing plan discussions, data preparation)?
	Community partner benefit	What are the intended outcomes of this project? Will project data be available in formats that are useful to community partners?
	Institutional review board (IRB) requirements	Is there a single IRB? Which institution(s) require IRB approval? What information is needed to obtain IRB approval? Was data sharing incorporated in the IRB approval?
Data management and use		
	Data ownership and access	At what point are data management and use addressed with community partners? What are the community partner's expectations regarding data use? Who owns the data? Who has access to the data? How is access to the data obtained? Who determines who has access to the data?
	Requirements for data deposits and access	Are the community partners aware/agreeable that the data will be made publicly available? Who is responsible for preparing the data for deposit? Do the community partners have a role or input into data preparation? Who approves the data deposit? Who has access to the deposited data?

(continued)

Table 16.4 (continued)

	Topics of importance	Questions to consider
	What is disseminated and in what form	Are there any data that should not be shared? Are there any potential unwanted outcomes? How should data be disseminated (e.g., de-identified, aggregate form)? Who determines what data should be disseminated? How are community partner preferences for data dissemination determined? Is the research team responsible for analyses desired/required by community partners and other stakeholders?

respected and that trust is sustained (Banks et al., 2013; Glass & Kaufert, 2007; Holkup et al., 2004; Wang et al., 2016; Minkler, 2005; Prehoda et al., 2019).

Developing and executing MOUs can be time-consuming and cause delays to projects. To address this issue, some institutions are turning toward "accelerated research agreements," because starting from scratch and negotiating each detail leads to a lot of delays and inconsistencies (National Center for Advancing Translational Sciences, 2022). In principle, these agreements also educate community partners on things they might want to think about. Accelerated research agreements can provide efficiency and transparency, and they can protect the interests of partners (Clinical and Translational Science Awards Consortium, 2022; National Center for Advancing Translational Sciences, 2022). However, often, less time and flexibility exist to negotiate elements that individual community partners might want that are tailored to specific details or components of a project.

References

Adhikari, B., Pell, C., & Cheah, P. Y. (2019). Community engagement and ethical global health research, *31*(1), 1–12. https://doi.org/10.1080/11287462.2019.1703504

Ansley, F., & Gaventa, J. (1997). Researching for democracy & democratizing research, *29*(1), 46–53. https://doi.org/10.1080/00091389709603114

Balls-Berry, J. E., & Acosta-Pérez, E. (2017). The use of community engaged research principles to improve health: Community academic partnerships for research. *Puerto Rico Health Sciences Journal, 36*(2), 84.

Banks, S., Armstrong, A., Carter, K., Graham, H., Hayward, P., Henry, A., Holland, T., et al. (2013). Everyday ethics in community-based participatory research. *Contemporary Social Science, 8*(3), 263–277. https://doi.org/10.1080/21582041.2013.769618

Black, G. F., Davies, A., Iskander, D., & Chambers, M. (2018). Reflections on the ethics of participatory visual methods to engage communities in global health research. *Global Bioethics, 29*(1), 22. https://doi.org/10.1080/11287462.2017.1415722

Blum, C. (2015). Access to, sharing and retention of research data: Rights & responsibilities. Council on Governmental Relations, Washington, DC. https://www.cogr.edu/sites/default/files/access_to_sharing_and_retention_of_research_data-_rights_%26_responsibilities.pdf

Bodison, S. C., Sankaré, I., Anaya, H., Booker-Vaughns, J., Miller, A., Williams, P., & Norris, K. (2015). Engaging the community in the dissemination, implementation, and improvement of health-related research. *Clinical and Translational Science, 8*(6), 814–819. https://doi.org/10.1111/cts.12342

Boyer, B. B., Mohatt, G. V., Pasker, R. L., Drew, E. M., & McGlone, K. K. (2007). Sharing results from complex disease genetics studies: A community based participatory research approach. *International Journal of Circumpolar Health, 66*(1), 19–30. https://doi.org/10.3402/ijch.v66i1.18221

Broom, A., Cheshire, L., & Emmison, M. (2009). Qualitative researchers' understandings of their practice and the implications for data archiving and sharing. *Sociology, 43*(6), 1163–1180. https://doi.org/10.1177/0038038509345704

Carroll, M. W. (2015). Sharing research data and intellectual property law: A primer. *PLoS Biology, 13*(8), e1002235. https://doi.org/10.1371/journal.pbio.1002235

Chauvette, A., Schick-Makaroff, K., & Molzahn, A. E. (2019). Open data in qualitative research, *18*(January), 1–6. https://doi.org/10.1177/1609406918823863

Clinical and Translational Science Awards Consortium. (2022). *Accelerated Clinical Trial Agreement (ACTA)*. https://www.ctsacentral.org/articles/accelerated-clinical-trial-agreement-acta/

Coats, J. V., Stafford, J. D., Thompson, V. S., Javois, B. J., & Goodman, M. S. (2015). Increasing research literacy: The community research fellows training program. *Journal of Empirical Research on Human Research Ethics, 10*(1), 3. https://doi.org/10.1177/1556264614561959

Coburn, C. E., & Turner, E. O. (2011). Research on data use: A framework and analysis. *Measurement, 9*(4), 173–206. https://doi.org/10.1080/15366367.2011.626729

de Montjoye, Y. A., Radaelli, L., Singh, V. K., & Pentland, A. S. (2015). Unique in the shopping mall: On the reidentifiability of credit card metadata. *Science, 347*(6221), 536–539. https://doi.org/10.1126/science.1256297

DuBois, J. M., Strait, M., & Walsh, H. (2018a). Is it time to share qualitative research data? *Qualitative Psychology (Washington, D.C.), 5*(3), 380. https://doi.org/10.1037/qup0000076

DuBois, J. M., Walsh, H., & Strait, M. (2018b). It is time to share (some) qualitative data: Reply to Guishard (2018), McCurdy and Ross (2018), and Roller and Lavrakas (2018). *Qualitative Psychology, 5*(3), 412–415. https://doi.org/10.1037/qup0000092

Fienberg, S. E., Martin, M. E., & Straf, M. L. (Eds.). (1985). *Sharing research data*. National Academy Press.

Flicker, S., Travers, R., Guta, A., McDonald, S., & Meagher, A. (2007). Ethical dilemmas in community-based participatory research: Recommendations for institutional review boards. *Journal of Urban Health: Bulletin of the New York Academy of Medicine, 84*(4), 478–493. https://doi.org/10.1007/S11524-007-9165-7

Freymann, J. B., Kirby, J. S., Perry, J. H., Clunie, D. A., & Carl Jaffe, C. (2012). Image data sharing for biomedical research – Meeting HIPAA requirements for de-identification. *Journal of Digital Imaging, 25*(1), 14–24. https://doi.org/10.1007/s10278-011-9422-x

Gilbert, S. G. (2006). Supplementing the traditional institutional review board with an environmental health and community review board. *Environmental Health Perspectives, 114*(10), 1626. https://doi.org/10.1289/ehp.9005

Glass, K. C., & Kaufert, J. (2007). Research ethics review and aboriginal community values: Can the two be reconciled? *Journal of Empirical Research on Human Research Ethics, 2*(2), 25–40. https://doi.org/10.1525/jer.2007.2.2.25

Gone, J. P. (2017). "It Felt Like Violence": Indigenous Knowledge Traditions and the Postcolonial Ethics of Academic Inquiry and Community Engagement. *American Journal of Community Psychology, 60*(3–4), 353–360. https://doi.org/10.1002/ajcp.12183

Goodman, M. S., Gbaje, E., Yassin, S. M., Dias, J. J., Gilbert, K., & Thompson, V. (2018). Adaptation, implementation, and evaluation of a public health research methods training for youth. *Health Equity, 2*(1), 349. https://doi.org/10.1089/heq.2018.0077

Guishard, M. A. (2018). Now's not the time! Qualitative data repositories on tricky ground: Comment on DuBois et al. (2018). *Qualitative Psychology, 5*(3), 402–408. https://doi.org/10.1037/qup0000085

Gymrek, M., McGuire, A. L., Golan, D., Halperin, E., & Erlich, Y. (2013). Identifying Personal Genomes by Surname Inference. *Science (New York, N.Y.), 339*(6117), 321–324. https://doi.org/10.1126/science.1229566

Han, H. R., Xu, A., Mendez, K. J. W., Okoye, S., Cudjoe, J., Bahouth, M., Reese, M., Lee, B., & Dennison-Himmelfarb, C. (2021). Exploring community engaged research experiences and preferences: A multi-level qualitative investigation. *Research Involvement and Engagement, 7*(1). https://doi.org/10.1186/s40900-021-00261-6

Holkup, P. A., Tripp-Reimer, T., Salois, E. M., & Weinert, C. (2004). Community-based participatory research: An approach to intervention research with a Native American community. *Advances in Nursing Science, 27*(3), 162.

Holt, C. L., & Chambers, D. A. (2017). Opportunities and challenges in conducting community-engaged dissemination/implementation research. *Translational Behavioral Medicine, 7*(3), 389–392. https://doi.org/10.1007/s13142-017-0520-2

International Committee of Medical Journal Editors. (2022). *Defining the role of authors and contributors*. http://www.icmje.org/recommendations/browse/roles-and-responsibilities/defining-the-role-of-authors-and-contributors.html

Israel, B., Schulz, A., Parker, E., & Becker, A. (1998). Review of community-based research: Assessing partnership approaches to improve public health. *Annual Review of Public Health, 19*, 173–202. https://doi.org/10.1146/annurev.publhealth.19.1.173

Jansen, P., van den Berg, L., van Overveld, P., & Boiten, J.-W. (2019). Research data stewardship for healthcare professionals. In P. Kubben, M. Dumontier, & A. Dekker (Eds.), *Fundamentals of clinical data science* (pp. 37–53) https://library.oapen.org/bitstream/handle/20.500.12657/22918/1007243.pdf?sequence=1#page=42

Jarquín, P. B. (2012). Data sharing: Creating agreements in support of community-academic partnerships. Colorado Clinical and Translational Sciences Institute & Rocky Mountain Prevention Research Center, Aurora, CO. http://trailhead.institute/wpcontent/uploads/2017/04/tips_for_creating_data_sharing_agreements_for_partnerships.pdf

King, K. F., Kolopack, P., Merritt, M. W., & Lavery, J. V. (2014). Community engagement and the human infrastructure of global health research. *BMC Medical Ethics, 15*(1). https://doi.org/10.1186/1472-6939-15-84

Komaie, G., Ekenga, C. C., Sanders Thompson, V. L., & Goodman, M. S. (2017). Increasing community research capacity to address health disparities: A qualitative program evaluation of the community research fellows training program. *Journal of Empirical Research on Human Research Ethics, 12*(1), 55. https://doi.org/10.1177/1556264616687639

Komaie, G., Goodman, M., McCall, A., McGill, G., Patterson, C., Hayes, C., & Thompson, V. S. (2018). Training community members in public health research: Development and implementation of a community participatory research pilot project. *Health Equity, 2*(1), 282. https://doi.org/10.1089/heq.2018.0043

Kouper, I., Raymond, A. H., & Giroux, S. (2020). An exploratory study of research data governance in the U.S. *Open Information Science, 4*(1), 122–142. https://doi.org/10.1515/opis-2020-0010

Langat, P., Pisartchik, D., Silva, D., Bernard, C., Olsen, K., Smith, M., Sahni, S., & Upshur, R. (2011). Is there a duty to share? Ethics of sharing research data in the context of public health emergencies. *Public Health Ethics, 4*(1), 4–11. https://doi.org/10.1093/phe/phr005

Mauthner, N. S., Parry, O., & Backett-Milburn, K. (1998). The data are out there, or are they? Implications for archiving and revisiting qualitative data. *Sociology, 32*(4), 733–745. https://doi.org/10.1177/0038038598032004006

McCurdy, S. A., & Ross, M. W. (2018). Qualitative data are not just quantitative data with text but data with context: On the dangers of sharing some qualitative data: Comment on DuBois et al. (2018). *Qualitative Psychology, 5*(3), 409–411. https://doi.org/10.1037/qup0000088

McDavitt, B. (2019). Dissemination as dialogue: Building trust and sharing research findings through community engagement. *Preventing Chronic Disease, 13*(3). https://doi.org/10.5888/pcd13.150473

McGowan, L. D., Stafford, J. D., Thompson, V. L., Johnson-Javois, B., & Goodman, M. S. (2015). Quantitative evaluation of the community research fellows training program. *Frontiers in Public Health, 3*(July), 179. https://doi.org/10.3389/fpubh.2015.00179

McLeod, J., & O'Connor, K. (2020). Ethics, archives and data sharing in qualitative research, *53*(5), 523–535. https://doi.org/10.1080/00131857.2020.1805310

Meyer, M. N. (2018). Practical tips for ethical data sharing, *1*(1), 131–144. https://doi.org/10.1177/2515245917747656

Mikesell, L., Bromley, E., & Khodyakov, D. (2013). Ethical community-engaged research: A literature review, *103*(12). https://doi.org/10.2105/ajph.2013.301605

Minkler, M. (2004). Ethical challenges for the 'outside' researcher in community-based participatory research. *Health Education & Behavior: The Official Publication of the Society for Public Health Education, 31*(6), 684–697. https://doi.org/10.1177/1090198104269566

Minkler, M. (2005). Community-based research partnerships: Challenges and opportunities. *Journal of Urban Health: Bulletin of the New York Academy of Medicine, 82*(Suppl 2), ii3. https://doi.org/10.1093/jurban/jti034

National Center for Advancing Translational Sciences. (2022). *Accelerated research agreements*. https://www.ara4us.org/

National Institutes of Health. (2003a). *Final NIH statement on sharing research data*. https://grants.nih.gov/grants/guide/notice-files/NOT-OD-03-032.html

National Institutes of Health. (2003b). *NIH data sharing policy and implementation guidance*. https://grants.nih.gov/grants/policy/data_sharing/data_sharing_guidance.htm

National Institutes of Health. (2020). *NOT-OD-21-013: Final NIH policy for data management and sharing*. https://grants.nih.gov/grants/guide/notice-files/NOT-OD-21-013.html

National Institutes of Health. (2021). *NIH grants policy statement: 8.2.1 rights in data (publication and copyrighting)*. https://grants.nih.gov/grants/policy/nihgps/html5/section_8/8.2.1_rights_in_data__publication_and_copyrighting_.htm

National Institutes of Health Office of Data Science Strategy. (2022). *Biomedical data repositories and knowledgebases*. https://datascience.nih.gov/biomedical-data-repositories-and-knowledgebases#repositories

National Science Foundation. (2022). *Dissemination and sharing of research results*. https://www.nsf.gov/bfa/dias/policy/dmp.jsp

Office of Science and Technology Policy. (2013). *Increasing access to the results of federally funded scientific research*. https://obamawhitehouse.archives.gov/sites/default/files/microsites/ostp/ostp_public_access_memo_2013.pdf

Pearce, N., & Smith, A. H. (2011). Data sharing: Not as simple as it seems. *Environmental Health, 10*(1), 1–7. https://doi.org/10.1186/1476-069X-10-107

Prehoda, E., Winkler, R., & Schelly, C. (2019). Putting research to action: Integrating collaborative governance and community-engaged research for community solar. *Social Sciences, 8*(1), 11. https://doi.org/10.3390/socsci8010011

Reynolds, L., & Sariola, S. (2020, June). The ethics and politics of community engagement in global health research. In *The ethics and politics of community engagement in global health research* (pp. 1–12). https://doi.org/10.1201/9781003011187-1

Shelby, R. (2000). Accountability and transparency: Public access to federally funded research data. *Harvard Journal on Legislation, 37*(2), 369–389.

Sturges, P., Bamkin, M., Anders, J. H. S., Hubbard, B., Hussain, A., & Heeley, M. (2015). Research data sharing: Developing a stakeholder-driven model for journal policies. *Journal of the Association for Information Science and Technology, 66*(12), 2445–2455. https://doi.org/10.1002/asi.23336

Tenopir, C., Rice, N. M., Allard, S., Baird, L., Borycz, J., Christian, L., Grant, B., Olendorf, R., & Sandusky, R. J. (2020). Data sharing, management, use, and reuse: Practices and perceptions of scientists worldwide. *PLoS One, 15*(3), e0229003. https://doi.org/10.1371/journal.pone.0229003

Terry, R. F., Littler, K., & Olliaro, P. L. (2018). Sharing health research data – The role of funders in improving the impact. *F1000Research, 7*. https://doi.org/10.12688/f1000research.16523.2

U.S. Department of Education. (2021). *Family Educational Rights and Privacy Act (FERPA)*. https://www2.ed.gov/policy/gen/guid/fpco/ferpa/index.html

U.S. Department of Health and Human Services. (2016). *Federal policy for the protection of human subjects ('common rule')*. https://www.hhs.gov/ohrp/regulations-and-policy/regulations/common-rule/index.html.

U.S. Department of Health and Human Services. (2020). *Attachment A – NIH data sharing policy: Implications of the NIH draft policy for data management and sharing on data derived from human participants*. https://www.hhs.gov/ohrp/sachrp-committee/recommendations/august-12-2020-attachment-a-nih-data-sharing-policy/index.html#_ftnref9

United Nations Educational Scientific and Cultural Organization. (2022). *What is open access?* https://en.unesco.org/open-access/what-open-access

United States Department of Health and Human Services. (1996). *Summary of the HIPAA privacy rule*. http://www.hhs.gov/ocr/hipaa

Wallerstein, N. B., & Duran, B. (2006). Using community-based participatory research to address health disparities. *Health Promotion Practice, 7*(3), 312–323. https://doi.org/10.1177/1524839906289376

Wang, C. C., Cash, J. L., & Powers, L. S. (2016). Who knows the streets as well as the homeless? Promoting personal and community action through photovoice, *1*(1), 81–89. https://doi.org/10.1177/152483990000100113

Wash. Univ. v. Catalona, 437 F.Supp.2d 985, 1002 [E.D.Mo.2006]. (2006).

Wilkins, C. H. (2011). Communicating results of community-based participatory research. *Virtual Mentor, 13*(2), 81–85. https://doi.org/10.1001/virtualmentor.2011.13.2.ccas1-1102

Wilson, E., Kenny, A., & Dickson-Swift, V. (2017). Ethical challenges in community-based participatory research: A scoping review, *28*(2), 189–199. https://doi.org/10.1177/1049732317690721

Wing, S. (2002). Social responsibility and research ethics in community-driven studies of industrialized hog production. *Environmental Health Perspectives, 110*(5), 437. https://doi.org/10.1289/ehp.02110437

Zimmer, M. (2010). 'But the data is already public': On the ethics of research in Facebook. *Ethics and Information Technology, 12*(4), 313–325. https://doi.org/10.1007/s10676-010-9227-5

Melody S. Goodman is the Vice Dean for Research and Professor of Biostatistics. She is a biostatistician and research methodologist. Her research interest is on identifying origins of health inequities and developing, as necessary, evidence-based primary prevention strategies to reduce these health inequities. She is a Fellow of the American Statistical Association (2021) and the inaugural recipient of the societal impact award from the Caucus for Women in Statistics (2021).

Kristyn A. Pierce is a Research Scientist and a biostatistician. She is interested in the application of statistical machine learning methodologies to understand and address health disparities for individuals with substance use disorder and other mental health disorders.

James M. DuBois is the Steven J. Bander Professor of Medical Ethics and Professionalism, Professor of Medicine and Psychology, and Director of the Center for Clinical and Research Ethics. He is an expert in bioethics and is focused on ethics across mental health research and organ transplantation, professional integrity, and moral development and education. He is the director of the NIH-funded Professionalism and Integrity in Research Program and a founding Editor of *Narrative Inquiry in Bioethics: A Journal of Qualitative Research*.

Vetta Sanders Thompson is the E. Desmond Lee Professor of Racial and Ethnic Diversity and a licensed clinical psychologist, educator, and health service provider. Her research is focused on racial identity, health services access, and socio-cultural determinants of health in diverse communities. She is the inaugural Associate Director of Diversity, Equity, and Inclusion in the Siteman Cancer Center at Washington University School of Medicine and recipient of The St. Louis American's 2022 Lifetime Achiever in Health Care award.

Part IV
Research Ethics Oversight

Chapter 17
Applying the *Belmont* Principles to Stakeholder-Engaged Research: Adaptions and Limitations

Elisa A. Hurley

17.1 The *Belmont Report* in Context

The *Belmont Report* has shaped regulation, practice, and collective thinking about research with human beings in the United States for over 40 years, since its publication in 1979. *Belmont* was a product of a specific time and historical context, a response to revelations of a series of egregious research abuses during the first half of the twentieth Century involving individuals from vulnerable and disadvantaged populations, such as the poor, the sick, and the incarcerated. A primary goal of *Belmont* was to protect such "populations of convenience" from being systematically selected as research subjects, often without their knowledge and with little to no benefit to them. The framework provided by the *Belmont Report* sought to prevent this sort of abusive human subjects research in the future and, thereby, restore public confidence in the research enterprise.

To that end, *Belmont* laid out three "basic ethical principles that should underlie the conduct of biomedical and behavioral research involving human subjects" (National Commission, 1979): (1) respect for persons, which entails treating individuals as autonomous (i.e., self-determining) agents and protecting individuals with diminished autonomy; (2) beneficence, which entails refraining from harming people and maximizing the potential for benefit and minimizing the possibility of harm; and (3) justice, which requires the fair distribution of the benefits and burdens of research among individuals.

Belmont provides the philosophical foundations for the federal regulations governing human subjects research in the United States. Yet in the four decades since *Belmont* was published, the research landscape has changed significantly. One of

E. A. Hurley (✉)
Boston, MA, USA
e-mail: elisa.hurley@gmail.com

E. E. Anderson (ed.), *Ethical Issues in Community and Patient Stakeholder–Engaged Health Research*, Philosophy and Medicine 146,
https://doi.org/10.1007/978-3-031-40379-8_17

those changes involves the emergence of efforts and imperatives to engage the communities in which research is to be conducted, or from which participants will be drawn, in the research. Community engagement can be seen as a product and beneficiary of larger social trends over the past several decades, including the democratization of knowledge production; increasing skepticism of authority and expertise, including that of the medical profession; and growing demands that institutions of power be more transparent about their activities so they can be better held to account. The 1980s saw the rise of patient and disease advocacy groups, including HIV/AIDS activists and breast cancer advocates, organizing to demand access to the benefits of research participation, challenging what was seen as the overly protectionist framework of *Belmont*. Around that time, individuals and communities began to realize the "value of their data, samples, and information that they provided at all stages of discovery," and to demand a greater degree of benefit-sharing and of engagement not just as research participants, but as research partners (Ross, 2010; Ross et al., 2010). Simultaneously, over the past two to three decades, the research enterprise began to focus more on the translation of research discoveries into health practices and outcomes—rather than on the discoveries themselves—and to appreciate the importance of engaging communities as stakeholders in achieving successful translation of research findings into real-world settings (Ross, 2010; Ross et al., 2010; Yarborough et al., 2013).

Community-engaged research (CEnR) is a reflection of these changes. For the purposes of this chapter, CEnR refers broadly to the full continuum of research activities that involve some sort of collaborative partnership with communities, from, on one end of the spectrum, community outreach and consultation on research activities that are primarily controlled by academic researchers, to, on the other, Community Based Participatory Research (CBPR), a general approach to research in which researchers and the community are "equal partners in all phases of research," from formulating study questions to study design and conduct (Thompson et al., 2021; Anderson & Spellecy, 2021; CTSA, 2011; Ross et al., 2010).

The question of what constitutes a "community" in the context of community-engaged research is complex; for some purposes, it is important to ask what (and who) defines a community, who is part of a community, and who speaks for that community, among other questions. For my purposes here, a "community" refers to any group of people affiliated by geographic proximity, by shared traits or characteristics (e.g., race, ethnicity, disease, or diagnosis), or by shared interests, beliefs, or history. Lainie Friedman Ross and colleagues have pointed out the difference between groups of individuals who happen to share traits, geography, or history, but do not have a defined internal structure or leadership—people living with HIV or the Black community, for instance—and established communities that may be organized around any of these characteristics *and also* have their own pre-existing organizational structure and leadership—the Black teachers association of Smithville, for example (Ross et al., 2010). I use the term "community" to refer to both types of groups, but agree with Ross and colleagues that, in order for an unstructured group to be *engaged* in research *as a community*, it must develop a structure and leadership, even if only for that research purpose (Ross et al., 2010, 5). This definition of "community" is intended to be capacious enough to cover what most people mean or are referring to when they talk about "community engaged research."

While the framework provided by the *Belmont Report* is flexible and adaptable in ways I discuss below, it is ultimately an imperfect fit for the ethics of CEnR. Its limitations fall along two dimensions. First, it fails to recognize communities as objects of ethical concern in their own right. Second, it does not countenance a role for individuals and their communities in research other than being a subject of that research. In what follows I explore these limitations and how *Belmont* might be "adapted" to address them and conclude with some practical implications and recommendations.

17.2 Applying *Belmont*'s Principles to CEnR: Flexibility in the Applications

In addition to laying out the three basic ethical principles of respect for persons, beneficence, and justice, *Belmont* articulates the application of these principles in three core requirements for ethical research, respectively: (1) seeking and obtaining individuals' informed consent for involvement in research; (2) conducting a systematic assessment of risks and benefits of the research project to ensure risks to individuals are minimized and the balance between those risks and any benefits that might result is reasonable; and (3) selecting the individual subjects of research fairly (both in terms of procedures and outcomes) (National Commission, 1979). The discussion of the application of the principles illuminates how *Belmont's* focus was squarely on protecting the rights and welfare of *individual* research subjects (Castro-Reyes et al., 2015; Ross, 2010).

This brings us to the first dimension of the limitations of *Belmont* as an ethical framework for CEnR: *Belmont* does not have within its purview communities, or groups of people, as entities of ethical concern in research. Engaging communities in research processes as consultants or partners entails recognizing that communities, as such, have interests in the research—what is asked, who is asked, how it is conducted, and its outcomes—which can be advanced or set back by the research. This entails, in turn, that those communities are in and of themselves deserving of ethical consideration. CEnR recognizes that communities, qua groups, can be *harmed* by research participation, for instance, by study findings that undermine a community's collective beliefs about itself, as in the case of the Havasupai Tribe (Garrison, 2013), or that threaten to stigmatize the community by exploring traits that are socially devalued (Ross et al., 2010). Research can also disrespect communities, for instance, by failing to get buy in to the research questions or recruitment plan before approaching individuals within the community to participate in the research as designed. Communities can also benefit from research, beyond the collective benefit of the individuals within the community, for instance, by gaining new infrastructure or capacity as a result of the research, or by emerging with greater understanding of a characteristic or experience within the community that will help the community thrive in the future. These sorts of benefits and harms, which affect communities as such, do not feature in *Belmont*.

To be sure, *Belmont* does recognize that individuals may be treated unfairly *because* they are members of certain identifiable classes or groups—specifically, that individuals from certain already disadvantaged socioeconomic or ethnic backgrounds, or from certain geographies, may be unfairly targeted for burdensome research, or unfairly excluded from research and its benefits. But the harms it is concerned with are harms to individuals. *Belmont* does not countenance that communities, whether defined by geography, characteristics, or self-identification, can themselves be harmed or benefited, respected or disrespected, treated justly or unjustly, by research. Nor does it countenance the idea that individual members of an identifiable group whose members are involved in research can be harmed, whether or not they themselves are participants in the research, for instance, when research findings threaten to stigmatize all members of that group. CEnR practitioners point out the importance of recognizing and grappling with these kinds of potential harms (Ross et al., 2010).

Nevertheless, some have suggested the *Belmont* principles are broad and flexible enough that their application can be expanded to include communities (Castro-Reyes et al., 2015; Shore, 2006). Indeed, according to *Belmont's* authors, the three principles were designed to be "comprehensive" and are "stated at a level of generalization that should assist scientists, subjects, reviewers, and interested citizens to understand the ethical issues inherent in research involving human subjects" (National Commission, 1979). Furthermore, there are other examples of the application of the *Belmont* principles in research oversight practices evolving over time to respond to changes in the research enterprise and social norms. For example, while justice as conceived in *Belmont* is primarily a matter of *protecting* individuals from certain disadvantaged groups from being unfairly targeted for research, in more recent years, justice has come to be understood as just as much a matter of ensuring people from some of those same groups have equitable *access* to the benefits of research participation, that is, are not unfairly excluded from research participation. The application of the principle of justice as fair distribution of benefits as well as burdens has evolved. Similarly, respect for persons, which *Belmont* applies exclusively through the requirement to obtain informed consent, is now often taken to demand attention to policies and practices around returning research results to participants (HHS, 2016; Shalowitz & Miller, 2005), compensating participants for their time and effort (Anderson, 2019; Largent & Lynch, 2017), and providing access to post-research care (Cho et al., 2018; MRCT, 2017).

Applying to CEnR the idea that the *Belmont* principles are broad and flexible enough to allow for new applications, some have suggested that the principle of respect for persons can be broadly interpreted and applied to encompass respect for communities as autonomous social groups (Castro-Reyes et al., 2015; Mikesell et al., 2013). (Also see Chap. 3, in this volume.) And beneficence can be interpreted not just as a matter of balancing the risks and benefits to individuals of participating in research, but, in the context of CEnR, as demanding efforts to minimize risks—to reputation, to group identity, to group safety, to group structure--to the communities engaged in research, and to balance those risks against considerations of what benefits might flow to those communities as a result of the research (Castro-Reyes et al., 2015; Mikesell et al., 2013; Shore, 2006). This does not mean that community benefit should be weighed on the same scale as, or against, individual benefit, but rather that, in the context of CEnR, the application of the principle of beneficence entails going beyond thinking about risks and benefits to individual research participants and includes the requirement to consider the relative risks and benefits to the community engaged in the research. Justice, in turn, should be seen as a matter of more than fairly distributing the burdens and benefits of research among individual potential research participants, but as encompassing and addressing the unfair under-representation in research of some communities as a whole and calling for efforts to build the capacity of communities to serve as research partners (CIOMS Guideline 82,016; Castro-Reyes et al., 2015).

Expanding the application of the *Belmont* principles to incorporate communities as entities to whom respect, beneficence, and justice are owed captures many of the ethical imperatives of CEnR. However, there is, a second dimension to the limitations of *Belmont* as applied to CEnR: *Belmont's* framework does not countenance the idea of communities as *partners* in the research, rather than mere objects of study.

17.3 The Limitations of *Belmont*: Communities as Research Partners

Belmont's framework assumes a "vertical" relationship between researcher and research participant (Shore, 2006)—the researcher determines the research question and articulates its significance, designs the study, making sure along the way, and perhaps with the help of an IRB, to minimize risks and maximize relative benefits and consider how to select subjects fairly; and approaches the subject for their free and informed consent. The participant, then, has the opportunity to decide, based on what has been presented to them regarding what the study involves, its benefits and risks, and the alternatives to participation, whether or not they want to participate in the study so planned and described. Built into the model are asymmetries of knowledge, authority, and control. The person who agrees to participate is, in the *Belmont* model, acted upon, as a research subject, according to the study as designed by the researcher. In this model, there is no conception of the research participant, other members of their community, or their community as a whole, as being stakeholders in the research in any other capacity than as objects of study.

CEnR, on the other hand, envisions a more "horizontal" relationship between participants and their communities, on the one hand, and researchers, on the other. Communities are not just the sites of research and the "sources" for research participants, but are partners who may, depending on the study, be involved in one or more of the following: Defining the research question, designing the research study and its recruitment plan, recruiting participants from within the community, analyzing results, disseminating study findings, and determining or implementing policy or practice changes within the community given those findings. CEnR entails a complex, multi-faceted relationship between participant communities and researchers whose ethical contours are therefore different from the standard researcher-subject relationship assumed by *Belmont*. This fact both complicates the application of the *Belmont* principles and may, furthermore, demand the articulation of additional ethical principles that better fit these complexities.

Consider, again, respect for communities as an expansion of the *Belmont* principle respect for persons. We can now see that respect for communities goes beyond respect for their autonomy and agency as entities that are being asked to *participate* in research as subjects, but also respect for the community as a research *partner* and for the partnership itself (Shore, 2006). Respect for communities thus entails respect for the community's self-definition and self-understanding and the interests, needs, expertise, and values it brings to the partnership, as well as respect for the community's internal structures, including who speaks for the group and how decisions are made (Castro-Reyes et al., 2015; Mikesell et al., 2013). It entails respecting the communities' role and voice in decision-making, per the scope for community input and involvement that has been determined for a particular study. In other words, within the context of CEnR, respect for communities is not just a matter of, for instance, getting community-level buy in to conduct a study with its members, or getting community leadership's permission to seek individuals' informed consent for participation; it entails respecting who the community is, what they value, and what goals they bring to the research partnership in every aspect of study design, implementation, and dissemination of findings.

Recognizing that community engagement entails a multi-faceted partnership role for the community reveals additional dimensions to the principle of beneficence applied to CEnR. For instance, the benefits that can accrue to communities from being engaged as partners in research include capacity-building or enhanced infrastructure that will help address a community-identified need or priority, a new understanding of the community's negotiating power as a group, or new appreciation of the value of their information to science (Ross et al., 2010). Similarly, risks to communities in CEnR include not just risks to the group's self-conception or reputation as a result of research findings, as discussed earlier. They include risks to the group's internal structure, such as when partnering in the research causes dissension between a group and its leadership regarding the direction and extent of that community's participation in the research. They also include risks to the community partners on the "front lines" of the research, for instance, risks to their reputations and relationships within the community if academic researchers fail to follow through on promises, or from having to "defend" potentially controversial research to others in their community (Ross et al., 2010; see Chap. 8, in this volume).

Furthermore, it is widely agreed that an important feature of CEnR is that communities have a key role in determining what constitutes benefits and risks of the research, as well as what is a reasonable balance between them (Castro-Reyes et al.,

2015; Shore, 2006). This includes a role in defining what research is important, relevant, and valuable in the first place, including, specifically, what research questions are significant to the community itself (Castro-Reyes et al., 2015; Mikesell et al., 2013). This is a notable departure from the *Belmont* model, in which the "value of research is taken as a given" (Shore, 2006), and the risks and benefits are defined by the investigator, reviewed by the IRB, and communicated to potential participants as fixed input to their decision-making. Furthermore, *Belmont* focuses on *individual* research studies—it answers the question, "can, or should, this particular study be done?" given its expected scientific or social value, the procedures it involves, and its risk/benefit profile. *Belmont* provides no guidance for deciding *among* possible studies, in a context of limited resources and competing needs and priorities, which would be *most* beneficial. And yet those are the types of decisions that communities who are engaged in research often need to make. The principle of beneficence, broadened to apply to CEnR, requires that risks and benefits, the appropriate relationship between them, and the appropriate tradeoffs between studies when resources are limited, be defined and negotiated in partnership with the community that will be affected.

As discussed, *Belmont* is primarily concerned with justice as a matter of distributive justice—the fair distribution of the benefits and burdens of research; above I noted how this notion of justice can be expanded from thinking about fair distribution among individuals to fair distribution among communities. But CEnR demands a broader conception of justice, one encompassing social justice, which involves "ensuring that research priorities reflect the health needs of all socioeconomic communities, particularly vulnerable communities; and promoting institutions and social practices that support capacities for self-determination and ensure respectful interactions" (Ross et al., 2010).

CEnR is at its core concerned with the question of who gets to set research priorities, and holds that justice in research requires that communities—especially those whose needs have been historically understudied in research—should be at the table for setting the research agenda. Much community-based participatory research is motivated by a desire to change the social conditions that lead to communities having health problems, being neglected by healthcare systems, or having their needs and voices ignored in health and other policy decisions. CBPR seeks to "generate knowledge that leads to social change and enhancement of community well-being and knowledge that reveals and challenge systemic problems rather than reinforcing relations of dominance" (Mikesell et al., 2013). The idea of empowering communities to set research agendas that change the conditions for social inequalities goes far beyond *Belmont's* conception of justice.

So far, I have proposed how we might interpret the three core *Belmont* principle to capture the multi-faceted relationships between communities and researchers posted by CEnR. Some CEnR practitioners and scholars have suggested that even so broadly construed, the *Belmont* principles may be insufficient as a framework for ethical CEnR, and must be supplemented by additional principles, including the following:

- **Reciprocity,** the "ongoing process of exchange with the aim of establishing and maintain equality between parties" (Maiter et al., 2008)
- **Trust** among all parties to the partnership
- **Transparency**, or open communication between research teams and communities as partners about the relevant stages of research
- **Shared power and decision-making** about various aspects of the research, from design to results dissemination, guided by the specific community engagement arrangement
- **Joint data ownership**, giving the community control of the data it generates and who has access to it, or the ability to negotiate what the data ownership arrangement looks like (Mikesell et al., 2013). (Also see Chap. 16, in this volume.)

Castro-Reyes and colleagues, in their 2015 proposed revisions to *Belmont* and the Common Rule, put forth a "revision of the articulation and operationalization of the original *Belmont* principles" for CEnR, but with the addition of three "core capacities [...] integral to all research involving human participants and [...] expected of researcher as they engage in research practices," namely, humility, relational integrity, and accountability (Castro-Reyes et al., 2015, 4). Others have added cultural competence or cultural humility—efforts to seek information that fosters cross-cultural understanding—as another key component of ethical CEnR (Shore, 2006).

Some CEnR practioners might argue that the *Belmont* principles are sufficiently broad and general that these various additional ethical considerations, rather than being distinct principles, can be derived from the *Belmont* principles themselves (Shore, 2006)—for instance, that accountability can be derived from respect for communities, or that joint data ownership is an application of beneficence. In the end, though, it may not matter if they *could* be derived from those principles or are principles in their own right. In either case, articulating these additional norms and standards requires additional conceptual work that goes far beyond the applications imagined by *Belmont*.

Finally, some have suggested that within the context of CEnR, what counts as ethical research is "emergent and situation specific": "Whereas ethical procedures in traditional research are approved ahead of time, CBPR practitioners view ethics as involving a fluid, negotiable, iterative process requiring continual reflection" (Mikesell et al., 2013; see also Chaps. 3, 5, and 6, in this volume). For instance, how to demonstrate respect for a community and the individuals within it may vary significantly community to community, depending on cultural norms around hierarchy, independence and interdependence, and the like. Within certain scientific and regulatory parameters, what is ethical research should be defined in collaboration with the community itself (Shore, 2006, 20; Mikesell et al., 2013). Some involved in CBPR, specifically, have gone so far as to suggest that the ethical principles involved in such research are themselves "principles in evolution," rather than comprising a fixed, static framework to be applied, top down, to each new project (Mikesell et al., 2013). This set of critiques raises an additional challenge for the application of the *Belmont Report* to CEnR, because it calls for finding a role for the community in defining the specific ethical concerns of the research, in an ongoing, iterative manner.

17.4 Conclusion

There are practical implications of *Belmont's* imperfect fit for CEnR. Community-engaged research presents special challenges to investigators, sponsors, and IRBs/research ethics committees (Anderson & Spellecy, 2021; Shore, 2007). Ensuring the ethical conduct of such research requires thinking beyond the individualistic framework presented by *Belmont* and the regulations based on them and understanding the specific goals and unique ethical dimensions of CEnR. Investigators can apply the principles outlined above by seeking training in the methods of CEnR, as well as taking responsibility for developing core capacities for building the robust partnerships at the heart of CEnR, including cultural competence and humility, accountability, and a relational stance.

To ensure adequate and appropriate review of CEnR research protocols, in turn, IRBs/research ethics committees and the institutions and sponsors that support them should consider the following strategies:

- Determine and utilize appropriate training for IRB personnel on community engaged research and its oversight. To the extent that community representatives are engaged as research partners, those individuals, too, should, under the authority of the IRB, receive appropriate human subjects research training (Anderson & Spellecy, 2021).
- Ensure the IRB has appropriate expertise to review CEnR. This might include making sure researchers with CEnR experience are represented on the committee; increasing the number of nonaffiliated members of the IRB beyond the regulatory minimum and making efforts to recruit members that truly represent the lay community; and making ample use of consultants and other outside experts when needed to supplement internal expertise on community engagement strategies or on a particular community (Anderson & Spellecy, 2021; Serpico et al., 2022)
- Put in place mechanisms for the institution/IRB to communicate with Community Advisory Boards (CABs), when they exist, to inform and supplement the IRB's review of research, for example, helping the committee understand areas like the community's values and interests in the service of better evaluating risk and benefit.

We have seen that the *Belmont Report*, the foundational document for research ethics in the United States, has limitations as a comprehensive, guiding ethical framework for stakeholder-engaged research. At the very least, the *Belmont* principles must be interpreted very broadly and applied in novel ways, far beyond the scope envisioned by *Belmont*, to fit the challenges and contours of CEnR. Even so expansively construed, the *Belmont* principles may need to be supplemented with additional ethical principles to adequately address the multi-faceted relationships between researchers and communities envisioned and championed by CEnR.

We need not take a stand on this point to see that *Belmont*, as we've inherited it, is an imperfect fit for CEnR. This is not a condemnation of *Belmont*—it was a product of a very different time and place, and has, I think we can agree, served the research oversight community remarkably well for the past 40 years. It does, however, mean that the ethical design and evaluation of CEnR requires additional conceptual work. The CEnR community will benefit from a shared articulation and appreciation of CEnR's guiding ethical principles. The chapters in this volume represent a significant step in that direction.

References

Anderson, E. E. (2019). A proposal for fair compensation for research participants. *American Journal of Bioethics, 19*(9), 62–64.

Anderson, E. E., & Spellecy, R. (2021). Patient and community engagement. In E. A. Banker, B. G. Gordon, E. A. Hurley, & S. P. Shriver (Eds.), *Institutional review board management and function* (3rd ed.). Jones and Bartlett Learning.

Castro-Reyes, P., Cooks, J., Drew, E., Edwards, K., Freeman, E., Isaacs, M.-L., Park, A., Sablan-Santos, L., Seifer, S. D., Shore, N., & Wat, E. (2015). *Research ethics reconsidered in the context of community-engaged research: Proposed revisions to the Belmont report and Federal Regulations Guiding the protection of research participants*. Campus-Community Partnerships for Health. Retrieved April 28, 2021 from https://ccphealth.org/2021/02/22/research-ethics-reconsidered-in-the-context-of-community-engaged-research-proposed-revisions-to-the-belmont-report-and-federal-regulations-guiding-the-protection-of-research-participants-2/

Cho, H. L., Danis, M., & Grady, C. (2018). Post-trial responsibilities beyond post-trial access. *The Lancet, 391*, 10129. Retrieved Sepetember 21, 2021 from https://www.ncbi.nlm.nih.gov/pmc/articles/PMC6010308/

Clinical and Translational Science Awards Consortium Community Engagement Key Function Committee Task Force on the Principles of Community Engagement (CTSA). (2011). *Principles of Community Engagement*. In *Centers for Disease Control and Prevention Agency for Toxic Substances and Disease Registry* (2nd ed.) Retrieved May 4, 2021 from https://www.atsdr.cdc.gov/communityengagement/pce_what.html#figure1

Department of Health and Humans Services (HHS). (2016). Secretary's Advisory Committee on Human Research Protections. *July 21, 2016 SACHRP Letter to HHS Secretary, Attachment B: Return of Individual Research Results*. Retrieved September 7, 2021 from https://www.hhs.gov/ohrp/sachrp-committee/recommendations/attachment-b-return-individual-research-results/index.html

Garrison, N. A. (2013). Genomic justice for native Americans: Impact of the Havasupai case on genetic research science. *Technology, and Human Values, 38*(2), 201–223. https://doi.org/10.1177/0162243912470009

Largent, E. A., & Lynch, H. F. (2017). Paying research participants: Regulatory uncertainty, conceptual confusion, and a path forward. *Yale Journal of Health Policy Law and Ethics, 17*(1), 61–141.

Maiter, S., Imich, L., Jacobson, N., & Wise, J. (2008). Reciprocity: An ethic for community-based participatory action research. *Action Research, 8*(3), 305–325. https://doi.org/10.1177/2F1476750307083720

Mikesell, L., Bromley, E., & Khodyakov, D. (2013). Ethical community-engaged research: A literature review. *American Journal of Public Health., 102*(12), e7–e14. https://doi.org/10.2105/AJPH.2013.301605

Multi-Regional Clinical Trials Center (MRCT). (2017). *Post-trial responsibilities: Continued access to investigational medicines guidance document, version 1.2*. The MRCT Center of Brigham and Women's Hospital and Harvard. Retrieved September 7, 2021 from: https://mrctcenter.org/wp-content/uploads/2017/12/2017-12-07-Post-Trial-Responsibilities-Guidance-Document-Version-1.2.pdf

National Commission for the Protection of Human Subjects of Biomedical and Behavioral Research. (1979). *The Belmont Report: Ethical principles and guidelines for the protection of human subjects of research.* Retrieved June 11, 2021 from https://www.hhs.gov/ohrp/regulations-and-policy/belmont-report/read-the-belmont-report/index.html#xethical

Ross, L. F. (2010). 360 degrees of human subjects protections in community-engaged research. *Science Translational Medicine, 2*(45). https://doi.org/10.1126/scitranslmed.3001162. Retrieved May 4, 2021 from https://www.ncbi.nlm.nih.gov/pmc/articles/PMC4261185/

Ross, L. F. et al. (2010). Human subjects protections in community-engaged research: A research ethics framework. *Journal of Empirical Research on Human Research Ethics, 5*(1), 5–17. https://doi.org/10.1525/jer.2010.5.1.5

Serpico, K., Rahimzadeh, V., Anderson, E., Gelinas, L., & Fernandez Lynch, H. (2022). Institutional review board use of outside experts: What do we know? *Ethics & Human Research, 44*(2), 26–32.

Shalowitz, D. I., & Miller, F. G. (2005). Disclosing individual research of clinical research—Implications of respect for participants. *Journal of the American Medical Association, 294*(6), 737–740.

Shore, N. (2006). Re-conceptualizing the Belmont report: A community-based participatory research perspective. *Journal of Community Practice, 14*(4), 5–26. https://doi.org/10.1300/J125v14n04_02

Shore, N. (2007). Community-based participatory research and the ethics review process. *Journal of Empirical Research on Human Research Ethics, 2*(1), 31–41. https://doi.org/10.1525/jer.2007.2.1.31

Thompson, V. L., Ackerman, N., Bauer, K. L., Bowen, D. J., & Goodman, M. S. (2021). Strategies of community engagement in research: definitions and classifications. *Translational Behavioral Medicine, 11*(2), 441–451. Retrieved September 7, 2021 from https://www.ncbi.nlm.nih.gov/pmc/articles/PMC8135186/

Yarborough, M., Edwards, K., Espinoza, P., Geller, G., Sarwal, A., Sharp, R., & Spicer, P. (2013). Relationships hold the key to trustworthy and productive translational science: Recommendations for expanding community engagement in biomedical research. *Clinical and Translational Science, 6*(4), 310–313.

Elisa A. Hurley is the former executive director of Public Responsibility in Medicine & Research (PRIM&R), an independent nonprofit organization dedicated to advancing ethical research.

Chapter 18
Stakeholder Engagement and (the Limits of) IRB Review

Stephanie Solomon Cargill

Both IRB review and patient and community stakeholder-engagement in research arose in response to the ethical failings of researchers, often perpetrated upon the most vulnerable and marginalized members of society. Both enterprises fundamentally embrace the idea that research that is conducted ethically ultimately achieves its scientific ends more completely. At their core, IRB review and stakeholder engagement both aim to ensure that research is safe, respectful, beneficial, and fair. With these similarities, one might assume harmony between IRBs and researchers doing stakeholder-engaged work, but unfortunately, this has not often been the case. The relationship between stakeholder-engaged research and IRB review has historically been contentious.

Researchers who conduct stakeholder-engaged research frequently complain that IRBs impose inappropriate obstacles and restrictions to their work. Over 20 years ago, Downie and Cottrell (2001, 9) referred to the process of submitting a community-engaged study for IRB review, "frustrating and sometimes demoralizing." A more recent survey of community-based participatory researchers (Shore, 2007) found that they encountered multiple challenges with IRBs, including a sense of disconnect between their projects and IRB standards as well as inappropriate feedback that misunderstands the expertise, legal constraints, and other commitments in place in the community context.

Two specific published examples further illustrate this disconnect. Brown and colleagues report on the challenges of obtaining IRB approval for several environmental health community-based participatory research (CBPR) projects, specifically due to aspects of stakeholder involvement (Brown et al., 2008). The authors reported on two major barriers to IRB approval: (1) designating and qualifying

S. S. Cargill (✉)
Albert Gnaegi Center for Health Care Ethics, Saint Louis University, Saint Louis, MO, USA
e-mail: stephanie.cargill@slu.edu

E. E. Anderson (ed.), *Ethical Issues in Community and Patient Stakeholder–Engaged Health Research*, Philosophy and Medicine 146,
https://doi.org/10.1007/978-3-031-40379-8_18

non-academic stakeholders as researchers on the study and (2) providing individual results to participants. Involving community partners as co-researchers in projects and providing research results to stakeholders are two key commitments of CBPR, and they represent two key ways that stakeholders can be engaged in the research process.

Another illustration of tensions between IRBs and stakeholder-engaged research is provided by Malone et al. (2006) in their article, "It's like Tuskegee in Reverse," in which they report on their struggle to obtain IRB approval for a CBPR study of cigarette sale practices in a predominately Black community in San Francisco. In this case, the IRB and the study team disagreed about the risks of the study as well as what constitutes adequate risk minimization for participants. They also disagreed more fundamentally about who was a research participant versus who was a research partner.

In this chapter, I will analyze the tensions that can occur between IRBs and researchers that engage with patient and community stakeholders and demonstrate how these tensions can be better understood as reflecting specific ways in which IRBs and stakeholder-engaged research are applying two different, but largely complementary, approaches to ethical research. I will first discuss four categorical differences between the ethical approach of patient- and community-stakeholder engaged research and IRB ethical review of research within the required regulatory constraints. As such, communication between researchers and IRBs is central in order for each side to understand the perspectives, priorities, and processes of the other and most importantly, to ensure ethical research. Then I will discuss current strategies available to IRBs and stakeholder-engaged researchers that could help facilitate a more collaborative understanding of research ethics review. Finally, I will acknowledge the limits of these strategies until or unless there is change at the structural levels of research funding and research regulations that create tension between IRBs and researchers who engage community and patient stakeholders in their work.

18.1 Whence the Divide?

IRB processes are outlined in federal regulations at 45 CFR 46 that determine the criteria by which research with human subjects can be approved and continue. These regulations focus on the protection of individual participants. Ethical guidelines developed for community- and patient-engaged research, on the other hand, focus on fair, ethical processes and respectful relationships throughout the life of a research project, from conception of the research question through dissemination of results (CTSA Consortium, 2011). The differences between research regulations and principles of community engagement can lead to conflict between IRBs and stakeholder-engaged research teams regarding what constitutes ethical research (Downie & Cottrell, 2001; Malone et al., 2006). Shore (2007) breaks these ethical differences down into three categories: the meaning and purpose of research; assumptions about relationship dynamics between the researcher and the "researched"; and methodological choices (Shore, 2007). To these categories, I will add a fourth, which is presupposed by the other three: differences in ethical frameworks. Understanding where stakeholder-engaged research and IRB review diverge along these four categories will help to better articulate where these approaches are consistent, where they may be different yet compatible, and where they are ultimately contradictory. This will allow the generation of focused solutions.

18.1.1 Differences in Ethical Frameworks

The ethical landscape of stakeholder-engaged research is much broader than what is in the federal regulations for IRB review. In contrast to the procedural and individualistic ethics applied by IRBs, the ethical goals of CBPR and other forms of stakeholder-engaged research are relational and contextual (Guta & Voronka, 2020, 567). (Also see Chap. 3, in this volume.) These approaches place ethical significance in partnership, collaboration, and participation (Banks et al., 2013). While IRBs may attend to the power dynamics between those conducting research and those participating by aiming to protect participants from coercion and undue influence, stakeholder-engaged research commits to redress power imbalances through co-creation of knowledge, rather than merely protecting the powerless.

Another difference between how IRBs and stakeholder-engaged researchers envision ethical research is how the risks and benefits of research are defined. Federal regulations require that "[t]he IRB should not consider possible long-range effects of applying knowledge gained in the research (for example, the possible effects of the research on public policy) as among those research risks that fall within the purview of its responsibility" (Protection of Human Subjects, §46.111, 2018). However, research that engages communities focuses on risks to both individual participants and communities and views these risks as interconnected (see Chaps. 15 and 17, in this volume). Ross et al. (2010) distinguish between group-mediated risks that affect individuals (such as discrimination due to membership in a social group), and group-level risks (such as research that undermines a community's religious beliefs). Stakeholder-engaged researchers are concerned with both of these types of risks, while neither may be considered by an IRB.

IRBs are restricted in their review to "consider only those risks and benefits that may result from the research (as distinguished from risks and benefits of therapies subjects would receive even if not participating in the research)" (Protection of Human Subjects, §46.111, 2018). This restriction is often interpreted to disqualify considerations of the underlying risks of the context in which research is conducted, as long as those risks are not caused by the research itself. Stakeholder-engaged research frequently assumes a reciprocal relationship between researchers and the community in which research takes place, whereby researcher duties extend beyond the particular intervention, both at the time of the research and beyond. "From a purely ethical stand-point, personal and long-term relationships necessarily expand the nature and scope of ethical obligations to the community beyond the typical ethical considerations in research" (Cross et al., 2015, 1013). In stakeholder-engaged research, there is an obligation for researchers to provide *community-level* benefits such as capacity-building, infrastructure benefits, or the benefits of disseminating useful results of the research to the community (Israel et al., 1998; Seifer et al., 2010; Shore et al., 2011b). This is not a responsibility required by the IRB, and may even be interpreted by the IRB to be prohibited, as in the case report by Brown et al.

18.1.2 Differences in Meaning and Purpose of Research

According to the federal regulations that structure IRB oversight, "research" is defined as "a systematic investigation, including research development, testing and evaluation, designed to develop or contribute to generalizable knowledge"(Protection of Human Subjects, §46.102, 2018). Equating the goal of research with the generalizability of its results yields an assumption that generalizable knowledge is fundamentally what makes research valuable. Thus, a research study and the risks it poses to participants are justified by establishing that the research is scientifically well-designed to produce generalizable knowledge.

When community and patient stakeholders (who are not academic researchers) engage in research, their ultimate goal is rarely generalizable knowledge for its own sake, but rather knowledge in order to achieve community benefits (Brush et al., 2020; Shore, 2007; Shore et al., 2011a). (Also see Chap. 2, in this volume.) While a particular research project may meet the regulatory definition of an investigation designed to develop generalizable knowledge, as it generalizes from the specific participant population to the community to which they belong, this framing has distinct implications for the evaluation of risks, burdens, and benefits. While for IRBs, the risks and burdens of research are justified by the generalized knowledge produced, for stakeholder-engaged research the risks and burdens of research are justified by the community-level benefits provided. These benefits can be framed broadly to include capacity developed through partnering in the research, the knowledge of how to improve or eliminate problematic practices or behaviors in the community, or even the economic benefits that may accrue from the research being located there, such as jobs or money paid to research participants that is spent in the community (for example, by providing gift cards for a local business as compensation for research participation). Providing community-level benefits also requires useful dissemination and implementation of results; otherwise, stakeholder partners may not view research as valuable or as providing adequate benefit to outweigh its risks. Guiding frameworks for IRB review and stakeholder-engaged research consider differently what counts as a risk and a benefit, and whose definition of risks and benefits matters (see Chap. 15, in this volume).

18.1.3 Different Assumptions About the Relationship Between the Researcher and the Researched

Another source of tension between IRBs and stakeholder-engaged researchers is the assumption by IRBs that the researchers and participants are separate and distinct sets of stakeholders, and that researchers and participants are the only relevant stakeholders in the research enterprise. The National Bioethics Advisory Commission defines the researcher/researched dynamic in this way: "participants are used at least to some extent by investigators to achieve their research objectives, which might or might not benefit the participants" (National Bioethics Advisory Commission, 2001, 38). This distinction has several implications. First, while researchers are seen as the agents of knowledge production, participants are seen as (usually passive) sources of information. As a result, there is no expectation that participants or other community stakeholders have agency (outside of informed consent) in shaping the research, in determining what benefits should be provided, or in interpreting the risks. Further, given this distinction, it is assumed that the goals of the research align with the goals of the researchers, and insofar as they align with the goals of the participants, this is incidental. As a result, IRBs often interpret participants as people to be protected *from* research, as it is being done to them for others' purposes.

In contrast, in stakeholder-engaged research, community members, patients, and others frequently play a more active role; although a subset of stakeholders may serve as participants, they are more than merely passive participants in someone else's research agenda. Stakeholders can be agents of the research while also being sources of information that shape its results. In research that is patient or community stakeholder directed, non-academic research partners shape every aspect of the study, from conception, through design and implementation, and ultimately collaborate in interpreting and disseminating the results. Thus, as active agents of the research, patient and community stakeholders do not expect to be protected *from* research so much as they desire to be empowered to shape the research to benefit them. This shift from mere means or even potential victims to agents of research illuminates how a similar goal to avoid research abuses yields contrasting views about appropriate roles and responsibilities of participants and other stakeholders in the community. The responsibility for the ethics of research lies with those who design and implement it. Stakeholder research seeks to empower stakeholders outside of the academic research world to be involved in the design and implementation of research, sharing the role, and the responsibility, of agents of research with their academic partners. This reflects a greater shift from a protectionist model embraced by IRBs to an empowerment model embraced by stakeholder-engaged research.

IRBs at academic institutions have been perceived as putting up barriers to community and patient stakeholders serving as partners in research. One barrier is the requirement for research teams to complete trainings that have been designed for academic researchers, which require access to and comfort with online learning and use technical language (Anderson et al., 2012). These trainings cover many topics not relevant to stakeholder partners' research roles, while also failing to teach necessary and relevant skills and knowledge. For example, community partners do not need to know the full extent of institutional regulation of faculty members' financial conflicts of interest, but they do need to know how to navigate issues of nonfinancial conflicts of interest that emerge when recruiting participants who live in one's own community or clients served by one's own organization.

IRBs are tasked with ensuring that researchers are appropriately qualified to conduct research. However, they may apply different standards to stakeholder partners when evaluating their qualifications. While community partners may be burdened with proving their qualifications to conduct research by completing extensive trainings and having their resumes scrutinized, academic researchers rarely are challenged regarding training or (lack of) experience working with vulnerable populations and communities. Community research partners may be more qualified to evaluate risks and benefits, recruit participants, or obtain informed consent than their academic researcher partners due to their experience as community social service providers and community organization leaders.

18.1.4 Different Methodological Assumptions

The current regulatory framework requires that a research protocol be fully articulated prior to the initiation of a study; ethical research adheres to the outlined protocol. Deviation from the research plan requires either prospective approval of amendments or reporting of problematic deviations after the fact. Unapproved changes prior to IRB review and authorization constitute "protocol deviations," "protocol violations," "protocol variances," or even "non-compliance." These labels at best imply exceptions to the rule and at worst unethical behavior deserving of penalties.

Cross et al. (2015) discusses the inherent tension between IRB assumptions of acceptable research methodologies and the methodologies commonly used in stakeholder-engaged research. Stakeholder-engaged research challenges these methodological expectations in two ways: emergent ethics and emergent research design. First, representatives of the populations of interest are expected to provide ethical input into the research process starting with the conception and design of the research and throughout the project. In other words, the assumption is that "many of the ethical issues that emerge in CBPR are often difficult to anticipate and only surface later into the life of a project" (Haggerty, 2004).

Second, stakeholder-engaged research frequently uses emergent designs, which assume that the research will adapt to new ideas, concepts, or findings that arise while conducting the research (Pailthorpe, 2017). Emergent design presupposes that changes will be commonplace and that such changes are good research practice, that is, responsive to community needs and preferences, rather than deviations. Emergent designs pose challenges for IRB review, as the protocol and participant-facing documents require approval in their completed form at the outset of the study. Substantive changes as a result of adaptations to new information require burdensome and bureaucratic approval each time, and are framed as exceptions to the plan, rather than part of the plan at the outset.

18.1.5 Potential Bridges of the Divide

The four categories along which IRBs and stakeholder-engaged research differ are the source of tensions that may arise when stakeholder-engaged research seeks IRB review. These tensions are not inevitable though if they are approached as largely complementary (rather than unresolvable) and adaptations are made by both researchers and IRBs. Structurally, the timing and process of IRB review pose barriers for stakeholder-engaged research approaches. These barriers, I will argue, can be overcome by exploring existing flexibility available to IRBs in their review of research, while also respecting that research must remain within the framework of the regulations.

18.2 Structural Adaptations: Flexibility in IRB Processes[1]

18.2.1 Recognition and Oversight of Stakeholders as Part of the Research Team

IRBs may have difficulty distinguishing community members who are sources of data for a research study (participants) from community members who are part of the team collecting data for a research study (researcher). To be fair, these lines are often blurred in stakeholder-engaged research. (See Chap. 14, in this volume.) As Wolf (2010, 78) states, "if data is collected *about* community partners, as well as *by* community partners, then they may be *human subjects* under the federal regulations. If so, the REC has both a legal and ethical obligation to protect the rights and welfare of those human subjects." Wolf's proposed solution to this challenge is that IRBs be clear regarding what constitute a "human subject" for the purposes of the regulations and that the research team be clear regarding the roles the patient and community stakeholder partners will perform at each stage of the research, perhaps outlined in a cover letter or through direct communication.

Once it is determined clearly that a community partner is a member of the research team and not a research participant, the next hurdle is to determine that they are qualified and have the necessary research skills to fulfill this role.

[1] Parts of this section are adapted from Solomon, DeBruin, et al. "Community-engaged research ethics review: Exploring flexibility in federal regulations." *IRB* 38.3 (2016): 11.

Assumptions by IRBs that community members lack the qualifications to perform research is a manifestation of a bias against informal or nonacademic types of expertise; this bias seems not to be extended toward other research partners, such as clinical research organizations or other academic research institutions. IRBs should require evidence of qualifications for conducting the research appropriately and equally from both academic and community stakeholder research team members and evaluate the evidence similarly. When IRB applications require evidence of experience to conduct research, traditional CVs from academic team members may not be sufficient to establish experience in particular communities without further documentation, such as evidence of working with or researching that community specifically. It is within the IRB purview to require this evidence from academic researchers and should be done when experience with the communities at the focus of research is not established by existing materials. Likewise, IRBs can legitimately inquire into the research qualifications of community members but should recognize that many of their experiences do translate into research skills. For example, experience in clinical care or social work requires maintaining confidentiality. IRBs must be willing to recognize that this experience, even if not academically attained, provides justification that community partners have skills relevant to conducting the research.

IRBs should also recognize that training programs widely used in human research protections may not meet the needs of community members on research teams. Comprehensive training such as that required by most academic institutions (e.g., Collaborative IRB Training Initiative [CITI]), may not be relevant, feasible, adequate, or culturally or contextually appropriate for community partners, especially those with narrowly-defined roles in the project. Such training programs also often assume a fairly high level of familiarity with technology and biomedical research (Anderson et al., 2012; Anderson, 2013; Solomon & Piechowski, 2011). Given the flexibility of OHRP's training requirement, IRBs should accept (and increasingly are accepting) alternative trainings that are more appropriate to the roles and challenges faced by research teams that include non-academic stakeholders. These alternative trainings are growing in number and available from various sources (Anderson, 2015; Nebeker et al., 2015; Solomon et al., 2014a, b). Ultimately, there are ways for IRBs to manage their risk aversion to covering stakeholders as members of the research team by recognizing experience and utilizing trainings which may not be currently familiar to them, while proactively building familiarity with community partners to increase their comfort in this role.

18.2.2 Managing the Review of Emergent Research Designs

The recognition that emergent research designs are often the best approach to certain research questions is neither new nor unique to stakeholder-engaged research. Flexible research designs have been standard in the clinical trials domain for years. "Adaptive design" of clinical trials is defined by the FDA as "a clinical trial design that allows for prospectively planned modifications to one or more aspects of the design based on accumulating data from subjects in the trial" (FDA, 2019). The pharmaceutical industry has recognized that in certain contexts, such as oncology trials, these flexible designs are ethical because they increase the likelihood that participants will be assigned to more effective treatments as the trials continue, or because they allow participants to switch to more promising arms if their current treatment does not appear to be working. At the same time, like the emergent trial designs utilized by much stakeholder-engaged research, there is a recognition that these designs come with "heightened logistical challenges to ensuring appropriate trial conduct (ibid)".

IRBs increasingly acknowledge the built-in flexibility of adaptive trial designs, and lessons for review of clinical trials can be applied to emergent designs in stakeholder-engaged research. The Secretary's Advisory Commission on Human Research Protections (SACHRP) recommends that protocols can be written with built-in flexibility, as long as this does not adversely affect participants' safety or the quality of the science (Secretary's Advisory Committee on Human Research Protections, 2011). The underlying philosophy is that adaptations must be planned as much as possible ahead of time. This does not mean that the actual changes must be known at the outset, which is the assumption of linear research designs, but rather that the decision rules (i.e., what triggers revisiting of a study design) and the decision authorities (i.e., who will be responsible for judging the need to change the study design) are specified at the outset. For adaptive clinical trials, this manifests as complex statistical proposals for when interim analyses should be conducted on the emerging data and the thresholds by which that data would justify changing the study design. Likewise, it requires designating the reviewing bodies responsible for judging when these thresholds are met and why, such as a data monitoring committee and/or a dedicated adaptation committee. The IRB is then responsible for prospectively reviewing the decision rules and the decision authorities, rather than evaluating the changes themselves.

A similar model could be used to prospectively review emergent designs in stakeholder-engaged research. The study team would be responsible for prospectively providing the IRB with decision rules and naming decisional authorities. Rather than statistical plans and data monitoring committees, this would include, for example, periodic presentations of the status of the study, specifically in terms of experiences that raise the risk threshold or lower the benefit threshold, to a Community Advisory Board. Changes within a defined scope would not constitute deviations from the protocol. Researchers could also supply the IRB with materials that include topics and examples of questions to be used in questionnaires, surveys or focus groups, rather than a specific final list of questions. Then, if community feedback during implementation suggests that certain questions or wordings are insensitive, inappropriate, etc., these can be altered without additional IRB approval, but rather supplied to the IRB a report after the fact. Accepting a more flexible protocol and endorsing periodic reports of changes would not eliminate IRB authorization nor the need for a prospective research plan as required by the regulations;

rather, such an approach creates space for emergent designs to evolve and for the responsiveness required of many community-engaged research projects.

18.3 Content Adaptations: Communication and Representation

While these structural changes can do much to overcome the tensions between IRBs and stakeholder-engaged researchers, they do not themselves address the issue of whether and how the standards to which IRBs hold human subjects research should be adapted considering stakeholder-engaged research.

Some stakeholder-engaged research scholars have examined how the ethical questions that IRBs pose to research can incorporate stakeholder values into them. For example, Flicker et al. (2007) conducted a content analysis of forms and guidelines used by US IRBs and research ethics board (REBs) in Canada to examine whether they queried community participation in the research process and reflected other ethical priorities of community-engaged research. What is notable about their analysis is that they found considerable overlap in the queries, but also identified clear places where compatible questions may not be asked but could be (see Table 18.1 below). (It should be noted that this study set aside the question of whether these additions should be within or outside of the purview of IRBs).

Flicker et al.'s analysis points to three categories of ethical content at issue. First, some ethical concerns of clear importance to stakeholder-engaged research are already asked by a significant number of IRBs, such as questions about protecting vulnerable populations, data storage and access, and compensation. Better communication between stakeholder-engaged researchers and IRBs, both at the general level and for particular projects could make clearer the many ways in which stakeholders' views of ethics are consistent with IRBs. Further, this communication could add nuance and depth to IRB questions so that the ethical goals of both could be attained. For example, in assessing individual risks to study participants, IRBs could incorporate risks that participants are exposed to as members of distinct communities, such as stigma and coercion, that may not be obvious without insight from stakeholder partners who share characteristics with participants.

Second, some of these proposed questions reflect the process changes suggested above. For example, all the IRB forms Flicker et al. examined asked about the scientific rationale for the study, but none asked whether there was community involvement in the process of identifying the rationale for the study. Similarly, there is always a section of the IRB application that asks about the qualifications of the research team to conduct the research, but rarely are there questions about the capacity of the research team to work with a particular population or community, or which members of the research team hold this expertise. Further, very few IRBs ask about training in how to handle sensitive data, which is likely a skill held by community members who work in social or health services but may not be held by

Table 18.1 REB/IRB protocol content analysis

	Yes	No
Background		
Does the form ask about the "scientific" rationale for the research (e.g., literature review)?	30	0
Does the form ask explicitly about community involvement in identifying the rationale for the research?	0	30
Research methodology		
Is there a section on staff training and/or community capacity-building?	0	30
Are there questions that are concerned with minimizing barriers to community participation (e.g., that ask about language/literacy issues, culturally sensitive methods/approaches etc.)?	6	24
Participants		
Are there questions about protecting "vulnerable groups"?	19	11
Is there a justification section for sample selection (not just sample size, but inclusion and exclusion criteria)?	16	14
Conflicts of interest		
Do forms explicitly ask about "power" relationships between researchers and participants?	3	27
Do forms ask about conflicts of interests (e.g., financial or otherwise)	17	13
Risks and benefits		
Do forms ask about risks and benefits on an individual level?	30	0
Do forms ask about risks and benefits on a community/societal level?	4	26
Do the forms ask about how unflattering data might be handled?	1	29
Privacy and confidentiality		
Do the forms ask about where data will be stored?	20	10
Do the forms ask about who has access to the data?	18	12
Do the forms ask about what training will be provided for those with access to sensitive data?	5	25
Compensation and budget		
Do the forms ask about who is managing the budget?	5	25
Do the forms ask about who is getting compensated for their time (and how)?	16	14
Do the forms ask for a budget justification (e.g., what resources are in place to minimize barriers to participation such as childcare, food, transportation etc.)?	0	30
Do the forms ask about equitable distribution of resources between community and institutional partners?	0	30
Do the forms ask about monetary values (particularly in relation to the potential for compensation to be seen as coercion)?	13	17
Informed consent		
Is there a section on individual consent?	30	0
Do the forms ask about getting "informed consent" from marginalized groups?	17	13
Do the forms ask about "community" consent?	0	30
Do the forms ask how partners or advisory boards will define accountability or decision making structures?	1	29
Outcome and results		
Do the forms ask how research results will be disseminated?	5	25
Do the forms ask about commitment to action and follow-up based on results?	2	28
Is there a process for vetoing publication or ending the study based on community concerns?	0	30

Flicker et al. (2007, 484)

researchers. These questions could be added to better align stakeholder and IRB focus without a significant change to the content (or process) of IRB review.

A third type of question indicates the ethical differences between IRBs and stakeholder-engaged research approaches discussed above. While all IRBs surveyed asked about the risks and benefits to participants at the individual level, only four asked about risk and benefits at the community or population level, and only one asked about the risks of unflattering data to the communities involved. This clearly reflects the restrictions placed on IRBs for considering long-term and societal impacts of the research discussed above, as well as IRBs' focus, discussed in Wolf (2010) and others, on how individuals, and not groups, are impacted by research. Likewise, none asked about community consent or permission from formal or informal community leaders on behalf of the community, and only one asked about how partners or advisory boards define accountability or decision-making structures. These priorities of stakeholder-engaged research are clearly not scrutinized by IRBs. Finally, very few IRBs ask questions about dissemination, follow-up, or concerns about publication arising from communities. These issues are clearly central to stakeholders' understanding of the benefits of research but are outside the conception of research benefit as understood by IRBs.

The central issue regarding these ethical concerns is whether IRBs are the right place for these questions to be asked and the appropriate authority to hold researchers accountable. It is questionable whether IRBs have the requisite expertise to recognize and evaluate studies for their community benefit and thus any social concerns articulated by IRBs will have a highly speculative quality. Likewise, were IRBs to weigh in on the (lack of) necessity of community consent or the quality of community decision-making processes, this would not necessarily be informed by knowledge of the local considerations needed to make these determinations. IRBs have long been criticized for their lack of community representation (Cho & Billings, 1997; De Vries & Forsberg, 2002; Hayes et al., 1995; National Bioethics Advisory Commission, 2001; Office of the Inspector General et al., 1998; Veatch, 1975), and the "community" members that are on IRBs, defined negatively as *non*-scientists or people *not* affiliated with the institution, are neither expressly recruited for nor trained regarding the risks and benefits that research poses to specific communities where research takes place (Allison et al., 2008; Anderson, 2006; Anderson et al., 2012; Solomon Cargill, 2018). If IRBs encounter frequent projects in the same communities, this issue could be addressed by complying with §46.107(a), which suggests including "one or more individuals who are knowledgeable about and experienced in working with these categories of subjects" on the roster. At the same time, these members would still be constrained by the restrictions on IRB review stated above.

Fleischman et al. (2011) suggest that while IRBs are not the appropriate locus for questions about social risks and benefits, this does not mean that these questions should not be asked, and they propose a standing national advisory committee. While this solution seems appropriate to deal with broad societal issues raised by research democratically and transparently beyond the expertise of IRBs, it seems less appropriate for the more local concerns about community risks and benefits, or appropriate communication and dissemination. Such local concerns would be better dealt with by a community advisory board or local community review mechanisms (Key, 2017).

These groups have not only a stake but expertise in how the research will impact their community (Solomon, 2009). In these cases, it makes much more sense for evaluations of research to be made by an appropriately diverse group that represents the community at hand rather than society as a whole (see Chap. 7, in this volume).[2]

IRBs have experience engaging outside expertise with differing standards from their own in the research administration enterprise. These include data safety monitoring boards, conflicts of interest committees, biosafety committees, and others. Recognizing that stakeholders representing the individuals and groups impacted by research should have a distinct say in whether and how the research should proceed does not require reinventing the wheel. Community advisory boards or other similar groups should be seen as appropriate gatekeepers for research that implicates their communities, and IRBs should respect (and perhaps even demand) that they sign-off on research projects, for example by providing letters to IRBs. In this way, the assessment of ethical concerns central to stakeholders is incorporated into IRB review without the expectation that IRBs are the only arbiters of these concerns. The distinct ethical roles of IRBs and other reviewing entities, such as community advisory boards, could be recognized as cooperative, and complementary. Both ethical lenses are important and necessary.

The key to resolving tensions is communication. Hyatt et al. (2009) discusses a scenario where a research team, noticing rising suspicion among their community partners regarding the restrictions on research being imposed by IRBs, arranged an open dialogue between community partners and IRB administrators. Relationships and understanding need to be built between IRBs and stakeholder-engaged research teams to achieve compromises that respect the constraints and priorities of IRBs as well as the expertise and priorities of stakeholders.

18.4 Limitations and Conclusion

IRBs and stakeholder engaged research teams both aim to protect participants. While this chapter has hopefully provided constructive suggestions for resolving some of the tensions between the ethical concerns of stakeholder-engaged research and the regulatory (and ethical) concerns of IRBs, some of this divide is built into the institutions and structures that govern research at a much deeper and broader level. Bridging the divide between stakeholder-engaged research and IRBs will require change at the higher levels of research funders and research institutions.

[2]This does not solve the difficult question of who the appropriate representatives for a community should be, which depends on many factors. But these questions are not more clearly delineated, and probably even less so, for a national committee than a local one.

Stakeholder priorities such as community dissemination and follow-up, as well as equitable sharing of resources between academic and community members of research teams, require support from grant funders and academic institutions. Both have in recent years given lip service (and some money) to prioritizing stakeholder-engaged research, but without recognizing that research engagement requires larger structural changes to become a reality, these words are relatively toothless.[3]

Acknowledgements I would like to thank Emily Anderson for inviting me to contribute to this book and providing me with insightful feedback on earlier drafts. I would also like to thank those IRB professionals and community partners with whom I have worked with over the years, who taught me that in spite of the challenges of conducting and reviewing research in this space, everyone has the best interests of research participants at heart.

References

Protection of Human Subjects, 45 CFR §46 (2018)

Allison, R. D., Abbott, L. J., & Wichman, A. (2008). Roles and experiences of non-scientist institutional review board members at the National Institutes of Health. *IRB, 30*(5), 8.

Anderson, E. E. (2006). A qualitative study of non-affiliated, non-scientist institutional review board members. *Accountability in Research, 13*(2), 135–155.

Anderson, E. E. (2013). Views of academic and community partners regarding participant protections and research integrity: A pilot focus group study. *Journal of Empirical Research on Human Research Ethics, 8*(1), 20–31.

Anderson, E. E. (2015). CIRTification: Training in human research protections for community-engaged research partners. *Progress in Community Health Partnerships: Research, Education, and Action, 9*(2), 283.

Anderson, E. E., Solomon, S., Heitman, E., DuBois, J. M., Fisher, C. B., Kost, R. G., Lawless, M. E., Ramsey, C., Jones, B., & Ammerman, A. (2012). Research ethics education for community-engaged research: A review and research agenda. *Journal of Empirical Research on Human Research Ethics, 7*(2), 3–19.

Banks, S., Armstrong, A., Carter, K., Graham, H., Hayward, P., Henry, A., Holland, T., Holmes, C., Lee, A., & McNulty, A. (2013). Everyday ethics in community-based participatory research. *Contemporary Social Science, 8*(3), 263–277.

Brown, P., Morello-Frosch, R., Brody, J. G., Altman, R. G., Rudel, R. A., Senier, L., & Pérez, C. (2008). *IRB Challenges in multi-partner community-based participatory research.*

[3] For example, while IRBs may acknowledge and support community demands for dissemination (beyond academic publications) and commitment to follow-up with the community, if these activities are not funded as part of research grants, nor given time to occur by tenure and promotion guidelines, requiring them at the ethical review stage is relatively ineffective. Likewise, Flicker et al.'s study suggests that IRBs ask about equitable distribution of resources between community and institutional partners. This is a vital question, but economic arrangements regarding payment structures such as indirect costs are out of the hands of researchers as well as IRBs. At best, academic researchers committed to stakeholder priorities would work to satisfy these requirements in their own time and on their own dime, and at worst researchers would avoid engaging stakeholders in research if significant institutional and economic barriers existed.

Brush, B. L., Mentz, G., Jensen, M., Jacobs, B., Saylor, K. M., Rowe, Z., Israel, B. A., & Lachance, L. (2020). Success in long-standing community-based participatory research (CBPR) partnerships: A scoping literature review. *Health Education & Behavior, 47*(4), 556–568.
Cho, M. K., & Billings, P. (1997). Conflict of interest and institutional review boards. *Journal of Investigative Medicine, 45*(4), 154–159.
Cross, J. E., Pickering, K., & Hickey, M. (2015). Community-based participatory research, ethics, and institutional review boards: untying a Gordian knot. *Critical Sociology, 41*(7–8), 1007–1026.
CTSA Consortium. (2011). *Principles of community engagement* (2nd Edn.). NIH Publication No. 11–7782.
De Vries, R. G., & Forsberg, C. (2002). What do IRBs look like? What kind of support do they receive? *Accountability in Research, 9*(3), 199–216.
Downie, J., & Cottrell, B. (2001). Community-based research ethics review: Reflections on experience and recommendations for action. *Health Law Review, 10*, 8.
FDA. (2019). *Adaptive design clinical trials for drugs and biologics: Guidance for industry*. https://www.fda.gov/Drugs/GuidanceComplianceRegulatoryInformation/Guidances/default.htm
Fleischman, A., Levine, C., Eckenwiler, L., Grady, C., Hammerschmidt, D. E., & Sugarman, J. (2011). Dealing with the long-term social implications of research. *The American Journal of Bioethics, 11*(5), 5–9.
Flicker, S., Travers, R., Guta, A., McDonald, S., & Meagher, A. (2007). Ethical dilemmas in community-based participatory research: Recommendations for institutional review boards. *Journal of Urban Health, 84*(4), 478–493.
Guta, A., & Voronka, J. (2020). Ethical Issues in community-based, participatory, and action-oriented forms of research: State of the field and future directions. In *Handbook of research ethics and scientific integrity* (pp. 561–576).
Haggerty, K. D. (2004). Ethics creep: Governing social science research in the name of ethics. *Qualitative Sociology, 27*(4), 391–414.
Hayes, G. J., Hayes, S. C., & Dykstra, T. (1995). *A survey of university institutional review boards: Characteristics, policies, and procedures*. IRB: A Review of Human Subjects Research. http://psycnet.apa.org/psycinfo/1999-13798-001
Hyatt, R. R., Gute, D. M., Pirie, A., Page, H., Vasquez, I., & Dalembert, F. (2009). Transferring knowledge about human subjects protections and the role of institutional review boards in a community-based participatory research project. *American Journal of Public Health, 99*(S3), S526–S531.
Israel, B. A., Schulz, A. J., Parker, E. A., & Becker, A. B. (1998). Review of community-based research: Assessing partnership approaches to improve public health. *Annual Review of Public Health, 19*(1), 173–202.
Key, K. D. (2017). Expanding ethics review processes to include community-level protections: A case study from Flint, Michigan. *AMA Journal of Ethics, 19*(10), 989–998.
Malone, R. E., Yerger, V. B., McGruder, C., & Froelicher, E. (2006). "It's like Tuskegee in reverse": a case study of ethical tensions in institutional review board review of community-based participatory research. *American Journal of Public Health, 96*(11), 1914–1919.
National Bioethics Advisory Commission. (2001). *Ethical and policy issues in research involving human participants*. https://scholarworks.iupui.edu/handle/1805/25
Nebeker, C., Kalichman, M., Talavera, A., & Elder, J. (2015). Training in research ethics and standards for community health workers and promotores engaged in Latino health research. *Hastings Center Report, 45*(4), 20–27.
Office of the Inspector General, US Department of Health and Human Services Services, & Brown, J. G. (1998). *Institutional review boards: A time for reform*. BiblioBazaar.
Pailthorpe, B. C. (2017). Emergent design. In *The international encyclopedia of communication research methods* (pp. 1–2).
Ross, L. F., Loup, A., Nelson, R. M., Botkin, J. R., Kost, R., Smith, G. R., Jr., & Gehlert, S. (2010). Human subjects protections in community-engaged research: A research ethics framework. *Journal of Empirical Research on Human Research Ethics, 5*(1), 5.

Secretary's Advisory Committee on Human Research Protections. (2011). *SACHRP minutes* (pp. 40–46). http://www.hhs.gov/ohrp/sachrp/mtgings/mtg03-11/sachrp_mtg_march2011.html
Seifer, S. D., Michaels, M., & Collins, S. (2010). Applying community-based participatory research principles and approaches in clinical trials: Forging a new model for cancer clinical research. *Progress in Community Health Partnerships: Research, Education, and Action, 4*(1), 37–46.
Shore, N. (2007). Community-based participatory research and the ethics review process. *Journal of Empirical Research on Human Research Ethics, 2*(1), 31–41.
Shore, N., Brazauskas, R., Drew, E., Wong, K. A., Moy, L., Baden, A. C., Cyr, K., Ulevicus, J., & Seifer, S. D. (2011a). Understanding community-based processes for research ethics review: A national study. *American Journal of Public Health, 101*(S1), S359–S364.
Shore, N., Drew, E., Brazauskas, R., & Seifer, S. D. (2011b). Relationships between community-based processes for research ethics review and institution-based IRBs: A national study. *Journal of Empirical Research on Human Research Ethics, 6*(2), 13–21.
Solomon, S. (2009). Stakeholders or experts? On the ambiguous implications of public participation in science. In *The social sciences and democracy* (pp. 39–61). Springer.
Solomon Cargill, S. (2018). What can IRBs learn from CABs? A qualitative analysis of the experiences of recruitment and training of nonscientist members on research review boards. *Journal of Empirical Research on Human Research Ethics, 13*(1), 88–94.
Solomon, S., & Piechowski, P. J. (2011). Developing community partner training: Regulations and relationships. *Journal of Empirical Research on Human Research Ethics, 6*(2), 23.
Solomon, S., Bullock, S., Calhoun, K., Crosby, L., Eakin, B., Franco, Z., Hardwick, E., Leinberger-Jabari, A., Newton, G., Odell, J., et al. (2014a). Piloting a nationally disseminated, interactive human subjects protection program for community partners: Unexpected lessons learned from the field. *Clinical and Translational Science, 7*(2), 172–176.
Solomon, S., Eakin, B., Kirk, R., Piechowski, P., & Thomas, B. (2014b). Piloting a nationally disseminated, interactive human subjects protection program for community partners: Design, content, and evaluation. *Clinical and Translational Science, 7*(2), 177–183.
Veatch, R. M. (1975). Human experimentation committees: Professional or representative? *Hastings Center Report, 5*(5), 31–40.
Wolf, L. E. (2010). The research ethics committee is not the enemy: Oversight of community-based participatory research. *Journal of Empirical Research on Human Research Ethics, 5*(4), 77–86.

Stephanie Solomon Cargill is Associate Professor of Health Care Ethics. Her empirical and theoretical research explores the ethical and policy issues that face research review boards like IRBs and Community Advisory Boards, as well as more specific issues around informed consent and research with vulnerable individuals and communities. She is also the Chair of Castle IRB, a private IRB that specializes in reviewing gene and cell therapy research.

Chapter 19
Community Research Ethics Oversight: Place, Experience, and Expertise

Alize E. Gunay, Phoebe Friesen, and Emily M. A. Doerksen

19.1 Introduction

Around the world, a growing number of communities are demanding authority in the governance of research and research ethics (Shore et al., 2011a, b). Within the traditional system of research ethics, university-based research ethics boards (REBs) review and approve institutionally affiliated research projects involving human participants. This review process primarily relies on ethical and regulatory frameworks such as the Nuremberg Code, the Declaration of Helsinki, the *Belmont Report*, and the Common Rule, all of which recognize the rights of individual human subjects and the responsibilities of academic researchers (Tuck & Guishard, 2013). These models, while securing protections for individuals and the given institution, largely exclude community-level ethical considerations and community oversight from the research ethics review process. Within this research ethics review process, it is customary for research projects conducted on or with communities to be subjected solely to individual and institutional-level ethical considerations; as a result, many communities, especially those that are systematically marginalized, experience research as harmful, exploitative, and disruptive to communal life (Quinn, 2004). To

A. E. Gunay (✉)
Department of Family Medicine and Bioethics, McGill University, Montreal, QC, Canada
e-mail: ece.gunay@mail.mcgill.ca

P. Friesen
Department of Equity, Ethics, and Policy, Department of Social Studies of Medicine, McGill University, Montreal, QC, Canada
e-mail: phoebe.friesen@mcgill.ca

E. M. A. Doerksen
Centre of Genomics and Policy, McGill University, Montreal, QC, Canada
e-mail: emily.doerksen@mail.mcgill.ca

E. E. Anderson (ed.), *Ethical Issues in Community and Patient Stakeholder–Engaged Health Research*, Philosophy and Medicine 146,
https://doi.org/10.1007/978-3-031-40379-8_19

protect themselves from such research harms, many communities have developed strategies to have a say in the oversight of research affecting them. These strategies include community guidelines or codes of ethics (Jürgens, 2005; The Naomi Patients Association and Boyd, 2012; Bauer et al., 2019; Boilevin et al., 2019); community-based research ethics boards[1] (Watkins et al., 2009; Martin del Campo et al., 2013; Boilevin et al., 2019; Carroll-Scott, 2020); and formal research agreements, signed between the community and institutional researchers (Riddell et al., 2017; Hsieh et al., 2019; Neufeld et al., 2019; Bull et al., 2019). In addition to establishing independent research governance structures, many communities are also active in academic partnerships with neighboring universities to control how research is conducted in their communities (Jane-Finch Community Research Partnership; Albert Einstein College of Medicine, 2012). Communities identify a number of benefits associated with involvement in research ethics governance, namely empowering community organizations as equal partners in the research process, fostering trust between researchers and community members, and developing community capacity for meaningful, long-term involvement in institutional REBs (Shore et al., 2014).

These strategies draw inspiration from models formalized by Indigenous communities in their resistance to colonial and exploitative research practices (Friesen et al., 2017). Research in Indigenous communities has frequently violated community consent, perpetuated stigmatizing and racist representations of communities and Indigenous Peoples, disproportionately benefiting researchers over the community, and, at times, resulting in physical abuse and death. One of the most well-known cases is genetic research with the Havasupai Tribe of the Grand Canyon in Arizona. In this study, the Havasupai Peoples agreed to give blood samples to Arizona State University for a study on "the causes of behavioural/medical disorders," while under the impression that the blood was to be used solely for the purpose of understanding genetic links to type-II diabetes in the community. Once researchers could not find such a genetic linkage, they used Havasupai DNA to research the genetic basis of mental disorders and the tribal origins of Native Americans, without obtaining informed consent from participants or the community leaders (Levenson, 2010). Violating the most obvious ethical tenet of human participant research, informed consent, this study also resulted in many community-level harms, including the publication of research papers with racist representations and deficient understandings of addiction and mental disorders in the community. Further, theories of the tribe's "genetic origin" put forward by the study team contradict Havasupai beliefs and knowledge, risking its use in political discourse and colonial rhetoric to delegitimize Havasupai claims to sovereignty in the US (Sterling, 2011).

---

[1]Also known as (Tribal) Institutional Review Boards (IRBs), Community Research Review Committees (CRRC) Ethics Committees (ECs), and Research Ethics Committees (RECs), and Research Advisory Councils (RACs). In this chapter, for institutional review entities, we will be using the terms IRBs and REBs interchangeably; IRBs refer to the US context and REBs refer to the Canadian context.

Canada also has an extensive and ongoing history of harmful research with its Indigenous Peoples. From 1942 to 1952, Health Canada performed nutritional experiments on over 1000 children in residential schools without the informed consent of the children or the parents, including while the Nuremberg Code was in effect. These experiments denied already malnourished children adequate daily nutrition and dental care, resulting in a number of children dying (Mosby, 2013; Macdonald et al., 2014). In a recent class action lawsuit filed against the government, a group of Indigenous people claim they were subjected to unethical medical experimentation as children in state sanitoriums and residential schools (Dangerfield, 2018). The group also claims that doctors performed harmful surgeries without informed consent, including the removal of lung tissue for tuberculosis, despite antibiotics being the well-established standard of care at the time (Dangerfield, 2018). Even in the absence of such explicit cruelty and harm, researchers in Canada still commonly uphold a culture of "helicopter research" by, often forcefully, entering Indigenous communities, intruding on communal life, collecting data, and never reporting back to communities or sharing results (Cherokee Nation; Campbell, 2014). As shown by such examples, Canada's system and culture of research and research governance is, at large, inadequate when it comes to addressing the needs of Indigenous communities, including the structural health disparities that stem from ongoing settler colonialism within the country.

In order to prevent such harms and ensure that research produces desired benefits, many Indigenous communities across the world have published codes of ethics and research guidelines to direct how research is to be conducted with their communities and on their land (Hudson et al., 2010; Schroeder et al., 2019; Australian Institute of Aboriginal and Torres Strait Islander Studies, 2020). In Canada, many Indigenous communities have community REBs or tribal councils to ensure ethical protections for the community within the research ethics review process (Ktunaxa/Kinbasket Tribal Council, 1998; Aboriginal Health Research Review Committee, 2003; Kahnawake Schools Diabetes Prevention Project, 2007; Manitoba First Nations Education Resource Centre, Inc., 2014). These REBs operate on culturally grounded ethical principles and balance individual and community rights (Hayward et al., 2021). In the policy realm, Chap. 9 of the *Tri-Council Policy Statement 2: Ethical Conduct for Research Involving Humans* (TCPS) offers guidance for researchers and institutional REBs working with First Nations, Métis, and Inuit communities in Canada, mandating a process of community consultation and approval through the institutional research ethics review process. To secure community control over the governance of research data, First Nations Peoples of Canada developed the *Ownership, Control, Access, and Possession* (OCAP) principles, centering data sovereignty within discussions in the research ethics governance space (Schnarch, 2004; Bull, 2016). While both Chap. 9 of the TCPS and OCAP have played a significant role in advancing the inclusion and authority of Indigenous communities in research ethics governance, their interpretation and application in specific communities and research contexts remain dependent on consultation with tribal councils, community REBs, codes of ethics, research agreements, and other localized, community-based governance structures (Brunger &

Bull, 2011; Bull, 2019).[2] This allows for research oversight be tailored to the specific worldview, culture, and governance systems of different Indigenous communities, contributing to the advancement of Indigenous research sovereignty in Canada.

While these models are a significant step forward, non-Indigenous communities face several challenges in seeking a role in research governance. Crucially, Indigenous communities have a right to self-determination recognized in the United Nations Declaration on the Rights of Indigenous Peoples (United Nations, 2007), while non-Indigenous communities without a clear right to sovereignty often lack authority over the research process. Indigenous communities also tend to have leadership structures and boundaries in place through criteria underlying membership, but this is often not the case for non-Indigenous communities. It is also important to note that urban Indigenous Peoples, those belonging to several Indigenous communities, and those not recognized as a result of the Indian Act, which stripped status from women who married non-Indigenous men, may also be excluded from community-based protections similar to non-Indigenous communities. In research contexts, non-Indigenous or urban Indigenous communities, who tend to lack sovereignty and agency in research governance, often come into being through a shared patient identity, a shared experience of harm or disenfranchisement, or as we will consider here in this chapter, through a shared geography or sense of place. As such, when communities are not formally recognized as communities and lack clear representatives or membership criteria, this complicates their demands to oversee research that involves them.

Despite not having a claim to sovereignty, non-Indigenous and urban Indigenous communities seeking a voice in research governance often share many features with the Indigenous communities that have inspired them. In many cases, they have experienced extractive and exploitative research, face significant health disparities, and gain little benefit from research that involves them (Friesen et al., 2017, 2021). These similarities raise questions about how we might understand different types of communities and their unique claims to research governance. Here, we consider the role that place might play in answering these questions. We ask: How does the notion of place circulate and operate in community research ethics governance? How do place-based communities define their boundaries? How is a concept of place articulated in the demands, strategies, and justifications for community research ethics governance? To answer these questions, we examine three examples of place-based community-based research governance initiatives, all developed by communities that lack sovereign status: the Bronx Community Research Review Board, the Vancouver Downtown East Side (DTES) *Manifesto*, and the Philadelphia Promise Zone Research Connection. We describe the community, their strategies for oversight in research ethics governance, and the context in which such strategies were formed and operationalized. We also examine the demands and justifications for

---

[2]To apply OCAP in research with Inuit communities of Canada, some Inuit tribal councils have suggested adapting the OCAP principles to the Inuit *Qaujimajatuqangit*, the traditional laws that guide living and knowing for the Inuit (Mashford-Pringle & Pavagadhi, 2020).

community authority and how place functions as a way to organize community boundaries and expertise. Out of all three initiatives, we offer our most extensive reflections on the DTES, as we work in close collaboration with Scott Neufeld, a co-author on the *Manifesto* (see Chap. 20, in this volume). In light of these three examples, we explain why place-based strategies for research ethics oversight can sometimes better represent the diversity and expertise of communities than identity-based forms of representation. This is especially apparent in current practices related to the inclusion of a community member on institutional REBs. Recognizing that these place-based strategies rely on a claim to community expertise, we take up this concept in discussion using feminist standpoint theory. In doing so, we explain communities' claim to ethical expertise and explore how this can inform the inclusion of such strategies within current processes of research ethics review.

19.2 Case Studies

19.2.1 The Bronx Community Research Ethics Review Board

The Bronx is a borough of New York City where most people are racialized, specifically identifying as Hispanic and Black (Kaplan et al., 2006). Structural racism and disinvestment in public infrastructure in the borough underpin the higher rates of poverty and disproportionately poorer health outcomes for this population when compared to the White people living in the Bronx and neighbouring boroughs (Kaplan et al., 2006). Given these social and health disparities, the Bronx is a popular site for research and researcher driven health initiatives; however, the critical disconnect between such initiatives and the community's experiences of ill-health is a significant barrier to meaningfully addressing health disparities in the Bronx. The community's experiences with racism, sexism, ableism, homophobia, transphobia, and fatphobia within healthcare settings, and in the context of academic, "outsider"-driven research projects, negatively colour the residents' perceptions of and trust in such institutions (Galea et al., 2001; Guishard et al., 2021).[3]

In response to these experiences, the Bronx Community Research Ethics Review Board (BxCRRB) was established in 2010 as part of a community-academic partnership between the Albert Einstein College of Medicine (AECM) and the Bronx

[3] Guishard et al. (2021) in "What We Not Finna Do: Respectfully Collaborating with Skinfolk and Kinfolk in Black Participatory Action Research" further describes the geographical and historical context of research in the Bronx, and the upcoming, community-led Community Engaged Research Academy (CERA) project, aimed at addressing harmful research and developing research capacity in the community. CERA is described as a strategy that is not only focused on teaching research methods for its own sake but on "redress[ing] research and schooling as sites of trauma and humiliation for BIPOC (Black, Indigenous, and People of Color) persons by nurturing the capacity of participants to develop research projects without researchers" (4).

Health Link (BHL) to provide an oversight role for the research occurring in the community. Volunteers for the BxCRRB are recruited at community events and selected based on "community involvement, experiences, availability, and demographics of the Bronx" (Martin del Campo et al., 2013, 341). They receive training in bioethics and research methods from the BHL to review research protocols and educate residents about the research taking place in the community. The BxCRRB model is inspired by developments in Indigenous research ethics, namely the work of Dianne Quigley (2006), and focuses on ensuring that, broadly, researcher goals are compatible with community needs; research is designed and executed in partnership with community; and, that the community is involved in the process of knowledge collection and production. This model also encourages the Bronx community and researchers to reach an official agreement on research data stewardship, ownership, publication, and dissemination.

The reported benefits of the model include the ability to assess community-level risks, not merely risks to individual participants, educate the community about their rights and research participation, and provide space for community members to share their experiences with research. These features create a feedback loop between community members and researchers, building trust, and thus benefitting the entire research process. Challenges reported include obtaining adequate and secure funding, a lack of respect and interest from researchers, recruiting and training members, and a tendency to attract professionals as members. While the BxCRRB is a well-recognized and established community REB, it remains dependent on local institutions to recognize its authority in research ethics governance. Because the Bronx is a heterogenous, non-Indigenous urban community without a claim to sovereignty, the BxCRRB, without Federal-Wide Assurance, has no legal authority as a research review board.[4] Thus, only local institutions can mandate BxCRRB approval as a component of the formal research ethics review process. Justifying the importance of community-level review, BxCRRB members propose that "if communities share enough in common to enable them to claim certain rights, then researchers are obliged morally to respect the structural and cultural integrity of the group they study and would be breaching their duty if they disrupt existing solidarity or intrude on communal life without obtaining the community's informed consent" (Martin del Campo et al., 2013, 341). Members of the Bronx are diverse in racial, ethnic, gender, class, ability, and sexual identity; a heterogeneous and intersectional constellation of lived experience forms the structural and cultural integrity of the community. The shared experience of place among members who "live, work, and struggle" in the Bronx is considered foundational to how the community is organized (Casado, 2013, 353). This provides a direct, place-based justification for why

[4] Federal Wide Assurance (FWA) is "an assurance of [the institution's] compliance with the U.S. federal regulations for the protection of human subjects in research" (US Department of Health & Human Services, 2017). FWA is the main mechanism for compliance oversight by the Office for Human Research Protections in the US. An IRB must have FWA in order to be eligible for support from the Department of Health & Human Services.

the Bronx community demands authority in research governance, mandating BxCRRB review as part of formal research ethics review processes.

19.2.2 Research 101: A Manifesto for Ethical Research in the Vancouver Downtown Eastside

The Downtown Eastside (DTES) is one of Vancouver's oldest and most diverse neighbourhoods. Home to a large and growing population of urban Indigenous Peoples, Indigenous knowledge from all across Canada is cultivated and sustained in the DTES (Newham, 2005). The strong culture of activism in the DTES has also paved the way for much of Canada's most progressive movements, including Canada's opioid harm reduction efforts. For example, North America's first supervised injection site, Insite, was founded in the DTES as a result of strong community activism and organizing. However, despite the radical and brilliant work taking place in the community, the DTES is often framed in public discourse as a site of poverty, drug use, and tragedy. A majority of DTES residents are street-involved and experience housing insecurity because of market-driven urbanization and gentrification in Vancouver. The DTES is also historically the site of multiple HIV/AIDs and overdose epidemics, a symptom of Canada's discriminatory healthcare system. Given its negative public image, its culture of political activism, and its wealth of knowledge, the DTES is one of the most researched communities in the world (Damon et al., 2017). Many researchers come to the DTES to study poverty, drug use, and homelessness—and to extract community knowledge. Racialized residents of the DTES also face challenges with access to safe healthcare services, which can exacerbate distrust of research. In the recent report, *In Plain Sight* (2020), which documents discrimination towards Indigenous people within BC's health care system, one First Nations woman in her 50s who lives in the DTES described how she's afraid to seek care because of past experiences of discrimination and trauma. The report describes how the "only time she has been able to get respectful treatment, and not be assumed to be drunk or high or subject to racism, was when she had a non-Indigenous friend accompany her as an advocate and support person" (Turpel-Lafond, 2020). This history of over-research, stigma, and discrimination has left the DTES community heavy with research fatigue and distrustful of researchers (Neufeld, 2019).

To address the harmful research practices occurring in the DTES, community members published *Research 101: A Manifesto for Ethical Research in the Downtown Eastside*, the result of a series of six weekly community workshops that discussed research ethics in the DTES (Boilevin et al., 2019). The *Manifesto* provides researchers and REB members with a set of community values and ethical considerations for research on or with the DTES community. It also demands that the DTES community have governing authority over research, proposing two strategies: formal research agreements (e.g., a Memorandum of Understanding) for research projects, signed by both community representatives and research partners, and a community research ethics board (CREB), run by residents of the DTES. The proposed CREB would consist of a core scientific group, trained in research methods, and a rotating cast of community members to ensure that proposals are reviewed by members with adequate scientific and ethical expertise on the subject matter. The rotating cast of community members would provide the review with ethical expertise originating from lived experience, and as relevant to the research project. Ideally, approval by the CREB would be a required component of existing institutional review processes, allowing the community greater control over research and ensuring adherence to the ethical standards outlined in the *Manifesto*. The CREB would also provide researchers with the opportunity to join the ethical review; this way, researchers would be invited to discuss suggested modifications, collaborate on revisions, and receive community ethics training from the community (Boilevin et al., 2019). To realize this, some of the co-authors of the *Manifesto* are continuing the work from Research 101 as the Community Research Ethics Workshop (CREW), a group working in partnership with the DTES community and surrounding research institutions. Aspiring to develop a community research ethics review model in the DTES, the CREW has, to date, piloted a number of research reviews of proposals relevant to the community (Neufeld, personal communication, 2022; Neufeld, 2019; also see Chap. 20, in this volume).

Several community organizations in the DTES have since signed in support of the *Manifesto* and its principles of community ethics, including Hives for Humanity. Following the Research 101 workshops, Hives for Humanity produced the Informed Consent Card, a transportable tool informing individuals and community organizations in the DTES of their rights concerning research and other forms of cultural production. Within the institutional realm, the University of British Columbia (UBC)'s Behavioural Research Ethics Board (BREB) endorses the *Manifesto*, meaning that the board "agrees with the Manifesto principles of Researcher Transparency, Community-Based Ethical Review, Peer Empowerment in the Research Process and Reciprocity in the Research Exchange" (Manifesto Endorsement Form, 2019). These developments are occurring alongside a broader shift in research culture and conduct, namely towards greater community involvement; in Vancouver, shortly after the publication of the *Manifesto*, Simon Fraser University (SFU) established the Community-Engaged Research Initiative, and UBC the Making Research Accessible Initiative, both with the goal of making research projects and its publications more accessible to communities. The Research 101 process has also inspired urban communities elsewhere in Canada to produce their own Manifestos, including, most notably, the publication of *Research 102: Meaningful Activist Research in amiskwacîwâskahikan (City Centre Edmonton)* (2020).

The *Manifesto* explicitly highlights the gaps in current institutional research ethics review processes concerning the rights of communities. It brings to the fore the importance of community-level ethical considerations in research, unique to each community, as they are unique to the DTES. Researchers are asked to reflect on questions unlikely to be asked by an REB, but that are essential to the ethical conduct of research in a community with a history of exploitation by researchers: "What are the potential wider consequences of your research? What do you expect to find in your research, who else could use the findings of your research and in what ways? Is it possible that other people will use your research to harm our community, or advocate for its elimination? How are you going to address this?" (Boilevin et al., 2019, 14). Beyond its claims to authority and expertise, the DTES is also a community of resistance to the ongoing dispossession, colonization, and market-driven urbanization in Vancouver that seeks to remove the community from its physical and symbolic place.[5] As such, the demand for place-based research governance in the DTES is intimately linked with the community's ability to exercise the self-determination necessary to remain in place and, in doing so, sustain the existence of the DTES community. The *Manifesto* and the proposed CREB reify the DTES as a place with a history, further defining and asserting the boundaries and authority of the community. In securing this power in the research governance process, the DTES community re-imagines its political subjectivity and enables its citizens to demand their rights in the broader political arena.

19.2.3 The Philadelphia Promise Zone Research Connection

The Philadelphia Promise Zone (PPZ) is a geographic area that spans ten neighbourhoods in West Philadelphia that have the highest rates of poverty in the city, due to racial segregation, discriminatory redlining practices, and a legacy of disinvestment from such neighbourhoods (Carroll-Scott et al., 2017). The US Department of Housing and Urban Development gave this area "Promise Zone" designation in 2014 to promote economic development and improvements in public health (Carroll-Scott, 2020). The "Promise Zone" designees are thus given priority status in federal grants and, much like the Bronx and Vancouver DTES, this has resulted in an influx of disruptive research in the PPZ. Residents report that these projects rarely produce felt benefits within the community, as they often over-research certain issues while neglecting others. This is in part due to researchers not engaging

[5] Initially a residential area for loggers and fishermen working in Vancouver's natural resource economy, the DTES offered workers single-occupancy hotel rooms and services such as bars. From the 1950s to the 1960s, urban and commercial development surrounding the DTES eventually drove out public transportation, public services, and investors from this area, attracting low-income people seeking affordable housing (Newham, 2005). By the 1970s, the DTES was a refuge for de-institutionalized psychiatric patients and those who suffered through the Canadian residential school system, the 60s scoop, the foster care system, and the national war on drugs and war on the poor (Masuda et al., 2020). It is in this historical context that the DTES community continually resists the dispossession stemming from market-dependent "revitalization" policies aimed to develop the DTES for real estate investment, which inevitably leave many residents to forcibly disperse, or ultimately, be re-institutionalized through the psychiatric or carceral system (Schatz, 2010).

communities in decision-making, research design, or identifying research priorities, leading to duplicative, and essentially, ineffectual research (Carroll-Scott, 2020). This raises concerns of research exhaustion and coercion in the PPZ, as residents emphasize an increasing loss of control over their community: "This area used to be a quiet family community but now it has become a subject of somebody else's report" (The West Philadelphia Promise Zone, 2018).

Borne out of these concerns, PPZ residents founded the Promise Zone Research Connection (PZRC) in 2015. The PZRC is a community-led advisory committee consisting of 15 PPZ residents, research partners, and city representatives working to ensure research in the PPZ benefits the community. The PZRC has established partnerships with Drexel University, the University of Pennsylvania, and the Children's Hospital of Pennsylvania; the committee works to connect Promise Zone residents with institutional research taking place in the community, and in turn, relay community ideas and concerns to researchers (The West Philadelphia Promise Zone, 2018). Motivating the importance of this work, PZRC members raise concerns about the limitations of institutional IRBs in the governance of research: "this area has been so researched but there is no strong community voice to regulate it" (The West Philadelphia Promise Zone, 2018). PZRC members also highlight the limitations of including a single community member on an IRB, which is insufficient in terms of adequately representing the broad range of experiences, interests, and needs present within the community. Further, because IRBs do not routinely code research protocols by geography, researchers from different universities can essentially conduct the same research project in the PPZ. Thus, a reliable system to measure and assess research burden by geographic area for communities in urban cities is lacking (Carroll-Scott, 2020).

To address these gaps in research governance, the PZRC is currently developing its own Community Research Review Board (CRRB). The CRRB consists of community members, trained in research ethics, who will review and approve (or disapprove) research projects taking place in the PPZ community. The mandate of CRRB is to: advocate for the best interests of the community; ensure that data and results are shared with the community; establish a line of communication for future community-researcher partnerships; and, advocate for community-engaged research among institutional partners for research in the PPZ. With this mandate, the PZRC intends that the CRRB will transform the "negative culture of research that currently exists in the Promise Zone" (Carroll-Scott, 2020, 8). Notably, as a place-based system of oversight, the CRRB is also well-positioned to consider how the federal government's "Promise Zone" initiative places the community at an increased risk for over-research and research harm. While the potential benefits of this place-based research ethics governance system in the PPZ community are clear, sustainable funding to establish the CRRB is reported as a major challenge. Funder priorities tend to favour outcomes-based research focusing on a specific health problems over community research infrastructure and training, even though such infrastructure is often needed to secure program-based funding. These priorities reflect the limited knowledge of grant reviewers, as "comments from grant reviewers engaged in research-focused funding mechanisms suggest they are not aware of the failures of the current IRB system to protect communities or of the detrimental effects of the power imbalance between communities and research institutions" (Carroll-Scott, 2020, 9). Despite this, the CRRB system has the potential to hold researchers and city representatives accountable to the community and not just to their own institutions and funders, which can help to shift the balance of power in the research enterprise towards communities.

19.3 Discussion

Urban communities experiencing marginalization often disproportionately bear the risks and burdens of research and are often left out of research ethics governance processes. To address this, many such communities have created place-based and community-led research ethics governance initiatives to ensure that community voice is included in discussions surrounding research conduct. As showcased in this chapter, place-based strategies in the Vancouver Downtown Eastside, the Bronx, and the Philadelphia Promise Zone successfully mobilize community perspectives in research ethics, filling in a significant gap in our current system of institutional research ethics review and oversight. These cases strongly suggest that place-based research ethics governance, as it is embedded within the social and cultural context of place-based communities, has the potential to account for the community-level risks posed by research projects and to ensure communities receive more felt benefits.

In implementing these strategies, communities are voicing several demands. Firstly, communities are demanding to be formally acknowledged, by institutional bodies such as REBs/IRBs, funding agencies, and universities, and the public at large, as recognizable communities with authority in research ethics governance. This demand brings forward the possibility of extending such communities collective protections similar to the protections afforded to Indigenous communities by the TCPS. Secondly, in establishing independent, place-based research ethics governance structures, communities assume a degree of expertise. To better understand the nature of these demands and their justifications, we now explore how place functions in organizing community boundaries and claims to expertise in these examples.

19.3.1 Community and the Shared Experience of Place

In this chapter, we observe that, in many cases, place and community are mutually constitutive. The history, culture, and living conditions of a place intersect with the social locations of its residents to shape the community and its identity; in turn, communities continually (re)define their place and its physical and symbolic reality. In neighbourhoods such as the Bronx, the DTES, and the PPZ, there is no uniform identity shared by community members, as individuals occupy diverse social locations. Instead, the shared experience of place among residents plays a role in constituting the community. The *Right to Remain*, a community-based participatory action project exploring the impacts of urbanization in the Vancouver DTES, describes this relationship as "the continual re-building of a community, premised on an internally coherent, if precariously held, sense of place among a diverse social mix of racialized and oppressed peoples" (Masuda et al., 2020, 234). Similar to the DTES, the Bronx and the PPZ also define their community boundaries through a shared experience of place, where histories of harmful "outsider" research constitute a part of this experience.

In what has become known as "identity politics," shared identities, linked to characteristics such as race, gender, sexuality, or religion, come to define and organize communities and their political orientations. While identity politics can unite and empower oppressed peoples, it often foregrounds a singular, "primary" identity, subsuming other identities and intra-group differences (Crenshaw, 1991). Place-based communities, in delineating their boundaries through a shared experience of place, offer an alternative to such configurations of identity, however, complicating the notion of identity as singular and reducible. This aligns with the concept of intersectionality, which steps away from a view of identities as essential (e.g., all woman share the experience of X) and instead highlights how intersecting identities shape differences in experience (e.g., giving birth in the US may be experienced very differently by a Black woman and a White woman). As such, it is essential to acknowledge the way in which interconnected identities produce diverse individual social locations within systems of advantage and disadvantage (Crenshaw, 1991; Collins, 1990). Thus, groups defined by a singular social identity risk representing the experiences and interests of those who are the most privileged within the identity group, potentially rendering multiply oppressed persons invisible (Heyes, 2002).

This singular and privileged viewpoint is of central concern within current processes for research ethics review. In most countries, REBs are required to have one or two community representatives in order to represent the perspective of potential research participants within the community.[6] However, while having a community member on an REB may help secure some protections for research participants, it is well known that such members do not accurately represent those likely to be recruited into research overseen by the REB (Lawrence & Stewart, 2016; Cheah et al., 2010; Carroll-Scott, 2020). Community members on REBs tend to be White, highly educated, and, primarily, cis-gendered women, chosen primarily because they are not researchers and because they are not employed by the research institution (Solomon-Cargill, 2018; Anderson, 2006). This lack of representation of actual participants is likely in part due to the way recruitment of such members takes

[6] Although the reasons for the inclusion of community members on REBs is not always well understood or articulated; see (Solomon-Cargill, 2016) for a detailed examination of this concern in the US context.

place. For example, when Stephanie Solomon Cargill examined recruitment processes for community members (known as non-scientist/ non-affiliated members) on IRBs in the US, they described "a 'process' that was based on convenience and social connections" (Solomon-Cargill, 2018, 90). In this volume Solomon Cargill's chapter, "Stakeholder Engagement and (the Limits of) IRB Review," elaborates on the limitations of the structure of IRB/REB review in community-engaged research. Relying solely on the inclusion of a community member or two on REBs replicates worrisome assumptions related to identities and representation. Even though these community members may be part of the "community" outside the institution, they may represent a very singular and privileged perspective and may be unable to see relevant ethical concerns raised by research protocols from their social location.[7] As a result, they may fail to prioritize the concerns of the most marginalized within a given community, allowing research harms to occur at both the individual and collective levels.

Even in the context of community research governance with Indigenous communities, identity-based conceptions of community boundaries and community representation are often insufficient to justify the demands put forward by Indigenous communities for authority in research ethics governance. The portrayal of Indigenous Peoples as paradigmatic communities recognized through a singular racial identity is a normalized practice within institutional discourses, despite the fact that many Indigenous scholars fundamentally challenge this concept. In *Red Skins White Masks*, Glen Coulthard (2014) argues that 'Indigenous' as a formal identity is itself a colonial concept, constructed and recognized through dominant conceptions of history, laws, and policies to facilitate the subjugation of Indigenous Peoples by the colonial nation-state. This is echoed by Kim Tallbear in *Native American DNA* (2013, 10), who stresses the increasing influence of Western DNA science in defining understandings of race and Indigenous identity; these discourses complicate debates on Indigenous citizenship, as genetically defined 'race' often contradicts Indigenous historical-legal conceptions of community identity. This critique is particularly relevant in terms of understanding how policies like the TCPS structure the processes through which urban Indigenous Peoples or non-status Indigenous Peoples are considered (or, rather, excluded) in research ethics governance, as they lack the appropriate 'identity' recognized formally by the Canadian government. In contrast, some Indigenous residents of the Vancouver DTES feel that their right to sovereignty is stronger in the DTES than elsewhere in Canada, even on certain traditional territories, due to the high visibility of Indigenous cultural practice and claims to Indigenous territory in the DTES community (Masuda et al., 2020, 242). Therefore, questioning how community boundaries and community identity come to be officially recognized, and importantly, who has the power to recognize them, is integral to discussions of representation in community research ethics governance.

[7] Despite this privilege, it's worth pointing out that many community members on REBs experience role confusion and struggle to contribute meaningfully to committee discussions, instead focusing primarily on revising consent forms (see Solomon-Cargill, 2016; Lidz et al., 2012; Klitzman, 2012).

Representation also remains a challenge for community-based strategies for research ethics oversight. This is especially a concern for strategies such as community REBs with standardized mandates, review protocols, and criteria for membership akin to the bureaucratic structures of institutional REBs and ethical review (Watkins et al., 2009; Martin del Campo et al., 2013; Pratt et al., 2015; Carroll-Scott, 2020). In certain contexts, the representation of a given community may be further limited due to the political dynamics of a given region (e.g., fewer women or an ethnic group on a community advisory board), or due to the limited authority and independence of a community group from a research institution (Pratt et al., 2015; Cheah et al., 2010; Morina et al., 2008). As these community-led strategies are a significant investment of time and are, often, unpaid labour, the social conditions and everyday context of life in a given community may not be conducive for the adequate participation of all community members. However, as the case studies show, in transferring a degree of power and authority to place-based communities in research governance, the diversity of identities and experiences within them can be better represented. Through mechanisms of place-based oversight, communities formalize their physical and symbolic boundaries in their own terms, and in turn, develop strategies more conducive to the inclusion of less privileged community members. Often, community REBs work to expand their community engagement by including a rotating cast of community members on the board (Johnson et al., 2009; Boilevin et al., 2019; Tremblay et al., 2018), mandating participatory components to projects (Blumenthal, 2006; Martin del Campo et al., 2013), and undertaking community outreach and education (Watkins et al., 2009; Martin del Campo et al., 2013; Morton et al., 2013). Documents such as community codes of ethics and research guidelines are also often co-authored by the community, and are created through participatory processes (e.g., series of accessible, weekly work sessions) that focus on the lived experience of research in said community (Boilevin et al., 2019; Jane-Finch Community Research Partnership, 2021). Overall, these strategies ensure that community-based oversight mechanisms consistently enforce an ethical standard for research projects, while remaining accountable to the community and its evolving needs and experiences.

Ethical standards can allow communities to convey community values to researchers, and importantly, are more legible to institutions like universities with bureaucratic research ethics governance mechanisms. The possibility of integrating community processes as a mandatory step within the institutional research ethics review process is of central concern to all communities discussed in this chapter. For communities with established research ethics review and governance structures, this may entail a referral process that will direct researchers to the community, and an institutional requirement for community approval on a given project. Formalizing referral thus recognizes community authority in research ethics governance, encouraging a more balanced distribution of decision-making power. This could encourage transformation in the research enterprise as a whole, towards better funding opportunities that prioritize community-based participatory research and the financing of community research ethics governance itself. However, despite the potential benefits of integrating community-based research ethics governance within institutions, there is little known about the interactions and relationships between community groups and institutional REBs. We know from our communications with the DTES CREW that they have met semi-regularly with REBs at UBC, Providence Healthcare, and SFU, from 2018 to 2019. Such institutions have shown support for Research 101 and its aspirations for community research ethics governance in the DTES, although no formal partnerships or referral processes have since been established (Neufeld, personal communication, 2022). Given this insight, research on the interactions between communities and institutional REBs is important from a practical standpoint, as this knowledge can guide communities seeking to develop their own research governance processes and establish partnerships with local universities. It is also important from a conceptual standpoint, as information on the roles and interactions of different stakeholders can elucidate problematic patterns of power that prevent communities from participating in research ethics governance, thus requiring intervention.

19.3.2 "Community Expertise" and the Epistemological Significance of Place

The case studies in this chapter present three primary justifications for community research oversight: historical and ongoing research harms in communities, the insufficiency of the current REB system, and the importance of community ethics expertise. As described, the Bronx, DTES, and PPZ each have ongoing histories of harmful research taking place in their communities, warranting community involvement in oversight. These research harms stem directly from limitations in the current REB system, which has failed to protect them while reviewing research protocols centered on their communities. In part, this is because REBs rarely consider the community-level risks posed by research protocols. In a Canada-wide assessment of 89 REB ethics review protocol forms for community-based participatory research projects, only 20% asked about risks and benefits to communities, while all asked about risks to individuals (Guta et al., 2010). Another study assessing 30 IRB/REB review forms for health research from the US and Canada similarly found that none asked about community involvement in identifying the rationale for the research project, while only 13% asked about risks and benefits on a community and societal level (Flicker et al., 2007). These findings point to the limitations of the broader ethical frameworks operationalized by REBs, namely, the hegemony of the biomedical framework that does not take into account the experience of community-based research, and assesses risk to individuals and institutions rather than communities (Flicker et al., 2007). Importantly, these frameworks conceptualize risk from a particular point of view that, as pointed out in the DTES *Manifesto*, "makes more sense to middle or upper class, white, settler folks" than to community members (Boilevin et al., 2019, 13). Considering that the foundational documents guiding contemporary research ethics review processes were largely influenced by Western moral theories, which were developed by primarily White, male philosophers from a different time and place, it is imperative to question whether and how such documents are applicable to research with communities experiencing marginalization today.

Indigenous scholars and community experts have long criticized the use of Western frameworks when researching with Indigenous communities, as they institutionalize a colonial worldview that overlooks Indigenous sovereignty and community-level concerns (Smith, 1999). As colonialism is deeply connected with, and inextricable from, heteropatriarchy, white supremacy, and other socio-political structures of power, the uncritical use of such frameworks can also be harmful to many non-Indigenous communities experiencing marginalization. As articulated in the DTES *Manifesto*: "Research has long functioned as a tool of colonialism, and colonial research practices continue in the ways that researchers exploit, exhaust, and extract from Indigenous and other marginalized communities" (Boilevin et al., 2019, 3). Echoed elsewhere, the assumption of a universal set of ethical principles is argued to "advance narrow beliefs about who and what needs protection," wherein such narrow conceptualizations of ethics are "intended to veil scientific research's complicity in sustaining White supremacy, heteropatriarchy, racism, and settler colonialism" (Tuck & Guishard, 2013, 10). Community oversight can thus be seen as intervening on these narrow beliefs, taking into consideration the community context, values, and goals, as well as the broader relations of power that exist between the researcher, institution, and community. This stance suggests that, rather than a universal code of ethics, communities have unique expertise that they bring to research governance. As the Manifesto says:

> *You might be an expert on some things but you're not the expert on our lives or our community no matter how many years you've spent studying "addiction", "homelessness", "sex work" or anything else. Don't read us the book we wrote.* (Boilevin et al., 2019, 16)

Feminist standpoint theory is useful in explaining such claims to community expertise. Standpoint feminism contends that all knowledge is achieved from a social standpoint, limited by the experience of our social locations ordered within broader structures of power. These experiences shape our social, political, and moral beliefs, which then form the background assumptions and aims operating within scientific projects (Harding, 1995). Those belonging to social groups who are oppressed and who have engaged in critical reflection related to knowledge production are more likely to identify and have insight into such implicit beliefs and dynamics of oppression because of their familiarity with how such structures of power operate within knowledge production. In other words, in a given research context, some standpoints may have an "epistemic advantage" over others in recognizing "how reliable particular kinds of knowledge are likely to be given the social conditions of their production" (Wylie, 2003, 30). Furthermore, members of oppressed groups are required to be knowledgeable with regard to both their own experiences and the experiences of privileged groups in order to survive under societal power structures (Wylie, 2003, 32). Essentially, one's membership in an oppressed community does not automatically result in a standpoint; rather, critical consciousness of how dynamics of oppression influence epistemic production is required (Intemann, 2010).

The communities presented in this chapter have direct experience of marginalization and harmful research. For those community members who have engaged in critical reflection about knowledge production, this lived experience provides them with an epistemic advantage regarding problematic background assumptions and individual- and community-level risks that may exist within research projects. This is especially the case for place-based communities, given their diversity. Such diversity of individual experiences can provide access to different kinds of evidence; as a collective, communities can compare their experiences and identify patterns of oppression that account for those who are most marginalized within the community. Thus, place-based communities may be especially capable when it comes to recognizing how power structures shape knowledge production and research ethics governance. Specifically, communities may be able to identify the social, political, and moral beliefs behind background assumptions in research protocols as it pertains to them. Communities may also contribute to enhancing the scientific validity of research projects by ensuring that research methods are culturally appropriate and account for the contextual factors that may influence the data collection process. In the theoretical literature, it is suggested that the critical consciousness necessary to achieve a standpoint is a place-based process (Freire, 2000; Johnson, 2010). Critical consciousness involves recognizing the situated nature of knowledge and how it is shaped by our environments and everyday "taskscapes," defined as the places and environments in which we live and work (Johnson, 2010). In light of our examples, communities connected through a shared history and experience of place also share a knowledge grounded in a common environment; this, along with critical reflection, provides members of such communities with the ethical expertise to know and do what is best for community well-being. The communities developing place-based strategies of research ethics oversight presented in this chapter have moral authority over the governance of research that pertains to them, grounded in their unique ethical standpoints.

Through participating in community-led research ethics governance, researchers and REB members are better prepared to achieve the understanding and insights accessible to those who have achieved a standpoint. For example, the BxCRRB invites researchers to join the review discussion and mandates research partnerships throughout the lifespan of the project. This allows researchers to not only consider community recommendations within the scope of the project but to take part in this process along with community members and apply insights to future research. Researchers developing a self-reflexive practice is a key epistemic requirement for ethical research in many communities, and documents like the DTES *Manifesto* encourage this by asking researchers: "Who are you? Where are you from, what's your story, what's your connection to this land? What are the types of social privilege (e.g. White? Male? Settler? Cis-gendered? etc.) you experience and how might those limit your ability to think and act ethically in your research?" (Boilevin et al., 2019, 11). Similarly, committees such as the PZRC require researchers to develop a self-reflexive and participatory practice that encourages examining proposed research projects through the standpoint of the Philadelphia Promise Zone community members. By formalizing such discussions of social location and power in research ethics oversight, community-led strategies attune universal ethical principles with context-specific community diversity (see Chap. 6, in this volume).[8] This approach can recognize a wider range of ethical considerations relevant for a given context and facilitate the inclusion of ethical values coming from different perspectives in the knowledge production process (Longino, 1994).

19.4 Conclusion

While we often imagine communities as formed through a shared identity related to race, gender, or religion, community initiatives related to research governance illuminate the important role that place plays in forming communities consisting of many diverse, intersectional identities. Such initiatives are being developed in the Bronx, the DTES of Vancouver, and the Philadelphia Promise Zone, all of which share ongoing histories of exploitative and extractive research which existing structures of research oversight have failed to prevent. As such, these communities are demanding authority in the governance of research taking place in their communities and developing novel forms of place-based research ethics oversight to claim such authority. Place-based communities sidestep simplistic notions of identity based on single shared features and make space for intersectional analyses and diverse community viewpoints to be taken into account. Such communities, as we have shown, have a unique claim to expertise given their shared experience of place, which, through critical consciousness, grants them the ability to see problematic assumptions embedded in scientific projects as well as potential community-level risks within research. Despite this experience, currently marginalized communities are excluded from current research ethics oversight processes. This exclusion demands critical examination and a way forward to facilitate the integration of place-based community oversight strategies within research ethics governance. Importantly, this integration will require revisiting assumptions of universality embedded in institutional research ethics review to make space for community diversity and place-based knowledge.

[8] A paper by Msoroka and Amundsen (2018) presents two case studies of community-based, emancipatory research projects, one in a Tanzanian prison, and the other with Maori communities in New Zealand. Both of these case studies showcase researchers and communities attuning universal ethical principles to the cultural context in which the ethical deliberation is taking place. The authors conclude that this hybrid approach "preserves the tension and insights of both universalism and relativism to proactively empower emancipatory research" (14).

Acknowledgements We would like to acknowledge and thank Scott Neufeld of Brock University for his guidance on the *Research 101: A Manifesto for Ethical Research in the Vancouver Downtown Eastside* section of this chapter.

Statement of Funding The Community Research Governance Project is funded by the Social Sciences Research Council of Canada (SSHRC, grant # 430-2020-00327). We would like to state that this book chapter was made possible through the funding for this larger project.

References

Aboriginal Health Research Review Committee & Manitoulin First Nations. (2003). *Guidelines for Ethical Aboriginal Research: A resource manual for the development of ethical and culturally appropriate community-based research within the First Nations communities in the Manitoulin area*. Noojmowin Teg Health Centre. Retrieved from: https://www.noojmowin-teg.ca/programs-services/manitoulin-anishinabek-research-review-committee

Albert Einstein College of Medicine. (2012). *Community IRBs and research review boards: Shaping the future of community-engaged research*. The Bronx Health Link and Community-Campus Partnerships for Health. Retrieved from: https://ccphealth.org/community-irbs-research-review-boards-shaping-the-future-of-community-engaged-research/

Anderson, E. E. (2006). A qualitative study of non-affiliated, non-scientist institutional review board members. *Accountability in Research, 13*, 135–155.

Australian Institute of Aboriginal and Torres Strait Islander Studies. (2020). *AIATSIS code of ethics for Aboriginal and Torres Strait Islander research*. Retrieved from: https://aiatsis.gov.au/sites/default/files/2020-10/aiatsis-code-ethics.pdf

Bauer, G., Devor, A., Heinz, M., Marshall, Z., Sansfaçon, A. P., & Pyne, J. (2019). *CPATH ethical guidelines for research involving transgender people & communities*. Canadian Professional Association for Transgender Health. Retrieved from: http://cpath.ca/en/resources/

Blumenthal, D. S. (2006). A community coalition board creates a set of values for community-based research. *Preventing Chronic Disease, 3*(1), A16. PMID: 16356369.

Boilevin, L., Chapman, J., Deane, L., Doerksen, C., Fresz, G., Joe, D. J., Leech-Crier, N., Marsh, S., McLeod, J., Neufeld, S., Pham, S., Shaver, L., Smith, P., Steward, M., Wilson, D., & Winter, P. (2019). *Research 101: A manifesto for ethical research in the downtown eastside*. University of British Columbia Open Collections. Retrieved from: http://hdl.handle.net/2429/69264

Brunger, F., & Bull, J. (2011). Whose agenda is it? Regulating health research ethics in Labrador. *Études Inuit Studies, 35*(1–2), 127–142.

Bull, J. (2016). In W. C. Van den Hoonaard & A. Hamilton (Eds.), *The ethics rupture: Exploring alternatives to formal research ethics review* (pp. 167–186). University of Toronto Press.

Bull, J., & Hudson, A. (2019). Research governance in NunatuKavut: Engagement, expectations and evolution. *International Journal of Circumpolar Health, 78*(2), 1556558. https://doi.org/10.1080/22423982.2018.1556558

Bull, J., Beazley, K., Shea, J., MacQuarrie, C., Hudson, A., Shaw, K., et al. (2019). Shifting practise: Recognizing indigenous rights holders in research ethics review. *Qualitative Research in Organizations and Management: An International Journal, 15*(1), 21–35.

Campbell, T. D. (2014). A clash of paradigms? Western and indigenous views on health research involving aboriginal peoples. *Nurse Researcher, 21*(6), 39–43.

Carroll-Scott, A. (2020). Importance of a place-based and community-moderated system of research oversight to maximize benefits for social change. *Social Innovations Journal, 2*(2), 1–18.

Carroll-Scott, A., Kolker, J., Confair, A., Moore, K., Melly, S., & Joshi, R. (2017). *Community health profile: West Philadelphia Promise Zone*. Urban Health Collaborative Community Brief. Dornsife School of Public Health, Drexel University. Retrieved from: https://drexel.edu/uhc/resources/briefs/West-Philadelphia-Promise-Zone/

Casado, J. (2013). Ethical engagement of communities, institutions, and providers in research: Lessons from the community. *Progress in Community Health Partnerships: Research, Education, and Action, 7*(3), 353–355.

Cheah, P. Y., Lwin, K. M., Phaiphun, L., Maelankiri, L., Parker, M., Day, N. P., et al. (2010). Community engagement on the Thai-Burmese border: Rationale, experience and lessons learnt. *International Health, 2*(2), 123–129.

Cherokee Nation. *Helicopter research*. Retrieved from: https://irb.cherokee.org/media/rkknqeww/helicopter-research.pdf

Collins, P. H. (1990). Black feminist thought in the matrix of domination. In *Black feminist thought: Knowledge, consciousness, and the politics of empowerment* (pp. 221–238). Unwin Hyman.

Coulthard, G. S. (2014). Introduction: Subjects of empire. In G. S. Coulthard (Ed.), *Red skin white masks: Rejecting the colonial politics of recognition* (pp. 1–24). University of Minnesota Press.

Crenshaw, K. (1991). Mapping the margins: Intersectionality, identity politics, and violence against women of color. *Stanford Law Review, 43*(6), 1241–1299.

Dangerfield, K. (2018, May 11). Canada subjected indigenous people to 'cruel' medical experiments, lawsuit claims. *Global News Canada*. Retrieved from: https://globalnews.ca/news/4202373/indigenous-people-medical-experiments-canada-class-action-lawsuit/

Damon, W., Callon, C., Wiebe, L., Small, W., Kerr, T., & McNeil, R. (2017). Community-based participatory research in a heavily researched inner-city neighbourhood: Perspectives of people who use drugs on their experiences as peer researchers. *Social Science & Medicine, 176*, 85–92.

Flicker, S., Travers, R., Guta, A., McDonald, S., & Meagher, A. (2007). Ethical dilemmas in community-based participatory research: Recommendations for institutional review boards. *Journal of Urban Health, 84*(4), 478–493.

Freire, P. (2000). *Pedagogy of the oppressed* (30th anniversary ed.). Continuum.

Friesen, P., Kearns, L., Redman, B. K., & Caplan, L. C. (2017). Extending ethical strides: From tribal IRBs to the Bronx community research review board. *The American Journal of Bioethics, 17*(11), W5–W8.

Friesen, P., Doerksen, E., & Gunay, A. (2021). Solidarity without sovereignty: Extending the Belmont principles further? *The American Journal of Bioethics, 21*(10), 25–27.

Galea, S., Factor, S., Bonner, S., Freudenberg, N., Latka, M., Palermo, A., & Vlahov, D. (2001). Collaboration among community members, local health service providers, and researchers in an urban research center in Harlem, New York. *Public Health Reports, 116*, 530–539.

Guishard, M. A., Heyward, D. A., Brown, J. T., & Stoddard-Pennant, M. (2021). What we not finna do: Respectfully collaborating with skinfolk and kinfolk in black participatory action research. *Global Journal of Community Psychology Practice, 12*(2), 1–35.

Guta, A., Wilson, M. G., Flicker, S., Travers, R., Mason, C., Wenyeve, G., & O'Campo, P. (2010). Are we asking the right questions? A review of Canadian REB practices in relation to community-based participatory research. *Journal of Empirical Research on Human Research Ethics, 5*(2), 35–46.

Harding, S. (1995). "Strong objectivity": A response to the new objectivity question. *Synthese, 104*(3), 331–349.

Hayward, A., Sjoblom, E., Sinclair, S., & Cidro, J. (2021). A new era of indigenous research: Community-based indigenous research ethics protocols in Canada. *Journal of Empirical Research on Human Research Ethics, 16*(4), 403–417. https://doi.org/10.1177/15562646211023705

Heyes, C. (2002). Identity politics. In E. N. Zalta (Ed.), *The Stanford encyclopedia of philosophy* (Fall 2020 ed.). Retrieved from: https://plato.stanford.edu/archives/fall2020/entries/identity-politics

Hsieh, J., Chang, E. Y. T., & Lakaw, S. (2019). From collective consent to consultation platform: An experience of indigenous research ethics in Makota'ay. *Junctures, 2019*(20), 71–86.

Hudson, M., Milne, M., Reynolds, P., Russell, K., & Smith, B. (2010) *Te Ara Tika. Guidelines for Māori research ethics: A framework for researchers and ethics committee members*. Retrieved from: https://www.hrc.govt.nz/resources/te-ara-tika-guidelines-maori-research-ethics

Intemann, K. (2010). 25 years of feminist empiricism and standpoint theory: Where are we now? *Hypatia, 25*(4), 778–796.

Johnson, T. J. (2010). Place-based learning and knowing: Critical pedagogies grounded in indigeneity. *GeoJournal, 77*, 829–836.

Johnson, J. C., Hayden, U. T., Thomas, N., Groce-Martin, J., Henry, T., Guerra, T., Walker, A., West, W., Barnett, M., & Kumanyika, S. (2009). Building community participatory research coalitions from the ground up: The Philadelphia area research community coalition. *Progress in Community Health Partnerships, 3*(1), 61–72.

Jürgens, R. (2005). *"Nothing about us without us" – Greater, meaningful involvement of people who use illegal drugs: A public health, ethical, and human rights imperative*. Canadian HIV/AIDS Legal Network.

Kahnawake Schools Diabetes Prevention Project. (2007). *Code of research ethics*. Retrieved from: http://qimnp.com/wp-content/uploads/2018/04/Appendix-A-ksdpp_code_of_research_ethics2007.pdf

Kaplan, S. A., Calman, N. S., Golub, M., Davis, J. H., Ruddock, C., & Billings, J. (2006). Racial and ethnic disparities in health: A view from the South Bronx. *Journal of Health Care for the Poor and Underserved, 17*(1), 116–127.

Klitzman, R. (2012). Institutional review board community members: Who are they, what do they do, and whom do they represent? *Academic Medicine: Journal of the Association of American Medical Colleges, 87*(7), 975.

Ktunaxa/Kinbasket Tribal Council. (1998). *Ktunaxa Nation's code of ethics for research*. Indigenous Child Well-being Research Network. Retrieved from: https://icwrn.uvic.ca/ethics/

Lawrence, C., & Stewart, K. (2016). The challenge of community representation: Lessons from six HIV clinical research community advisory boards in Uganda. *Journal of Empirical Research on Human Research Ethics, 11*(4), 311–321.

Levenson, D. (2010). After Havasupai litigation, native Americans wary of genetic research. *American Journal of Medical Genetics, 152A*(Part A), IX.

Lidz, C. W., Lorna, J. S., Antonia, V. S., Suzanne, M., William, G., Philip, J. C., Robert, A., & Paul, S. A. (2012). The participation of community members on medical institutional review boards. *Journal of Empirical Research on Human Research Ethics, 7*(1), 1–8.

Longino, H. E. (1994). In search of feminist epistemology. *The Monist, 77*(4), 472–485.

Macdonald, N. E., Stanwick, R., & Lynk, A. (2014). Canada's shameful history of nutrition research on residential school children: The need for strong medical ethics in aboriginal health research. *Paediatrics & Child Health, 19*(2), 64.

Martin del Campo, F., Casado, J., Spencer, P., & Strelnick, H. (2013). The development of the Bronx Community Research Review Board: A pilot feasibility project for a model of community consultation. *Progress in Community Health Partnerships: Research, Education, and Action, 7*(3), 341–352.

Mashford-Pringle, A., & Pavagadhi, K. (2020). Using OCAP and IQ as frameworks to address a history of trauma in indigenous health research. *AMA Journal of Ethics, 22*(10), E868–E873.

Masuda, J. R., Franks, A., Kobayashi, A., & Wideman, T. (2020). After dispossession: An urban rights praxis of remaining in Vancouver's Downtown Eastside. *Environment and Planning D: Society and Space, 38*(2), 229–247.

Morton, D. J., Proudfit, J., Calac, D., Portillo, M., Lofton-Fitzsimmons, G., Molina, T., Flores, R., Lawson-Risso, B., & Majel-McCauley, R. (2013). Creating research capacity through a tribally based institutional review board. *American Journal of Public Health, 103*(12), 2160–2164.

Mosby, I. (2013). Administering colonial science: Nutrition research and human biomedical experimentation in aboriginal communities and residential schools, 1942–1952. *Histoiresociale/Social History, 46*(1), 145–172. https://doi.org/10.1353/his.2013.0015

Msoroka, M. S., & Amundsen, D. (2018). One size fits not quite all: Universal research ethics with diversity. *Research Ethics, 14*(3), 1–17.

Neufeld, S. D. (2019). *Manifesto endorsement form: Support the research 101 manifesto!* [Google form]. Retrieved from: https://docs.google.com/forms/d/1bRMlpbKID7SzORYnKsG8T2JkVjpoTzLfIrmsBeK9dm4/viewform?edit_requested=true

Neufeld, S. D., Chapman, J., Crier, N., Marsh, S., McLeod, J., & Deane, L. A. (2019). Research 101: A process for developing local guidelines for ethical research in heavily researched communities. *Harm Reduction Journal, 16*, 41.

Newham, J. (2005). *An overview of Vancouver's downtown eastside for UBC learning exchange trek program participants*. UBC Learning Exchange.

Pratt, B., Lwin, K. M., Zion, D., Nosten, F., Loff, B., & Cheah, P. Y. (2015). Exploitation and community engagement: Can community advisory boards successfully assume a role minimising exploitation in international research? *Developing World Bioethics, 15*(1), 18–26.

Quigley, D. (2006). A Review of Improved Ethical Practices in Environmental and Public Health Research: Case Examples From Native Communities. *Health Education & Behavior, 33*(2), 130–147. http://www.jstor.org/stable/45055734

Quinn, S. C. (2004). Protecting human subjects: The role of community advisory boards. *American Journal of Public Health, 94*(6), 918–922.

Riddell, J. K., Salamanca, A., Pepler, D. J., Cardinal, S., & McIvor, O. (2017). Laying the groundwork: A practical guide for ethical research with indigenous communities. *International Indigenous Policy Journal, 8*(2). https://doi.org/10.18584/iipj.2017.8.2.6

Schatz, D. (2010). *Unsettling the politics of exclusion: Aboriginal activism and the Vancouver downtown east side.* Annual meeting of the Canadian Political Science Association (2010), session M10(b) beyond statistics: Urban indigenous politics.

Schnarch, B. (2004). Ownership, control, access, and possession (OCAP) or self-determination applied to research: A critical analysis of contemporary first nations research and some options for first nations communities. *Journal of Aboriginal Health, 1*(1), 80–94.

Schroeder, D., Chatfield, K., Singh, M., Chennells, R., & Herissone-Kelly, P. (2019). The san code of research ethics. In *Equitable research partnerships* (SpringerBriefs in research and innovation governance). Springer. https://doi.org/10.1007/978-3-030-15745-6_7

Shore, N., Drew, E., Brazauskas, R., & Seifer, S. D. (2011a). Relationships between community-based processes for research ethics review and institution-based irbs: A national study. *Journal of Empirical Research on Human Research Ethics, 6*(2), 13–21.

Shore, N. P., Brazauskas, R. P., Drew, E. P., Wong, K. A., Moy, L., Baden, A. C., et al. (2011b). Understanding community-based processes for research ethics review: A national study. *American Journal of Public Health, 101*(S1), S359–S364.

Shore, N., Park, A., Castro, P., Wat, E., Sablan-Santos, L., Isaacs, M. L., Freeman, E., Cooks, J. M., Drew, E., & Seifer, S. D. (2014). *Redefining research ethics review: Case studies of five community-led models*. Community-Campus Partnerships for Health.

Smith, L. T. (1999). *Decolonizing methodologies: Research and indigenous peoples*. Zed Books.

Solomon-Cargill, S. (2016). Too many rationales, not enough reason: A call to examine the goals of including lay members on institutional review boards. *Accountability in Research, 23*(1), 4–22.

Solomon-Cargill, S. (2018). What can IRBs learn from CABs? A qualitative analysis of the experiences of recruitment and training of nonscientist members on research review boards. *Journal of Empirical Research on Human Research Ethics, 13*(1), 88–94.

Sterling, R. L. (2011). Genetic research among the Havasupai – A cautionary tale. *Virtual Mentor, 13*(2), 113–117. https://doi.org/10.1001/virtualmentor.2011.13.2.hlaw1-1102

Tallbear, K. (2013). An indigenous Feminist approach to DNA politics. In *Native American DNA: Tribal belonging and the false promise of genetic science*. University of Minnesota Press.

The NAOMI Patients Association, & Boyd, S. (2012). *NAOMI research survivors: Experiences and recommendations*. Retrieved from: https://drugpolicy.ca/wp-content/uploads/2012/03/NPAreportMarch5-12.pdf

The West Philadelphia Promise Zone. (2018). *The Promise Zone research connection takes first place!* Retrieved from: http://www.sharedprosperityphila.org/promise_zone_blog/the-promise-zone-research-connection-takes-first-place/

Tremblay, M., Martin, D. H., McComber, A. M., McGregor, A., & Macaulay, A. C. (2018). Understanding community-based participatory research through a social movement framework: A case study of the Kahnawake schools diabetes prevention project. *BMC Public Health, 18*(487), 1–17.

Tuck, E., & Guishard, M. (2013). Uncollapsing ethics: Racialized scientism, settler coloniality, and an ethical framework of decolonial participatory action research. In *Challenging status quo retrenchment: New directions in critical research.* (Chapter 1). Information Age Publishing.

Turpel-Lafond, M. E. (2020). *In plain sight: Addressing indigenous-specific racism and discrimination in B.C. health care.* Government of British Columbia.

U.S Department of Health & Human Services. (2017). *Federalwide assurance instructions.* Retrieved from: https://www.hhs.gov/ohrp/register-irbs-and-obtain-fwas/forms/fwa-instructions/index.html

United Nations. (2007). United Nations Declaration on the Rights of Indigenous Peoples. Retrieved from: https://www.ohchr.org/en/indigenous-peoples/un-declaration-rights-indigenous-peoples

Watkins, B. X., Shepard, P. M., & Corbin-Mark, C. D. (2009). Completing the circle: A model for effective community review of environmental health research. *American Journal of Public Health, 99*(Suppl 3), S567–S577. https://doi.org/10.2105/AJPH.2008.149369

Wylie, A. (2003). Why standpoint matters. In R. Figueroa & S. G. Harding (Eds.), *Science and other cultures: Issues in philosophies of science and technology* (pp. 26–48). Routledge.

Alize E. Gunay is a Turkish, first-generation immigrant settler currently living in Tiohtià:ke (Montreal), on the unceded territories of the Kanien'kehá:ka Nation. Her experiences as a member of Turkish and Muslim im/migrant communities in the Middle East and Canada shape her perspective on the topic of community research ethics oversight. As a Master's student in the Department of Family Medicine and Bioethics at McGill, her research interests center on power as it pertains to health equity, and her theoretical focus includes social constructivist, interpretivist, and intersectional feminist theoretical paradigms that recognize the situated and political nature of knowledge production.

Phoebe Friesen is a Caucasian (Ukrainian, Dutch, and Scottish) settler, raised by hippies on the unceded Coast Salish territories of Vancouver Island. She now lives in Tiohtià:ke (or Montreal) on unceded territories of the Kanien'kehá:ka Nation. Phoebe is a cis, White, able-bodied woman and this social location inevitably informs her work and her way of being in the world. As an Assistant Professor in Biomedical Ethics and Social Studies of Medicine, she is always grappling with what it means to hold such a position and how she might produce scholarship that is worthwhile and impactful.

Emily M. A. Doerksen is a White settler currently living in Tiohtià:ke (Montreal). She grew up among the Rocky Mountains and on the traditional territories of the Blackfoot Confederacy, the Tsuut'ina First Nation, the Stoney Nakoda, and the Region 3Métis Nation of Alberta. She is a cis, able-bodied, and neurotypical woman with a background in philosophy currently working towards a Masters in Human Genetics and Bioethics at McGill University. Her research interests are informed by feminist and intersectional theory. These theoretical approaches were fostered during her time in the humanities, where she first came to question academic epistemology. As a member of the academic institution, she tries to maintain a healthy degree of criticism and self-awareness as she confronts the pedagogy of her discipline and her own approach to knowledge production.

Chapter 20
Introducing the Downtown Eastside Community Research Ethics Workshop: Notes on a Process for Community Ethics Review

Scott D. Neufeld, Jule Chapman, Nicolas D. Leech-Crier, Samona Marsh, and Jim McLeod

Almost all university-based research with human subjects must receive ethical approval before researchers can begin data collection. While university research ethics boards (REBs[1]) play an important role in making researchers consider and address the ethical issues raised by their research, they are not a guarantee of ethical research, at least by community standards. REBs are not equipped to keep researchers accountable to actually follow their proposed research protocols, REB members may not have much experience evaluating ethical issues in community-based (as opposed to laboratory) settings, and the ethical codes REBs use to guide their evaluations typically prioritize ethical care for individual research participants over ethical care for communities or social groups. They also might be using ideas of "risk" that make more sense to middle or upper class, white, settler folks than they do to community members (Tuck & Guishard, 2013). Ultimately, we recog-

[1] Research Ethics Board (REBs) is the term used most often in Canada and internationally whereas "Institutional Review Board" (IRB) is the term used in the United States. Since we write from a Canadian context we will use the term "REB" throughout.

S. D. Neufeld (✉)
Psychology Department, Brock University, St. Catherines, ON, Canada
e-mail: sneufeld@brocku.ca

J. Chapman · S. Marsh
Sex Workers United Against Violence (SWUAV), Vancouver, BC, Canada

N. D. Leech-Crier
Transformative Health & Justice Research Cluster, University of British Columbia, British Columbia Mental Health and Substance Use Services, PHS Community Services Society/ Vancouver Coastal Health Mobile Overdose Prevention Unit, Megaphone Magazine, Vancouver, BC, Canada

J. McLeod
Hives for Humanity, Vancouver, BC, Canada

E. E. Anderson (ed.), *Ethical Issues in Community and Patient Stakeholder–Engaged Health Research*, Philosophy and Medicine 146,
https://doi.org/10.1007/978-3-031-40379-8_20

nize that different people can have very different understandings of what "ethical" means. The ethical concerns of university REB members may not be the same as the ethical concerns of community members.

Excerpt from a section titled "Ethical Review: Whose Ethics?" in "Research 101: A Manifesto for Ethical Research in the Downtown Eastside" (Boilevin et al., 2018, 6–7).

We are a group of community members, drug policy activists, storytellers, poets, beekeepers, trauma survivors, and experts of lived experience and academic scholarship. In this chapter, we want to share our process of working together in Vancouver's Downtown Eastside (DTES) neighborhood to develop what we call a "community ethics" for research. As outlined in the quote above from our co-authored *Manifesto for Ethical Research in the Downtown Eastside* (Boilevin et al., 2018), how members of a community understand key components of "research ethics" may sometimes differ from how formal ethics policies and institutional Research Ethics Boards (REBs) understand or apply ethics concepts. We built on our experiences creating a set of community guidelines for "ethical" research (the *Manifesto*) and piloted a form of community ethics review in the DTES that we came to refer to as the "Community Research Ethics Workshop" or CREW. In this chapter, we share our experiences with this process of "community ethics review."

20.1 Research in the DTES and Our Experiences with "Research 101"

In our experience, there are too many stories of DTES communities and individuals who have felt misrepresented, exploited, disrespected, or exhausted by research. There is a very large volume of research and researchers in the DTES at any given time (see Linden et al., 2013; McKay, 2021). This community is often described by those of us who live here as one of the most heavily-researched communities in the world and a place that has been "researched to death" (see Culhane, 2011; Damon et al., 2017; Goodman et al., 2018).

Together, over the past four years, we have had many discussions about the role and impact of "research" in Vancouver's DTES. We have co-authored a *Manifesto* (Boilevin et al., 2018), published an academic paper together (Neufeld et al., 2019), taken road trips to conferences (see Neufeld & Leech-Crier, 2020), and co-presented our work in countless community organizations, graduate research methods classes, and other university spaces. The start of our work together was in the lead-up to a series of workshops called "Research 101" (Spring 2018) held in the DTES and hosted by an organization called "Hives for Humanity." There were many different issues raised. Some of us wanted to get more involved and learn more about how research was being conducted in our neighborhood and what it was being used for. There is little to no safety net and little accountability, or even tracking of research conducted in DTES with marginalized people who also continue to face an ongoing health crisis, housing crisis, and extensive stigmatization.

After the series of Research 101 workshops, the five of us continued meeting to discuss how we can be part of positive changes and put "peers" (i.e., community members, people with lived experience) in positions that historically have only been held by academics (e.g., ethics reviewers). Over several months of meetings and collaborations with different organizations and individuals, many of whom were familiar with or have worked or lived in the DTES, the five of us developed our understanding of how much research has affected our community, our friends, and even ourselves. Given the sheer volume of research being conducted, we felt it necessary to continue our work as a means of promoting community safety and working in solidarity with neighbors and colleagues across the DTES. We all face the constant frustration of having to deal with outside researchers and then often feeling misrepresented or exploited by research. Since developing, releasing, and sharing our *Manifesto* (Boilevin et al., 2018) widely, we have continued our work by exploring what a process for "community ethics review" could look like in the DTES.

20.2 What Is a Community Ethics Review Process and Why Is It Important?

As many before us have pointed out, institutional REB review processes routinely underemphasize ethical issues that communities like the DTES consider to be very important. Examples include not appropriately considering how research can stigmatize groups (e.g., "damage-centered" research, see Tuck, 2009), inadequate knowledge of community norms and practices of respect and care, and not being mindful of sensitive histories of research harms in a community (see Anderson et al., 2012; Bungay et al., 2022; Flicker et al., 2007; Tuck & Guishard, 2013). While many REBs are required to include a "community member" who is neither affiliated with the institution nor a "scientist," these individuals are hardly a stand-in for direct representation of the many diverse communities impacted by over-research or harmful histories of research abuse. "Community members" on REBs may not be academics but they are frequently recruited through academic social networks, often highly educated, and mostly from dominant groups (e.g., cis, white, male, able-bodied), enabling them to navigate the academic space of an REB with ease (Anderson, 2006; see Chaps. 18 and 19, in this volume). Even still, "community members" on REBs report a lack of clarity in their roles and challenges intervening their outsider perspective into academic discourse surrounding research ethics review (Anderson, 2006; Klitzman, 2012; Solomon, 2016; Solomon-Cargill, 2018).

Rather than attempting to reform institutional REBs to better reflect community concerns with research in the DTES, we (like many other communities before us) chose an alternative and complementary approach to ethics review of research proposals: community ethics review (e.g., del Campo et al., 2013; Guishard et al., 2021; Shore et al., 2011a, b; Solomon-Cargill, 2018). There is now a growing literature on community research ethics boards. Among the most useful is a U.S. study of institutional review boards (IRBs) based on a 2008 online survey of 109 community groups and community-institutional partnerships, including non-profit organizations, health centres, and tribal organizations (Shore et al., 2011a). The authors note that IRBs are designed to protect individual study participants, and therefore do not routinely assess issues of consent, risks, or benefits for groups and communities. When asked their reasons for conducting a research ethics review process of their own, the groups surveyed emphasized the need to ensure that the community directly benefits and is protected from risks, and that members are directly engaged at each stage of research. They also highlighted factors considered very important in reviewing research proposals such as ensuring that methods, recruitment strategies, communicating findings, and obtaining informed consent are appropriate to community needs, values, and histories.

In the DTES, we have piloted a process where members of the community in which the proposed research will take place are empowered to perform a kind of "ethics review." Community ethics reviewers are guided primarily by their personal knowledge of community norms of respectful practice, personal and community histories of interactions with outsider researchers, and their personal understandings of vulnerabilities, risks, and protocols for protecting the well-being of their fellow community members. By applying our lived experience and lens of what constitutes ethical and respectful practice in our community to an independent community ethics review process, community ethics reviewers may be able to identify ethical issues and suggest proposal revisions that institutional REB members may never consider, let alone understand how to integrate or implement in the research process itself.

20.3 Introducing the CREW

In the *Research 101 Manifesto* (Boilevin et al., 2018) we included a key recommendation that local universities and community organizations in the DTES support the development of a "Community Research Ethics Board" or CREB in the DTES. From our initial conversations about strategies for changing an extractive and exploitative culture of research in the DTES, we knew that simply creating and sharing a set of guidelines for more ethical and respectful research practice in the neighborhood would not be enough to compel researchers to take community requests for change seriously (see Neufeld et al., forthcoming, for a greater discussion of the limitations of the *Manifesto* as a community ethics strategy). The only way we could envision being able to more systematically empower members of the DTES community to have a say in deciding how research should proceed in the neighborhood was to assert community governance at the level of research ethics review. We aspire to work together in a spirit of genuine collaboration and peaceful negotiation. Community members provide an incredible amount of time and energy to the constant influx of researchers yet ultimately experience very little in the way of reciprocity, respect, or return for their sincerely concerted and conscientious efforts. Worse still, community members who engage with researchers are often virtually abandoned and ignored by those same "ethically approved" researchers; them now having surreptitiously acquired the necessary data collection, the prestigious academic journal publication credit, the PhD and the ticket to their upper-class futures, far removed from the "terror and tragedy" of the DTES.

Creating a CREB modelled after other successful examples such as the Bronx Community Research Review Board (see https://bxcrrb.org but also del Campo et al., 2013; Guishard, 2015; Guishard et al., 2021) seemed to us an effective way of moving beyond mere "hopes and dreams" for positive treatment shared with researchers through the *Manifesto* and towards a strategy with some "teeth" that might actually compel researchers to follow the guidance of DTES community members and hold researchers accountable. We envisioned a system, operating in a physically communal space we had ownership of, in which community ethics reviewers could gather, organize, and review outsider research proposals through the critical lenses of community-adapted TCPS2 training (standard research ethics training modules in Canada), community reviewers' personal lived experience, and a healthy suspicion of research and researchers in the DTES. Given the naturally cooperative impetus of the community itself, the system would also provide feedback and direction to researchers on how to adjust their proposals to reduce harm to participants, conform to community expectations of respectful treatment, and promote maximum benefits through research for the DTES.

In 2019, we applied for a small grant from Simon Fraser University's "Community Engagement Initiative" and received $5000 in funding for "Piloting a Community Research Ethics Board in the Downtown Eastside." Whereas university-based REBs apply formal ethics policy to their reviews of research proposals, we proposed that the CREB would train DTES community members to contribute their local expertise on what constitutes ethical and respectful engagement in their community to the proposed projects of student and faculty researchers from SFU and other local institutions. We hoped this grant would support ongoing capacity building within the DTES community to build towards a full-fledged CREB capable of reviewing research proposals from student/faculty researchers. This would include exploring existing models of CREBs in other locations, developing a web presence for the CREB, providing training for an initial cohort of DTES community members on how to review research proposals, and supporting honoraria payments for community members to review several voluntarily submitted research proposals related to the DTES.

With funding secured we set out to work together with a variety of community and academic partners to learn more about other successful models of community research ethics governance while also developing and piloting our own model. An important initial step was changing the name of the thing we were trying to develop from "CREB" to "CREW" or "Community Research Ethics Workshop." We made this change because a local "Clinical REB" had already taken the acronym CREB, we were unsure if we really wanted to develop a full-fledged "REB," and the term "workshop" better reflected how we saw this work as in process or under construction. We were a small and by no means representative group of community members and academics keenly aware that we do not and never will speak for the

"Downtown Eastside" in all its diversity. We did not want to convey that we felt we could simply declare ourselves an official REB working on behalf of an entire neighborhood.

We continued meeting as a group to further clarify our goals and mission as a "CREW" and co-wrote a mission statement to express how we understood the purpose of our work together (see Fig. 20.1).

The CREW humbly offers its services to researchers, as it has become apparent that the DTES is indeed a heavily-researched population with much vulnerability. Co-author Nick described our proposed process as developing a mechanism for the community-led examination and articulation of incoming academic research

The Downtown Eastside (DTES) "Community Research Ethics Workshop" (CREW) is a group made up of some of the co-authors of Research 101: A Manifesto for Ethical Research in the Downtown Eastside (DTES). We all have very close connections to the DTES, in many different capacities. We are activists, board members, workshop facilitators, writers, journalists, researchers, beekeepers, and public speakers. We also have lived experience of many things that researchers who come to the DTES are interested in studying: using illicit substances, poverty, sex work, criminalization, stigma and most of all, being a part of the DTES community.

The CREW builds on the work of the "Community Ethics in Cultural Production" project initiated by Hives for Humanity and SFU's Vancity Office of Community Engagement. We want to extend the guidelines laid out in the Manifesto for more ethical and respectful research in the DTES (Boilevin et al. 2018) by ***working to develop a local ethics review body that can provide oversight, suggestions, requests for revision and accountability for research taking place in, or on, our DTES community.*** *This body will primarily consist of DTES community members like us with lived experience of the topics and identities researchers are interested in studying. We want to develop a community review model that empowers community members to review and offer suggestions on research proposals in collaboration with researchers. Ultimately, we want to work towards reducing the harms associated with research and make it easier for researchers to collaborate in our community in a positive, respectful way.*

We are currently exploring existing models for community research ethics reviews that exist elsewhere and also working on developing our own local process for community ethical review by piloting several research reviews this year. We are developing locally-adapted university (i.e. TCPS2) ethics training and ethics reviewer training to supplement our existing local expertise on ethical and respectful research to do this work.

Fig. 20.1 CREW mission statement

interests, in as far as they relate to our community and its members and their variable needs and interests. This optional process may or may not include: a panel of review, a survey or questionnaire process, a personal interview with the research team, and/or a possible offer/request to have either one or all of our committee members present as an informal liaison throughout the research process. Members of the CREW have all been trained in the various aspects of ethics review and are competent enough, we feel, to "workshop" a project. This may include an informal cost/benefit consideration of the project's trajectory in terms of community member involvement as research subjects and/or as data collectors/compilers and within our common capacity for expert advisory skills as Persons with Lived Experience. We may also examine a project's long-term relevance to its ongoing development in this, a highly sensitive time of major social and infrastructural transition for the DTES. We also felt it is important that the CREW is not in any capacity affiliated with any official research institution, body, board, or ideology and at no time intends any influence, bias, harm, or preconceived effect on research efforts.

Review by CREW may or may not also include a follow-up report for researchers outlining suggestions or questions. Such reports will address ethical aspects of a research project as they relate to our community. Wherever possible the process concludes with an actual event hosted for the community by the research team. This event should include territorial land acknowledgements, food, visual aids, demonstrations, and/or participation of committee members in some capacity, to share results, findings, and intentional goals and/or perceived outcomes of the planned research.

20.4 Research Ethics Training for Community Reviewers

A next step in the journey towards developing the CREW was determining what additional training community ethics reviewers should complete. This stage of our project coincided with some colleagues in Vancouver asking us to help them develop a series of "community-engaged research ethics training" (CERET) workshops for peer research assistants working on their participatory action research project. They wanted to integrate content from the Manifesto into these trainings, which we agreed to do (see Morgan et al., 2023 for more detail on CERET). We also engaged with the CERET training as both presenters and workshop participants and considered this as the first step in our "community ethics reviewer" training for the CREW.

As we considered what further training would be important for community members to take before embarking on practice ethics reviews, we reflected on two things. First, local REB staff and board members informed us that it was common practice for institutional REB members to receive no more training than we had just completed through the CERET workshops, which were modelled on the federally prescribed TCPS2 CORE Tutorial (https://tcps2core.ca/welcome). Second, we realized that just as we had co-authored the *Manifesto* out of peoples' place-based lived experience of research and ethics in the Downtown Eastside, the key source of expertise for community reviewers was the lived expertise and community wisdom they already had—they did not need further training in ethics. We felt that the purpose of community ethics review should not simply be to make community members better resemble institutional REB members. Rather, we should embrace and elevate peoples' existing knowledge of their community's strengths and challenges, the informal codes of respect and reciprocity, and the unique risks and vulnerability experienced by their friends and neighbors in the DTES. As others have pointed out (see Banks et al., 2013; Westfall et al., 2017), matters of "ethics" in community settings are more rooted in everyday understandings of community norms and unique vulnerabilities than in abstracted, rigid, "universal" principles of ethics. We decided to embrace this existing strength of CREW members and did not pursue any further "reviewer training."[2]

20.5 Piloting Practice Reviews

Beginning in December 2019, we collaboratively started a process of "piloting" community ethics reviews of three proposals for research in the DTES. All three "CREW Reviews" were facilitated by co-author Scott as the academic ambassador/translator and included the other four co-authors (JC, NC, SM, JM) as community reviewers. In each case, we printed copies of the university REB application (all three had already gone through the University of British Columbia (UBC) Behavioral REB review process) and read through them as a group together while making notes and discussing any concerns or questions that arose. The first practice review involved the four community reviewers meeting with Scott to read through and critique Scott's own doctoral research proposal to conduct focus groups with people who use(d) opioids in the DTES. As a joke, and because he thought of Scott as a highly ethical person given our prior collaborations on Research 101, Jim suggested that Scott should "put something unethical in there" before the group reviewed his ethics application "so we'll have something to talk about." Scott did not do this, but the group still had lots to talk about! Our second review was of a study on which we were also listed as collaborators: a series of interviews about the Research 101/CREW project that would form the basis of a short documentary film (now available online: www.dtescrew.ca). Our third, final, and most rigorous practice review involved a project Nick was a collaborator on that proposed a series of storytelling and writing workshops with formerly incarcerated people which would also be a basis for research. In each practice review, we took detailed notes during our discussions on the questions that were raised and any recommendations made, then summarized these for the applicants. Our third practice review took the form of a more

[2] Though see Anderson et al., 2012 for a more in-depth discussion of the uses and varieties of research ethics training in community-engaged research for REB/IRB members, community organizations, and community members.

formalized 11-page review summary with recommendations and elicited a formal response from the researchers detailing the revisions they had made to their application and their responses to our specific recommendations. In general, feedback on our community reviews was highly positive, with one applicant reporting, "thank you all for what I can honestly say is the most valuable ethics feedback that I have ever received—a sentiment that I know is shared amongst our team."

20.6 The Potential of Community Ethics Review: Notes from Three Pilot CREW Reviews

In this section, we summarize some themes that arose from our shared experience as "community reviewers" in our three pilot CREW reviews. This responds to calls for detailed case studies of the "nitty gritty" of community ethics review processes and further describes the differences between institutional and community conceptualizations of research ethics (Anderson et al., 2012; Tuck & Guishard, 2013). Community reviewers critiqued the academic and difficult to understand language and format of institutional ethics applications, raised concerns about problematic notions of "risk" and "vulnerability" in the DTES that were implied in the ethics applications we reviewed, identified unintentionally stigmatizing assumptions and protocols written into the research proposals, noticed when researchers' limited understanding of "lived experience" was apparent, and flagged indications that future community ethical oversight might be needed (e.g., the proposal hinted at future uses of data or secondary data analysis).

20.6.1 Identifying Inaccessibility and the Need for Language and Formats That Everyone Can Understand

A persistent theme across all three CREW reviews was the need for Scott to play the role of academic translator. In this role, he attempted to define and clarify obscure academic language as well as explain the institutional process of ethics review and the many (sometimes strange) questions an REB asks a researcher to answer. In general, we found that a typical ethics application (in these cases from UBC) is not presented in an accessible format or in accessible "plain language" that everyone could easily understand. Because we knew Scott well and trust had been established between us, reviewers felt comfortable asking him to define jargon words and phrases that showed up in ethics applications (e.g., "ethnography," "participant observation," "minimal risk"). It is not always easy to admit that you are not familiar with a word or concept someone else is using, and it can make you feel like your intelligence is in question. However, in this context Scott had repeatedly emphasized a basic value of plain language and accessibility: if you cannot understand the message then the *messenger* is at fault for not communicating in a way their audience can understand. This created a context where it was normal, and encouraged, to call out jargon and ask for definitions. The hard-to-comprehend language and format of the ethics applications reflected poorly on the researchers and the institutions that had created and written them, not the community reviewers who had a hard time understanding them.

Scott's role as the academic "translator" or "interpreter" for the group also suggested to us that this could be a focus for further "community ethics reviewer" training. Having a better understanding of the process of conducting research, research method terminology, and REB review could enhance community reviewers' ability to apply their lived expertise in community ethics to an application as usefully as possible, with less need for translation along the way. This would likely get easier with more practice doing community ethics reviews as well.

More generally, community ethics review provided an excellent context to hold researchers (and institutions) accountable for the language and formats they use to communicate their goals and intentions in research. Plain language that community members can understand is essential throughout an entire research project for ensuring good working relationships between academic and community collaborators, facilitating truly informed consent for participants, ensuring participants comprehend survey or interview questions, and promoting valuable and comprehensible knowledge translation. The process of plain language writing and accessible format should extend into the ethics application phase, especially when engaging with a community ethics review process.

20.6.2 Critiquing Institutional Assumptions About Quantifying Risk and Vulnerability on Behalf of Communities

In each of the applications that we reviewed, community reviewers had very strong reactions to a three-by-three matrix the UBC BREB application form used to assess the study's "risk" to participants (low, medium, high) and participants' "vulnerability" (low, medium, high). If a researcher deemed their study to be in the lowest three cells of this matrix (e.g., low risk, medium vulnerability) then it would potentially be approved more quickly under a minimal risk, "delegated review" process and not proceed to the dreaded "full board review." In general, reviewers had many questions about how the abstract concepts of "risk" and "vulnerability" could be quantified on a three-point scale. More importantly, we marveled at the strangeness of an institutionalized process where researchers who do not live in the DTES, or who are not a part of the communities they want to research, assess that community's level of vulnerability and how risky they think the research methods they propose will be for the participants. We also noted that there is a motivation for researchers to make this rating fall within the lowest three boxes of the three-by-three chart, potentially downplaying either the risks or vulnerability to avoid full board review and speed up REB approval. In one of our practice reviews, we felt that the proposed research (which involved eliciting and promoting public storytelling about incarceration experiences) was actually riskier than the researchers had assessed. Reviewers suggested the researchers increase its rating, pushing it above "minimal risk" and likely triggering a full board review, feedback that the researchers accepted.

To us, this felt like the first very clear example of why subjective judgements about risk and vulnerability should not be made by non-experts who are not a part of the community. We pondered the strange image of PhD student Scott sitting in a coffee shop somewhere in Vancouver several months prior, writing his ethics application, drinking a cappuccino, and imagining how risky his proposed research was and how vulnerable marginalized people who use(d) opioids in the DTES were as he completed his three-by-three matrix. As he wrote an accompanying argument to the REB about the anticipated well-being of people he had never met in a community he was still very unfamiliar with, what qualified him to make those judgements? Why would those truly interested in protecting research participants think this practice of subjectively assessing risk and vulnerability as an outsider and from afar is normal, okay, or actually protective of participants?

Of course, researchers are not only motivated to downplay risk and vulnerability. They also may often overstate both research risk and participant vulnerability out of a misguided sense of paternalism and stigma towards marginalized people (Anderson & McNair, 2018). As community reviewers, we hated the assumption (often conveyed through ethics applications) that all people who live in the DTES (including us) are automatically "vulnerable" when we see ourselves as resilient, strong, activists fighting for our community. As Nick pointed out, institutional ethics codes and researchers may be operating with assumptions about people in the DTES through their lens of being middle or upper class, white, settler-identifying people, whereas DTES community members often experience economic poverty, practice substance use, have substance use disorders/addictions, experience social and self-stigmatization, discrimination, displacement, marginalization, criminalization and/or incarceration, each of which carry their own varying ideas of "risk." Each of these lived experiences and identities requires their own mitigation considerations regarding the potential for research "risks" or participant "vulnerability," as they relate to research being conducted in the DTES community. We agree with Bell and Salmon (2012) who argue that the right of marginalized people who use drugs (and in our case DTES residents more generally) to be "protected" from research should not be "emphasized at the expense of their rights to be included in research that reflects their concerns, interests and priorities, as well as their rights to benefit from the results of such research" (197). As Jule once explained to an REB member who asked the CREW if there was a better word to use than "vulnerable" to refer to the DTES, the best solution to preventing the further marginalization of the DTES through research is not paternalistic hand-wringing about "vulnerability" from outsiders but rather empowering the community to protect and care for itself. An empowered CREW review process is one way of taking steps towards this.

20.6.3 *Noticing Unintentional Stigmatization in Research Design*

Research can (and often does) produce descriptions of a social category or neighborhood that are stigmatizing by highlighting only the negatives, deficits, trauma or harm these people or places experience (Tuck, 2009). But stigma can also be found baked into research designs that assume certain deficiencies of proposed research participants. For example, while reviewing Scott's dissertation application, Nick noted with some disappointment that he had planned for one focus group to include both cis- and trans- women and another to only include cis-men. This proposed arrangement was justified with an appeal to past research in the DTES supposedly demonstrating the "hegemonic masculinity" present amongst men who use illicit drugs that could create danger for a trans-man in a mostly cis-male focus group. Nick felt this was stigmatizing and over-generalizing violent/oppressive attitudes and behaviors to all men in the DTES. He felt this was unfair and contrary to anecdotal examples he and other reviewers could share about trans folks who were not mistreated by cis-men in the DTES. We discussed how this had happened (there had been some back and forth with one of Scott's supervisors and the REB on this point, leading to the justification Nick was critiquing) but it was another good example of how strange (and inappropriate) it often is for outsiders like Scott to make fairly sensitive judgement calls about safety and the potential for harm within a community of which they are not a part. While these assumptions are usually based on our 'best evidence,' this evidence often comes from more research (i.e., "the literature") and not actual community relationships or experiences. Justified or not, this section of the application gave the stigmatizing impression that cis-men in the DTES would always create an unsafe environment for trans folks in a research setting. These kinds of harmful assumptions about community members' supposed deficiencies are much more likely to be noticed, flagged, and resisted when they are reviewed by the community members to whom they refer.

20.6.4 *Conceptualizing and Advocating for Strong Approaches to Ongoing Consent*

Central to many stories in the DTES of exploitative or damaging "research" (or art-making, news reporting, documentary film-making, or other forms of "cultural production" in the DTES, see Hives for Humanity, 2019) is a failure of ongoing consent. How and when does a community member get to decide what an outsider may do with the data and stories they have entrusted to a researcher, artist, or journalist? Ideally, we imagine the story-sharing (or "data extraction") process between DTES community member and outsider (e.g., an academic researcher) as a relationship of mutual benefit and respect. But too often there comes a moment in that exchange when the researcher "rips" the participant's story away from them and gains full control. Community reviewers were keenly aware of the subtle ways researchers normalize this extractive process in their ethics proposals, and were motivated to encourage and advise realistic approaches to strong forms of ongoing consent that could help minimize the damage of extraction.

For example, in one practice review the researchers stated that "consent shall be maintained throughout the research project" and gave a specific anticipated end date for the project. After that date, we wondered if researchers were suggesting they would retain the exclusive rights to participant data, stories, or images produced through the research. Perhaps consent should be maintained beyond the project? Perhaps it is important to maintain participants' consent for as long as the materials collected or shared from the project are planned to be used or kept in public circulation? We pushed the researchers to clarify when participant consent would naturally come to an end (e.g., if researchers lose contact with a participant). Would participant consent be assumed to continue indefinitely after the loss of contact, or would it be automatically extinguished? We also observed how so often in the DTES a failure of ongoing consent is really a failure of ongoing communication. How would researchers plan to maintain long term communication with marginalized participants who may not have consistent access to a single phone number or email address and may be difficult to contact in future? Ongoing consent requires a robust and collaborative plan for ongoing communication with participants who have entrusted their data and stories to others, particularly if those stories will be shared in public settings (e.g., lived experience videos, see Costa et al., 2012 for a critique).

Community reviewers discouraged one team of researchers from using their institution's standard "blanket consent" photo release form as it did not appropriately respect the need for greater care when representing marginalized peoples' stories, identities, and images to the public. Jim pointed out that people might want to review their images before they are used, especially if they are being cropped or modified in some way. Nick pointed out that people may not want to be associated with criminality (via the public products of the research project) down the road if their life situation changes. Will having the products of this project (that aimed to capture and publicly share formerly incarcerated peoples' stories) out in the world (especially digital spaces) make it harder for them to move on from a criminalized identity later in life? We recommended that the researchers ensure their participants knew the (future) risks of telling their story publicly, provide a clear and accessible option for participants to withdraw their story later if they chose, and consider how to ensure, from a practical standpoint, that online stories could always be modified/removed at any time in the future at the participants' request. Despite practical challenges, community reviewers were adamant that researchers needed to devise a process to ensure participants' ongoing, eternal, and irrevocable "editing power" over their story and image as captured by the researchers or workshop facilitators.[3]

[3] For more information on how some of us have approached thinking through processes of "ongoing informed consent" for a variety of forms of cultural production in the DTES please see the "Empowering Informed Consent" card we helped to co-produce as a companion resource with the *Research 101 Manifesto*: www.dtescrew.ca/resources

20.6.5 What Lived Experience? Clarifying Researchers' Vague Understandings of Key Community Roles

Because of their lived experiences in the DTES and interactions with researchers in this environment, community reviewers were very familiar with the nuances of concepts like "lived experience," "peer positions" and the complex nature of roles and relationships within a community setting. Whereas outsiders to the community often conceptualize "lived experience" in a vague and homogenized way (e.g., "anyone whose experiences are different than mine," "marginalized people"), community reviewers are much better prepared to identify and push researchers on the complex concerns and important ethical issues that elevating "lived experience" in community-based research may raise. In one example, it seemed to community reviewers that the researchers kept referring to one of their team member's "lived experience" with the prison system as if this alone would protect their project from all manner of ethical wrongdoing. We sensed a false equivalence being made across very different forms of "lived experience" with the prison system (e.g., three years in a provincial institution is not the same thing as the occasional night in the drunk tank). Community reviewers saw through this vagueness and asked specific questions about the type and duration of this team member's lived experience. We wondered if this person's lived experience within the prison system was relevant enough to potential participants (recently released from prison) that they would truly be considered a "peer" as the REB application suggested.

Shared experience with peers is the primary value of incorporating people with lived experience in community-based research projects. Researchers and REBs are much less likely to ask critical questions about the relevance and suitability of a team member's alleged "lived experience" since they may tend to see the inclusion of people with lived experience as a check box to be ticked rather than an issue that raises a host of new and complex ethical issues to be thought through.

20.6.6 Sustaining Community Oversight When Community Connections Grow Fuzzy

A final theme across practice reviews was concern around the possibility of "future uses of data" or secondary analyses. Whereas community reviewers appreciated the opportunity to look closely and critically at research ethics applications, we also noticed right away with some suspicion that each application contained a section where researchers could indicate to the REB if they had any future plans for doing "other things" with the data. Who would review those planned analyses or future uses of community data? Was this a kind of loophole for researchers to evade community or even institutional oversight of how they might use the data? Could researchers simply decide to take the project and framing of peoples' data in a different direction down the road? (See Chap. 16, in this volume).

This raised major concerns for community reviewers who felt that vaguely-defined, future, secondary analyses could be far less accountable to the community than the initially planned analyses that were rooted more firmly in the values and ethics of community-based research. The convenience of having access to previously collected data in the future might be too great a temptation for researchers to resist re-analysing and publishing in ways that might not have been approved by the initial community collaborators. What if those future analyses were used to make damaging, stigmatizing, or otherwise harmful claims about the DTES? Who would have a say in that?

The realization of the potential harms of secondary data analysis raised further issues with the challenge of "ongoing consent" in community-based research in the DTES, but also suggested a potential further role for the CREW review process. If a researcher was no longer in contact with their initial community-based research collaborators, a meeting with the CREW could potentially fill this gap by providing easily accessible and rigorous community oversight. We further imagined that the CREW could play an important role in providing community oversight for studies that sought to characterize people or aspects of the DTES but did not actually interact with any DTES organizations or community members (e.g., studies relying on linking administrative records). This seemed like an important gap to fill as we knew of several examples where administrative records research had been used to study or characterize the DTES with minimal institutional ethical oversight, no community oversight, and significant harmful repercussions for the DTES community (see McMartin, 2016).

20.6.7 Other Potential Benefits of Community Ethics Review in the DTES

While these did not come up extensively because of the small number and nature of the first three proposals we reviewed, several other important potential benefits of community ethics review were identified by community reviewers. These included:

- Raising critical questions about a research project's funders or flagging researchers with a history of disrespectful practice in the community for further scrutiny by the CREW.
- Drawing attention to inadequate plans for including and compensating community members as project collaborators that do not align with current best practices in the DTES (e.g., community standards of hourly pay, ensuring community collaborators are truly empowered to shape research agenda and analysis instead of merely being exploited for their access to "hard to reach" participants). In this sense, the CREW could serve as a kind of "ombudsperson" role as previously suggested by Damon et al. (2017) in their qualitative study of Peer Research Assistants' experiences contributing to community-based research in the DTES.

- Asking researchers if and how community collaborators (e.g., "Peer Research Assistants") had been trained in research ethics (see Anderson et al., 2012; Morgan et al., 2023) or what other forms of capacity-building and research training were being offered.
- Questioning the merit of a proposed study based on novelty or relevance in the context of the DTES. Nick noted that one component of the institutional ethics application forms was a question about external "scientific review" to confirm that this study was sufficiently novel in the wider scientific literature to justify the use of public funding. How much more relevant is this question in the context of a community that routinely experiences research as redundant, intrusive, and irrelevant? "No, we do not need another study that might produce a better description of how bad it is to be economically marginalized, thank you."
- CREW reviewers (and Jim especially) also relished the opportunity to identify spelling and grammar errors in academics' ethics applications, perhaps as a form of resistance to academics' relentless use of jargon words outside reviewers' vocabulary. Thus, community ethics review not only offers rigorous community oversight but may also ensure ethics applications are grammatically correct and typo-free!

20.7 Authority, Community Ethics Review, and the Possibility of Real Accountability in Research

Beyond mere ethics "review," we envision a future version of the CREW model that could serve a host of roles in mediating the relations between outsider academic researchers, institutional REBs, and the individual community members and organizations of the DTES who engage with these outsiders. Primarily, we feel it is essential for a community ethics review process to be empowered to actively hold researchers accountable to their promises of ethical practice with community members. While REBs may review project proposals and weigh in on ethical concerns before the start of a project, this is often the end of their ethical oversight of the project. They rely on an honor system; that is, researchers self-report protocol deviations, harms to participants, and other unanticipated events. The extent to which unethical behavior goes unreported is not really known; however, reports of unethical, exploitative, or harmful research practice continue to reverberate within communities like the DTES.[4] While research participants are required to be informed of their right to "complain" to the institutional REB if they have had a negative experience with a given research project, in our experience this information (e.g., the phone number of the director of the Office of Research Ethics) is typically provided

[4] See Bungay et al., 2022 for a recent qualitative study of the ethics of financial incentives from the perspectives of community service organization staff, researchers and people engaged in sex work (research participants), including clear evidence of ethical breaches by both institutional (i.e. TCPS2) and community standards.

by a member of the research team, rarely emphasized because unethical practice is not anticipated, and promptly forgotten or lost by participants. This is not real accountability.

Change to this ethical (un)accountability structure could come through the empowerment of local community ethics review processes. In our context in the DTES, and in line with the suggestions of Shore and colleagues (2011a), we have envisioned a model in which a community ethics review is both a complement to and a requirement of institutional REB review for DTES-specific research.[5] A researcher's proposal for research in the DTES would first be flagged by their institutional REB. This could resemble the current practice in Canada where proposals for research in Indigenous communities are flagged, thus initiating a process where researchers must respond to additional ethical considerations in line with the TCPS2 Chap. 9 guidelines on ethical research in Indigenous communities (Government of Canada, 2022). In our case, DTES-focused research could be flagged and then redirected to the DTES CREW for a community ethics review along the lines of what we have described above. Researchers could send their plain language research proposals to the CREW who would then have an opportunity to review and suggest revisions.

Researchers could also meet with CREW members, present their research proposal in an accessible format, and respond to questions and suggestions in person. Researchers would have the opportunity to revise their proposals and bring them back to the CREW for a second review and possible approval if changes are satisfactory. The CREW would also have the option to reject a research proposal outright, for example if it was determined to be overly redundant with previous research in the DTES, irredeemably harmful to research participants, or insufficiently respectful or responsive to expressed community expectations of ethical practice. Crucially, for this process to function as more than another community "consultation" body, it would need to be tied to the regulatory authority of an institutional REB. Institutional ethics clearance could be tied to a satisfactory CREW review process and "approval." Once the CREW approves a proposal the institutional REBs ethics review could continue with the revised ethics application (see Neufeld et al., forthcoming for more discussion of other changes needed in the DTES research infrastructure to reduce harms in the community).

An empowered community ethics review process with the authority to reject research proposals (Tuck & Wayne Yang, 2014) or compel revisions to a proposal holds the possibility of creating real and ongoing accountability between researchers and communities. REBs are not designed nor necessarily motivated to continually check in on specific researchers' ethics compliance (i.e., "Have you actually done what you said you were going to do?")—but empowered community research ethics review processes could be. Community review processes are much better positioned to keep tabs on actual researcher practice in a community setting, to

[5] See Shore et al. (2011b) for a helpful survey and review of the many challenges Community Research Ethics Review Processes often encounter in their interface with institutional REBs.

receive community complaints and initiate community (and/or institutional) censure of badly behaving researchers (see Yarbrough, 2020). This could reduce the chance of researchers deviating from their institutionally and/or community-approved ethics protocols, provide a useful and knowledgeable sounding board for working through community-specific ethical quandaries that arise once research has started (which disconnected REB members could only guess at), and facilitate meaningful forms of course correction or restorative justice when community members have been (unintentionally) harmed in the research process. It is unrealistic to ask REBs to perform this role in the multitude of community settings where institutionally-sponsored research takes place. Yet these forms of care and accountability for research participants in heavily-researched and marginalized communities are a necessary component of reducing and perhaps eliminating the harms of research.

20.8 Unresolved Challenges: Funding, Ownership, and Community Representation

As Shore and colleagues (2011a) have observed in their national review of community-based review processes, there are no clear sources of funding to support or build the "research ethics infrastructure" that effective and empowered forms of community research ethics review require. Other examples of successful community ethics review boards have been funded by their affiliated academic institutions, Indigenous tribal authorities, or one-off research or community-engagement grants. Funding from institutions raises questions about ongoing sustainability and independence of community research ethics review processes.[6] How much power will an academic institution give a community review process to hold its researchers accountable if it is also funding the community review process?

In our own experience, we have applied for and received small pockets of grant funding from "community engagement" initiatives of local universities in Vancouver (SFU and UBC) to fund our initial community-engagement work (e.g., Research 101 Workshops, knowledge translation of the *Manifesto*) and the pilot review process. The next stage of our planned work together will require a significant re-investment in community-engagement across the DTES to ensure that any community ethics review process that is developed would truly be a co-creation of representative groups from across the neighborhood. We have struggled with the issue of "community representation" in our work (see Neufeld et al., 2019; Neufeld et al., forthcoming) and sought to hold loosely our claims that the *Manifesto* or the CREW review process truly represents the diverse community of the DTES. To

[6] See (del Campo et al., 2013, Guishard, 2015, and Guishard et al., 2021) for some description of the Bronx Community Research Review Board and its ongoing struggle to assert its independence as a review body from the university and health organizations that founded and supported it initially.

attempt to move forward in a good way, we feel strongly that we must re-engage with a wider breadth of community organizations and community leaders from across the DTES to ensure there is community buy-in and support for the work. We feel this essential cross-community collaboration and co-creation would in turn lend authority to the review body itself once established. However, to date our applications for more funding have been unsuccessful and our collaboration together in community has been somewhat stalled by the COVID-19 pandemic, mixed priorities, and waning energy levels amongst key collaborators to keep doing the work. We offer this chapter in part as a reminder to ourselves of how far we have come and the potential we believe exists in this work. We also invite future collaborators and potential funders who could help us continue moving forward to contact us.

20.9 Conclusion

Piloting community ethics reviews has not only been a valuable learning experience for each of us, it has also been a lot of fun. Preparing this chapter has reminded us of the many adventures we have had together over the past few years. The road trip to a research ethics conference in Kelowna that Scott took with Samona and Nick (see Neufeld & Leech-Crier, 2020), figuring out how to get around UBC's expansive campus as a motley "CREW" of conference presenters, navigating the challenges of paying CREW members in cash (and online since COVID-19) when university bureaucracies resist this form of accessible payment with everything they have, Jule and Samona razzing Scott for his academese language no one understands and the time they thought he made up the word "reciprocity" (though as it turned out, they both already understood the meaning of "reciprocity" quite well). And who could forget our many meetings stuffed into the classic greasy spoon diner booths at the storied Ovaltine Café in the DTES? Or that time Scott made all the co-authors hoodie sweatshirts with our names on the sleeves, "Research 101" on the front and "Downtown Eastside Community Research Ethics Workshop" on the back.. except the printer messed up and wrote "Wokshop" instead.

But besides all the fun, we are also incredibly proud of what we have accomplished so far together. Our co-authored *Manifesto* has been read by people around the world, was made required reading for first year medical students at UBC and has been integrated into numerous other university course syllabi. We have been invited (and paid!) to present on our work together in countless places. We have seen our work inspire others beyond Vancouver and even had our process replicated in other cities (e.g., "Research 102," see Alook et al., 2021) just like we hoped it would be (Neufeld et al., 2019). We even filmed a whole documentary about this empowering journey through paradigm shifting and ethical struggles of the people, recently made available publicly on our newly-designed website (www.dtescrew.ca). Most important of all, we have seen our work ingested by actual target audiences (i.e., researchers in the DTES) and seen the first glimmers of change in a wider exploitative and extractive system of research in the DTES. Through this work, we have done some amazing things that will matter for years to come.

We, as a community, are on a collaborative journey of witnessing, observing, and communicating between the research community and the community of the Downtown Eastside. Ours is a pioneering effort to work in solidarity with researchers themselves, to give voice and opinion on research conducted in this neighborhood. We hope that our work together will one day make it possible for researchers to state, with integrity that community were not only consulted, but respected, learned from, treated with reciprocity and that every effort was made to protect the privacy, property (intellectual and physical), and persons of the DTES from exploitation, irrelevant examination, and exhaustion. We hope our work towards developing a local process for community ethics review will one day help ensure that research has been conducted respectfully, with reciprocity and return as core values in accordance with the community wisdom of those who reside in the DTES. We also hope others can learn from our initial experiences with community ethics review.

Acknowledgements The authors of this chapter would like to thank the many, many people and organizations who have funded, supported, offered wisdom, offered space, or spread the word about our work together over the years. These individuals include Am Johal, Sarah Common, Heather Holroyd, Janina Krabbe, Jean Ruiz, Jeffrey Morgan, Tara Taylor, Angela Towle, Kathleen Leahy, Alina McKay, Thomas Kemple, Kristina McDavid, Jeff Toward, Kalamity Hildebrandt, Michael Schmitt, Ryan McNeil, Lindsay Deane, Will Damon, Matt Heard, Margot Fuller, Jean Swanson, King Mong Chan, and many others including all of the original community co-authors of the 2018 *Research 101 Manifesto*. Special thanks to Professor Thomas Kemple for generously offering to review existing models of community ethics review for us as a volunteer "faculty research assistant," writing a summary of his findings, and allowing us to use some small snippets of his writing in this chapter. Organizations that have funded and supported us in important ways include Hives for Humanity, SFU Woodward's Vancity Office of Community Engagement, SFU's Community Engagement Initiative, SFU's Community-Engaged Research Initiative (CERi), the UBC Learning Exchange, VANDU, WAHRS, the Carnegie Community Action Project, the BC Centre on Substance Use and many other organizations that have invited us to present or formally endorsed the Manifesto (see http://bit.ly/R101Manifesto for a list of individual and organizational endorsements). Finally, we would like to thank the Ovaltine Café in the DTES for always being the place to meet and discuss our nefarious plot to rid the world of the evils of extractive research practices and for hosting our CREW reviews. They're such nice people. Great OREO shakes.

References

Alook, E., Bambrick, S., Beausoliel, C., Cardinal, K., Copley, T., Chen, C., Danyluk, L., Fafard, M., Hawryluk, C., Joseph, E., Kafara, R., Kakolak, B., Kaiser, R., Kennedy, N., MacDonald, M., Mackenzie, D., Mah, K., Mckie, A., Morris, L., Mulyk, J., Neis, B., Osman, A., Pereira, R., Pruden, D., Puddu, C., Quinn, B., Savidov, M., Siek, M., Twan, S., Vaughan, M., Woodruff, D., & Worm, H. (2021). Research 102: Meaningful activist research in amiskwacîwâskahikan (City Centre Edmonton). In *Treaty 6 territory, the territory of the Papaschase, and the homeland of the Métis Nation*. https://rylankafara.wordpress.com/2021/04/15/research-102-meaningful-activist-research-in-city-centre-edmonton/

Anderson, E. E. (2006). A qualitative study of non-affiliated, non-scientist institutional review board members. *Accountability in Research, 13*(2), 135–155.

Anderson, E., & McNair, L. (2018). Ethical issues in research involving participants with opioid use disorder. *Therapeutic Innovation & Regulatory Science, 52*(3), 280–284.

Anderson, E. E., Solomon, S., Heitman, E., DuBois, J. M., Fisher, C. B., Kost, R. G., Lawless, M. E., et al. (2012). Research ethics education for community-engaged research: A review and research agenda. *Journal of Empirical Research on Human Research Ethics, 7*(2), 3–19.

Banks, S., Armstrong, A., Carter, K., Graham, H., Hayward, P., Henry, A., Holland, T., et al. (2013). Everyday ethics in community-based participatory research. *Contemporary Social Science, 8*(3), 263–277.

Bell, K., & Salmon, A. (2012). Good intentions and dangerous assumptions: Research ethics committees and illicit drug use research. *Research Ethics, 8*(4), 191–199.

Boilevin, Louise, Jules Chapman, Lindsay Deane, Caroline Doerksen, Greg Fresz, DJ Joe, Nicolas Leech-Crier, Ramona Marsh, Jim McLeod, Scott Neufeld, Steven Pham, Laura Shaver, Patrick Smith, Martin Steward, Dean Wilson, and Phoenix Winter. *Research 101: A manifesto for ethical research in the downtown eastside* (2018). Report available online at http://bit.ly/R101Manifesto

Bungay, V., Guta, A., Slemon, A., Varcoe, C., & Comber, S. (2022). The ethics of financial Incentivization for Health Research participation among sex Workers in a Canadian Context. *Qualitative Health Research*, 1–10. 10497323221089877.

del Campo, F., Martin, J. C., Spencer, P., & Strelnick, H. (2013). The development of the Bronx community research review board: A pilot feasibility project for a model of community consultation. *Progress in Community Health Partnerships, 7*(3), 341–352.

Costa, L., Voronka, J., Landry, D., Reid, J., Mcfarlane, B., Reville, D., & Church, K. (2012). “Recovering our stories”: A small act of resistance. *Studies in Social Justice, 6*(1), 85–101.

Culhane, D. (2011). Stories and plays: Ethnography, performance and ethical engagements. *Anthropologica, 1*, 257–274.

Damon, W., Callon, C., Wiebe, L., Small, W., Kerr, T., & Mcneil, R. (2017). Community-based participatory research in a heavily researched inner city neighbourhood: Perspectives of people who use drugs on their experiences as peer researchers. *Social Science & Medicine, 176*, 85–92.

Flicker, S., Travers, R., Guta, A., McDonald, S., & Meagher, A. (2007). Ethical dilemmas in community-based participatory research: Recommendations for institutional review boards. *Journal of Urban Health, 84*(4), 478–493.

Goodman, A., Morgan, R., Kuehlke, R., Kastor, S., Fleming, K., Boyd, J., & Western Aboriginal Harm Reduction Society. (2018). “We’ve been researched to death”: Exploring the research experiences of urban indigenous peoples in Vancouver, Canada. *International Indigenous Policy Journal, 9*(2), 1–22. https://doi.org/10.18584/iipj.2018.9.2.3

Government of Canada (Canadian Institutes of Health Research, Natural Sciences and Engineering Research Council of Canada, and Social Sciences and Humanities Research Council of Canada). Tri Council Policy Statement: Ethical Conduct for Research Involving Humans. (2022). Accessed online at https://ethics.gc.ca/eng/policy-politique_tcps2-eptc2_2022.html

Guishard, M. A. (2015). *Nepantla and Ubuntu ethics Para nosotros: Beyond scrupulous adherence toward threshold perspectives of participatory/collaborative research ethics*. City University of New York.

Guishard, M. A., Heyward, D. A., Brown, J. T., & Stoddard-Pennant, M. (2021). What we not Finna do: Respectfully collaborating with Skinfolk and kinfolk in black feminist participatory action research. *Global Journal of Community Psychology Practice, 12*(2), 1–35.

Hives for Humanity. (2019). Empowering informed consent – Community ethics in cultural production. https://doi.org/10.14288/1.0381026

Klitzman, R. (2012). Institutional review board community members: Who are they, what do they do, and whom do they represent? *Academic Medicine: Journal of the Association of American Medical Colleges, 87*(7), 975–981. https://doi.org/10.1097/ACM.0b013e3182578b54

Linden, I. A., Mar, M. Y., Werker, G. R., Jang, K., & Krausz, M. (2013). Research on a vulnerable neighborhood—The Vancouver downtown eastside from 2001 to 2011. *Journal of Urban Health, 90*(3), 559–573.

McKay, A. (2021). Housing, building, and neighbourhood influences on the experience of home for long-term tenants of Vancouver's downtown eastside. *Unpublished doctoral dissertation.*

McMartin, P. (2016). The high cost of misery in Vancouver's downtown eastside. *The Vancouver Sun.*. http://www.vancouversun.com/health/pete+mcmartin+high+cost+misery+vancouver+downtown+eastside/11632586/story.html

Morgan, J., Neufeld, S. D., Holroyd, H., Ruiz, J., Taylor, T., Nolan, S., & Glegg, S. (2023). Community-Engaged Research Ethics Training (CERET): Developing accessible and relevant research ethics training for community-based participatory research with people with lived and living experience using illicit drugs and harm reduction workers. *Harm Reduction Journal, 20*(1), 86.

Neufeld, S. D., Chapman, J., Crier, N., Marsh, S., McLeod, J., & Deane, L. A. (2019). Research 101: A process for developing local guidelines for ethical research in heavily researched communities. *Harm Reduction Journal, 16*(1), 1–11.

Neufeld, S. D., Chapman, J., Leech-Crier, N., Marsh, S., & McLeod, J. (forthcoming). Changing the system: Steps towards empowering community governance of research ethics in the downtown eastside of Vancouver. *Book Chapter Under Review.*

Neufeld, S. D., & Leech-Crier, N. (2020). An illegal road trip: Drugs, friendship, and following Jesus. *Geez Magazine Spring Issue #56, Disobedience.* https://geezmagazine.org/magazine/article/an-illegal-road-trip-drugs-friendship-and-following-jesus

Shore, N., Brazauskas, R., Drew, E., Wong, K. A., Moy, L., Baden, A. C., Cyr, K., Ulevicus, J., & Seifer, S. D. (2011a). Understanding community-based processes for research ethics review: A national study. *American Journal of Public Health, 101*(S1), S359–S364.

Shore, N., Drew, E., Brazauskas, R., & Seifer, S. D. (2011b). Relationships between community-based processes for research ethics review and institution-based IRBs: A national study. *Journal of Empirical Research on Human Research Ethics, 6*(2), 13–21.

Solomon, S. (2016). Too many rationales, not enough reason: A call to examine the goals of including lay members on institutional review boards. *Accountability in Research, 23*(1), 4–22.

Solomon-Cargill, S. (2018). What can IRBs learn from CABs? A qualitative analysis of the experiences of recruitment and training of nonscientist members on research review boards. *Journal of Empirical Research on Human Research Ethics, 13*(1), 88–94.

Tuck, E. (2009). Suspending damage: A letter to communities. *Harvard Educational Review, 79*(3), 409–428.

Tuck, E., & Guishard, M. (2013). *Uncollapsing ethics: Racialized sciencism, settler coloniality, and an ethical framework of decolonial participatory action research* (pp. 3–27). New directions in critical qualitative research.

Tuck, E., & Wayne Yang, K. (2014). Unbecoming claims: Pedagogies of refusal in qualitative research. *Qualitative Inquiry, 20*(6), 811–818.

Westfall, J. M., Zittleman, L., Felzien, M., Ringel, M., Lakin, A., & Nease, D. (2017). Institutional review board training when patients and community members are engaged as researchers. *Family Practice, 34*(3), 301–304.

Yarbrough, D. (2020). "Nothing about us without us": Reading protests against oppressive knowledge production as guidelines for solidarity research. *Journal of Contemporary Ethnography, 49*(1), 58–85.

Scott D. Neufeld, Psychology Department, Brock University, St. Catherines, Ontario, Canada. Scott wrote the bulk of this chapter, because he is an academic guy and was invited to contribute to the edited book through an academic collaborator. While he did his best to organize the ideas and get the words down on paper, the insights, content, experiences and wisdom shared here are a collaborative product of all five co-authors' work together over the past several years. Many lines, phrases, paragraphs and sections were added by the other co-authors. Scott is a cisgender, able-bodied, heterosexual, male, university faculty member/PhD student, and dad to three kids who is racialized as White and grew up within a White, rural and culturally Christian environment in Langley, British Columbia on the unceded territories of the Kwantlen, Katzie and Semiahmoo First Nations. Importantly, he does not have lived experience of poverty, criminalized substance use, or significant childhood trauma, nor have he or his communities ever been the subject of the intense scrutiny by researchers that many marginalized communities experience. Participating in and being shaped by culturally dominant communities and identities his entire life has meant he has had much to unlearn as he has attempted to engage in equitable, respectful, and reciprocal knowledge exchange and collaboration with people and communities whose experiences and expertise have often gone unrecognized and unappreciated by people from his communities. Scott now resides in St. Catharines, Ontario on the ancestral territories of the Chonnonton, Missisaugas of the Credit, Anishinaabeg, Ojibway/ Chippewa and Haudenosaunee peoples in the Niagara Region under the terms of the Dish-With-One-Spoon and Two-Row Wampum Agreement as well as the Upper Canada Treaties. He is privileged to work as a tenure track Lecturer in Community Psychology at Brock University.

Jule Chapman, Sex Workers United Against Violence (SWUAV), Vancouver, British Columbia, Canada. Jule has been involved with research for many years, as a long-time research participant in drug use-related research. Born and raised in Vancouver, Jule has lived in the DTES for twenty years, though she was born and raised in the beach-side Vancouver neighborhood of Kitsilano. She identifies as a long-time drug user, but more importantly, she identifies as a survivor of childhood trauma. Jule volunteered on the board of directors of Sex Workers United Against Violence, (SWUAV), and worked as a peer support/outreach worker for the past eight years. Jule is an avid writer and poet with many pieces published in Vancouver's Megaphone Magazine. She has a co-authored publication in *AIDS and Behavior* and *Harm Reduction Journal*. She was an interviewer and co-author of, *'Me I'm Living It', The Primary Health Care Experience Research For Empowerment Study* and is co-author of *Opioids A Survivor's Guide*, the *Research 101 Manifesto*, and the *Empowering Informed Consent Cards*. She was recently one of the first two peers (alongside Nicolas) to complete The Fundamentals of Reporting course at Langara College.

Nicolas D. Leech-Crier, Transformative Health & Justice Research Cluster, University of British Columbia, British Columbia Mental Health and Substance Use Services, PHS Community Services Society/Vancouver Coastal Health Mobile Overdose Prevention Unit, Megaphone Magazine, Vancouver, British Columbia, Canada. Nicolas, an inter-racial adoptee of Cree ancestry, is a survivor of intergenerational, in utero and infancy traumas, and today, is well adjusted and greatly appreciated as a peer leader in Vancouver's Downtown Eastside community. He works with a number of progressive initiatives, including four full-time staff positions: Storytelling & Community Networking Liaison at Megaphone Magazine, Peer co-lead Writer and Research Assistant with the UBC Transformative Health and Justice Research Cluster, Lived Experience Strategic Advisor with BC Mental Health and Substance Use Services, and Peer Responder/ Outreach worker at the PHS/VCH Mobile Overdose Prevention Unit. He also attends a Continuing Studies course through Simon Fraser University called Community Capacity Building. In his spare time, Nicolas has begun writing the first draft script for a stage-play tentatively titled Unmarked, about the processing of individual and national grief and loss trauma in the shocking wake of the recent discovery of thousands of unmarked children's graves at former Residential School-era sites across Canada and how this process (including the massive impending research process required to identify the remains of these children and then have them returned to their rightful families) will by and large shape the relationship of Truth and Reconciliation efforts between Canada and its Indigenous peoples for at least the next 7 generations. In all he does, he sends love to his 11-year-old son, Money.

Samona Marsh, British Columbia Yukon Association of Drug War Survivors, Sex Workers United Against Violence, Canadian Association of People who Use Drugs, Coalition of Peers Dismantling the Drug War, Vancouver, British Columbia, Canada. Samona is a volunteer on many boards of peer-based organizations in the DTES and has had plenty of experience with research in the DTES, both as a participant and more recently as a peer researcher conducting interviews and analyzing data. Samona is a former president of the Vancouver Area Network of Drug Users (VANDU) and is currently the vice president of the BC/Yukon Drug War Survivors and on the board of the Coalition of Peers Dismantling the Drug War, all BC-based activist organizations. She is also on the editorial board for the award-winning podcast Crackdown (www.crackdownpod.com). Her 30 years of lived experience as a drug user make her a highly sought-after research collaborator in the DTES community. One role she is especially proud of is acting as an "ethical substance use navigator" ensuring peers can use substances safely when attending academic conferences. Samona has lived, worked, and played in the DTES of Vancouver for several decades and has been an advocate after losing her mother and father to fentanyl overdoses.

Jim McLeod, Hives for Humanity, Vancouver, British Columbia, Canada. Jim is an active community member in the DTES of Vancouver, working with Hives for Humanity, a non-profit focused on beekeeping, gardening and changing the narrative on the DTES. He has served on the boards of the Vancouver Area Network of Drug Users and the Drug Users Resource Centre. Jim believes the Downtown Eastside is brimming with talent the rest of the world overlooks. He is excited about his work with Megaphone Magazine's Speaker's Bureau project, working with audiences and participants to help them see People Who Use Drugs as just that—people. Jim is also a cast and research member of the Illicit Theatre project—a shadow play about peer first responders and the overdose crisis in the DTES. Jim notes that he is not a "functional addict" but that his functioning, all of his community advocacy, beekeeping and gardening, is possible because he is self-medicating with pain medication. Chemically dependent since elementary school, people are often surprised to learn that Jim has a spotless criminal record. Jim was born and raised in Vancouver and his ancestry is Açorean Portuguese on his dad's side, and on his mother's Haida, Kwakiutl and Inuit, with Irish and some British and French.

Index

E. E. Anderson (ed.), *Ethical Issues in Community and Patient Stakeholder–Engaged Health Research*, Philosophy and Medicine 146,
https://doi.org/10.1007/978-3-031-40379-8

R